Oral-Facial Evaluation for Speech-Language Pathologists

Oral-Facial Evaluation for Speech-Language Pathologists

Barbara Ann Johnson-Root, PhD, CCC-SLP

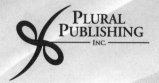

PLURAL
PUBLISHING
INC.

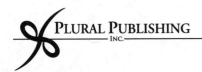

5521 Ruffin Road
San Diego, CA 92123

e-mail: info@pluralpublishing.com
Website: http://www.pluralpublishing.com

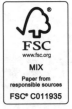

Typeset in 10.5/13 Palatino by Flanagan's Publishing Services, Inc.
Printed in the United States of America by McNaughton & Gunn, Inc.

Library of Congress Cataloging-in-Publication Data

Johnson-Root, Barbara Ann, author.
  Oral-facial evaluation for speech-language pathologists / Barbara Ann Johnson-Root.
    p. ; cm.
  Includes bibliographical references and index.
  ISBN 978-1-59756-575-2 (alk. paper)—ISBN 1-59756-575-X (alk. paper)
  I. Title.
  [DNLM: 1. Diagnosis, Oral—methods. 2. Language Disorders—diagnosis. 3. Evidence-Based Practice.
WL 340.2]
  RC423
  616.85'5—dc23
                              2014048788

Contents

Foreword

The orofacial examination (OFE), also known as the oral peripheral examination or speech mechanism examination, is one of the earliest components of clinical education in speech-language pathology. It is also one of the first examinations typically administered to a child or adult with a suspected problem of articulation, resonance, voice, or swallowing. Early instruction in this examination usually gives the student some basic pointers on how to conduct the examination, what to look for, and how to write a brief report summarizing the observations. The instruction is seldom deep or detailed because the student is just learning about the anatomic and motoric complexity of this system and has not been exposed to the array of clinical issues that can arise. This early clinical experience with the OFE is an essential introduction, but students who continue to learn the knowledge and skills required for independent professional practice become aware that the initial exposure to the OFE merely opens the door to a wider set of clinical observations and decision making. It is one thing to perform the examination on a typically developing child who is compliant in all facets of the examination but quite another thing to perform this examination on a child with a cleft palate or other craniofacial anomaly, an adult with a facial paralysis resulting from stroke, or an individual with autism. The OFE is not a cut-and-dry, one-size-fits-all procedure. Rather, it is an adaptive inquiry into a system that has numerous vulnerabilities and complex interactions.

The OFE broadly applied to the practice of speech-language pathology is multifaceted and multilayered. With experience, clinicians can and should go far beyond the basic principles typically learned in a first course. But this knowledge is personal and is usually won with substantial time in the clinic. Commonly, a curriculum addresses this need by incorporating extensions and elaborations of the OFE in various courses such as craniofacial disorders, speech sound disorders, voice disorders, neurogenic disorders, and birth-to-3. Although this approach is satisfactory for some purposes, it can fail to show the integrated nature of the OFE in its diverse clinical application. The OFE is a longstanding basic procedure in speech-language pathology, but it appears that it is often taught and practiced in a nonstandardized and fragmented way. That circumstance is about to change.

Oral-Facial Evaluation for Speech-Language Pathologists takes several significant steps toward a systematic and reasoned OFE. The first two chapters define the basic problems and guide the reader through the routine process of the examination. Methods of the examination are clearly tied to purpose and conclusions. Subsequent chapters consider the manifold issues of the OFE in relation to discretionary observations, adaptations for individuals with special needs, interpreting findings, and documenting findings. In this way, the book unfolds into an expanding coverage of the OFE that meets diverse needs in speech-language pathology. Illustrations, tabled summaries, a glossary, and companion videos make this a book that is highly informative in an inviting and supportive format.

This book consolidates clinical expertise to guide readers through an effective examination of the structural and functional integrity of a complex system in individuals with a variety of communication disorders. Author Barbara Johnson-Root has given the field of speech-language pathology an unparalleled resource in the logic and methods of the OFE. Her book is a *tour de force* that will be consulted repeatedly by clinicians with various levels of experience. *Oral-Facial Evaluation for Speech-Language Pathologists* is a milestone in the literature on clinical methods.

—Raymond D. Kent, PhD
Professor Emeritus
University of Wisconsin–Madison

Introduction: About *Oral-Facial Evaluation for Speech-Language Pathologists*

Practicing speech-language pathologists customarily inspect the oral-facial region whenever evaluating a person for communication disorder or difference. This time-honored tradition is carried out routinely, regardless of the reason for evaluation or age of the person being examined (Bankson, Bernthal, & Flipsen, 2009; Bauman-Waengler, 2011; Boone, McFarlane, Von Berg, & Zraick, 2010; Buckendorf, Gordon, & Goodwyn-Craine, 2007; Duffy, 2013; Dworkin & Culatta, 1996; Gordon-Brannan & Weiss, 2007; Haynes & Pindzola, 2012; Johnson, 1996; Kummer, 2008; Leder, Suiter, Murray, & Rademaker, 2013; Peña-Brooks & Hegde, 2007; Shipley &

McAfee, 2008; St. Louis & Ruscello, 2000; Tomblin, Morris, & Spriestersbach, 2002).

In fact, oral-facial inspection routinely appears on the list of activities to be completed whenever planning a comprehensive communication evaluation. Table 0–1 shows a sample evaluation protocol, illustrating the clinical context that normally surrounds oral-facial inspection.

Note that each evaluation activity shown in Table 0–1 has a particular clinical purpose and provides perspective on at least one aspect of communication that is under scrutiny. When analyzed as a whole, the evidence gathered through the overall

Table 0–1. Sample Protocol Showing the Full Context of the Evaluation Process

Evaluation Activity	Participants and Their Roles	General Objective(s)
Case history intake form	Examinee, a significant other, or both complete the case history intake form prior to attending the evaluation.	• Clarify interview and testing objectives for the full evaluation. • Generate clinical questions that are individualized and relevant to the examinee.
	Examiner reads the case history intake, identifies information relevant to interview and testing, and makes a preliminary decision about a plan of care.	• Identify specific information to be obtained or clarified during the opening interview. • Plan evaluation procedures according to the examinee's symptoms and needs.
Opening interview	Examiner asks questions of the examinee or a significant other, while also providing information about the procedures.	• Clarify information provided on the case history intake form. • Provide information that fosters the clinical relationship, while also facilitating a unified set of objectives for the evaluation session.
	Examinee and significant other respond to questions and have opportunity to ask questions of the examiner.	• Provide examiner with a clearer understanding of the examinee's needs and expectations. • Address any questions or concerns that the examinee brings to the table, so that they can be considered during testing and directly addressed during the closing interview.
		Begin to establish clinical rapport.

continues

Table 0–1. *continued*

Evaluation Activity	Participants and Their Roles	General Objective(s)
Formal or standardized testing	Examiner administers selected tests to the examinee.	Obtain numeric scores and descriptive information that are useful for ruling out disorder, diagnosing disorder, rating severity if a disorder is identified, and describing the disorder as it manifests in the examinee.
Informal testing and strategic observations	Strategically observe examinee during structured and nonstructured communication opportunities.	Obtain information about the examinee's communication performance to supplement evidence obtained through standardized or formal procedures.
Hearing screening	Examiner screens hearing using age-appropriate audiometry procedures.	Identify or rule out the need for audiometric evaluation.
Oral-facial inspection	**Examiner inspects the examinee's face, head, and speech mechanism for structure and function.**	**See this manual for details.**
Closing interview	Examiner summarizes results of testing.	Provide examinee and significant other with a summary of the findings, including results of testing, diagnosis, prognosis, and recommendations.
	Examiner verbally communicates diagnosis, prognosis, and recommendations to the examinee and/or significant other.	
	Examinee and significant other receive information about the results of testing, diagnosis, and recommendations, then seek clarification as needed.	Ensure that the examinee and significant other have opportunity to seek clarification and provide input.
	Examiner responds to questions.	Ensure that all examinee questions are either addressed or a plan is put in place so that they may be addressed.
Diagnostic report	Examiner writes the clinical report.	Formally document pertinent historical data, results of testing, results of hearing screening, results of oral-facial evaluation, and relevant clinical observations.
		Formally document the diagnosis, prognosis, and a series of recommendations for follow-up.

evaluation process comprises the key pieces of a diagnostic puzzle, allowing the diagnostician to gain understanding that, after taking the full matter into consideration, leads to a valid diagnosis, prognosis, and follow-up plan.

Although only a small part of the overall evaluation process, the oral-facial inspection's role cannot be minimized. That is, by carefully completing the inspection, clinicians gain insight into whether anatomic or physiologic challenges potentially influence perceptible speech symptoms. With this in mind, the focus of the inspection is to find out whether all anatomic parts necessary for speech are present, intact, and functioning satisfactorily and, furthermore, to verify whether any identified irregularities contribute to the perceived communication concerns.

Of course, the customary oral-facial inspection only detects overtly visible and audible symptoms, limiting the amount and type of information that can be gained from it. Consequently, although the inspection may shed superficial light on anatomic or physiologic matters that can ultimately lead to definitive findings, some resulting evidence is more useful for highlighting aspects of oral structure or function that demand more in-depth study. Moreover, in many cases, the inspection confirms that the person's communication idiosyncrasies lack physical explanation.

Significance of Oral-Facial Inspection

In most cases, a thorough inspection confirms that all anatomic parts are present, intact, and functioning, implying no physical barrier to spoken communication. For these examinees, inspecting the oral-facial region rules out readily discernible organic etiology. As a result, follow-up can generally ensue with the assumption that medical intervention or compensatory considerations are unnecessary.

Yet for fewer examinees, the inspection exposes or substantiates anatomic or physiologic irregularity that has potential to contribute to an identified communication concern. When this happens, the speech-language pathologist's responsibility is to ascertain whether the observed anomaly appreciably factors into the audible symptoms and, if so, describe the

associated features, clarify the extent to which the anomaly contributes to the speaking pattern, and create a follow-up plan that takes into account the person's anatomic or physiologic idiosyncrasies.

The follow-up plan may include but is not limited to specialist referral, recommendation for a particular approach to further assessment or treatment, or other considerations intended to enhance the likelihood of successful service delivery outcome. The discovery of irregularities with potential to influence treatment decisions can make a tremendous difference to the person whose communication is being evaluated.

The Need for a Thorough Inspection Tool

Checklists, textbook narratives, and screenings that focus on oral-facial inspection are available. Yet as a rule, they tend to be less structured, rendering them more useful to experienced practitioners than to students and newer clinicians. Furthermore, most focus on a particular target population, placing a boundary around their utility as a comprehensive tool (Andrianopoulos, n.d.; Bankson et al., 2009; Bauman-Waengler, 2011; Boone et al., 2010; Boshart, 2009; Buckendorf et al., 2007; Duffy, 2013; Dworkin & Culatta, 1996; Gordon-Brannan & Weiss, 2007; Kummer, 2008; Shipley & McAfee, 2008; St. Louis & Ruscello, 2000: Yorkston, Beukelman, Strand, & Hakel, 2010).

In addition, many speech-language pathologists are uncertain as to how to perform and interpret some parts of the inspection (Kummer, 2008). For example, a reminder to check for submucous cleft palate, tongue-thrust swallow, or gag reflex is useful to those who know how to perform the procedures. Nevertheless, those who are newer to the process or do not have experience in every area benefit from explicit instruction as well as precise descriptions of possible outcomes for a full range of procedures. Extensive details of this type are frequently absent from existing resources.

The Need for Confidence Beyond One's Clinical Comfort Zone

It is rare for a service provider or academician to have specialized preparation that sweeps across the full professional practice spectrum. Yet most practitioners are called upon at least occasionally to evaluate the needs of people who present some symptoms outside their area of expertise. Moreover, the odds are high that cases with symptoms crossing more than one area of expertise eventually find their way to each clinician's caseload. Knowing how to diagnose or at least when to recommend in-depth post-testing outside a specialty area is vital to competent service delivery.

Furthermore, whenever encountering an examinee with apparent physical symptoms beyond one's clinical comfort zone, the burden of cobbling together a meaningful inspection seems to fall on the evaluating clinician. Yet most speech-language pathologists carry heavy workloads (Rudebusch & Weichmann, 2011); for that reason, a thorough investigation of rarely seen anomalies is not always possible, hindering confident service delivery practices when practitioners manage diverse caseloads.

Why *Oral-Facial Evaluation for Speech-Language Pathologists*

It is incumbent on every speech-language pathologist to perform efficient and comprehensive oral-facial evaluations that yield reliable and clinically useful evidence, even when symptoms extend beyond the scope of the clinician's formal training and everyday practice. Without this precept, clinically relevant anomalies can be missed while resources may be spent investigating physical differences that in reality lack noteworthy impact to the individual. For this reason, one cannot underestimate the value of an efficient and accurate oral-facial inspection protocol.

A Comprehensive Oral-Facial Inspection Tool

Oral-Facial Evaluation for Speech-Language Pathologists offers a comprehensive collection of eight routine and 16 discretionary inspection procedures, all in a single resource, spanning a wide range of clinical practice areas. This feature minimizes the risk of overlooking relevant features simply because symptoms extend beyond the clinician's formal education or everyday practice.

An Efficient Oral-Facial Inspection Tool

The manual tactically guides a routine comprehensive oral-facial evaluation, applying principles of evidence-based practice throughout. Then carefully thought-out clinical questions steer examiners toward appropriate discretionary procedures on an *as-needed* basis. At the same time, the manual provides a framework that includes detailed information to support the process of interpreting the evidence, while also ensuring handy access to a rapid review of anatomy and physiology basics. With this compendium of resources, the rarely seen anomaly is less apt to go undetected, and clinicians expend less time on idiosyncrasies that are not directly relevant to the examinee's communication concerns. That is, *Oral-Facial Evaluation for Speech-Language Pathologists* is designed to offer some relief to busy clinicians who encounter a wide range of disorder types or even to those who occasionally see patients with a multiplicity of symptoms, some of which extend beyond their area of expertise.

An Oral-Facial Inspection Tool That Promotes Consistency Across Examiners

By offering a rigorous and coherent set of suggested practices and by accompanying it with a complement of support resources, *Oral-Facial Evaluation for Speech-Language Pathologists* stands to enhance clinician preparedness. Thus, the manual promotes consistency of practice across the discipline.

An Oral-Facial Inspection Tool That Is Useful for Both Teaching and Clinical Practice

The amount of detail and structure establishes *Oral-Facial Evaluation for Speech-Language Pathologists* as an exceptional resource that is useful for introducing newer clinicians to sound principles and practices that are fundamental to oral-facial inspection. Although most experienced clinicians do not necessarily require the same amount of guidance overall, the detail provided in the manual leaves little room for uncertainties that potentially lead even some experienced clinicians to rely on tradition and, in some cases, clinical folklore. Furthermore, the manual's broad scope validates it as a useful resource for professionals at any level who sometimes encounter examinees with symptoms outside one's education and everyday practice.

The Scope of the Manual

Oral-Facial Evaluation for Speech-Language Pathologists is a comprehensive manual that tactically guides clinicians through the process of preparing for, executing, interpreting, and documenting a meaningful, thorough, and uniformly applicable oral-facial inspection. The tool's overarching objective is to reveal and document evidence that enables the speech-language pathologist to distinguish between functional and organic communication concerns with the intent of promoting effective and appropriate recommendations and follow-up.

Brief Overview of the Manual

Chapter 1 provides key information that examiners need before beginning the inspection, including prerequisite qualifications, comments to examiners,

information on target populations, directions for readying the work area, and guidance for instructing the examinee or guardian.

Chapter 2 then conveys instructions for eight routine clinical observations that are universally administered for nearly all examinees; moreover, the chapter guides data collection while simultaneously focusing on a series of relevant clinical questions. Refer to Tables 0–2 and 0–3 for overarching and specific clinical questions.

Some evidence gathered through the Chapter 2 procedures exposes a need for a more in-depth inspection that, although not routinely administered, falls under the scope of oral-facial inspection; therefore, Chapters 3 and 4 provide 16 discretionary procedures that are only completed when routine procedures or special needs reveal additional clinical questions that mandate further exploration in a particular area.

Chapters 2 through 4 are intended to be used in conjunction with the proper recording form, as described below. The chapters guide the evidence-gathering process, while the recording forms are useful for documenting and organizing the data.

Chapter 5 outlines a generic process of clinical decision making, beginning with the most fundamental of clinical questions, in an effort to provide less experienced clinicians with a practical framework that can be applied across the board. The chapter also discusses potential implications for each clinical question proposed in Chapters 2 through 4, as well as some information on specific symptom patterns associated with readily identifiable diagnoses.

Table 0–2. Overarching Clinical Questions That Oral-Facial Inspection Addresses

	Overarching Clinical Questions
1	Are all anatomical parts presumed necessary for speech *present*, *intact*, and *functioning adequately*?
2	If not, which parts are not present, intact, or functioning?
3	According to the evidence gathered, what exactly is the problem with the identified atypical part or parts?
4	Does evidence suggest a link between the identified anatomical or physiological difference and the idiosyncratic speaking pattern?

Table 0–3. Clinical Questions Associated With Specific Clinical Observation Procedures

Routine and Discretionary Clinical Observations		The Clinical Question	Remarkable Response
Routine Clinical Observation 1: Conversational Speech Sample, Facial Region Inspection, Breathing Observations (Chapter 2)	1	Does the conversational speech sample reveal a specific atypical speaking pattern that should be further explored during a later portion of the inspection so as to discover whether the speaking pattern has an organic etiology, potentially affecting the plan of care?	Yes
	2	Is intelligibility rating in connected speech *fair*, *poor*, or *unintelligible*?	Yes
	3	Is a spontaneous swallow, while at rest or during speech, followed immediately by cough or noticeable change in vocal quality?	Yes
	4	Does the inspection reveal any externally observable anomalies of the face or head that may either interfere with speech or guide a specialist referral?	Yes
	5	Do observations of breathing reveal any pattern that may hinder normal, fluid, and properly resonant speech?	Yes
Routine Clinical Observation 2: Assess Lips and Tongue for Mobility and Strength (Chapter 2)	6	When inspecting lips and tongue for strength and mobility, does the examinee exhibit irregularities that potentially explain articulatory errors noted during speech?	Yes
Routine Clinical Observation 3: Assess Dental Bite and Alignment (Chapter 2)	7	Does a systematic inspection of dentition reveal bite or alignment irregularities that potentially influence an identified atypical speaking pattern or imply a need for a specialist referral?	Yes
Routine Clinical Observation 4: Assess Dental Occlusion (Chapter 2)	8	Does dental occlusion inspection reveal a maxillary-mandibular relationship that implies craniofacial anomaly?	Yes
	9	Does dental occlusion inspection reveal a maxillary-mandibular relationship that may be considered one symptomatic element of a syndromic cluster to be diagnosed by a specialist?	Yes
	10	Does dental occlusion inspection reveal a maxillary-mandibular relationship that seems to reduce intraoral space available for tongue excursion?	Yes
	11	Does dental occlusion inspection reveal a maxillary-mandibular relationship that seems to result in an improper alignment between the tongue and palatal surface, potentially affecting articulatory precision?	Yes

Table 0–3. *continued*

Routine and Discretionary Clinical Observations		The Clinical Question	Remarkable Response
Routine Clinical Observation 5: Assess Oral Interior (Chapter 2)	12	When asked to lower the jaw, does the examinee's mandible move with adequate excursion to allow for viewing the oral cavity?	No
	13	When lowering and raising the jaw while the examiner manually applies resistance, does the examinee exert adequate strength to overcome the resistance symmetrically?	No
	14	Does inspecting the oral interior expose any structural irregularities, such as missing, damaged, or malfunctioning parts, that may potentially explain or partially explain the examinee's idiosyncratic speaking pattern?	Yes
Routine Clinical Observation 6: Assess Velar Movement (Chapter 2)	15	When prompting velar movement through /ɑ/ phonation, does the velum appear to move symmetrically and with adequate excursion?	No
	16	Is the velar dimple observed to be properly located during /ɑ/ phonation?	No
Routine Clinical Observation 7: Assess Verbal Diadochokinesis (Chapter 2)	17	For speech-alternating motion, are the verbal diadochokinetic syllables produced with steady rate and articulatory precision?	No
	18	For speech-sequential motion, are the three distinctly different syllables produced accurately, rapidly, and in sequence?	No
	19	For speech-alternating motion and speech-sequential motion, are the syllables produced with rate, volume, and precision that do not deteriorate?	No
	20	For speech-alternating motion and speech-sequential motion, are approximately five syllables produced per second?	No
Routine Clinical Observation 8: Assess Vowel Prolongation (Chapter 2)	21	When sustaining a vowel, does the examinee exhibit vocal pitch, quality, loudness, and evenness that are perceived to be within normal limits?	No
	22	When sustaining a vowel, do duration and loudness suggest breath support that is adequate to sustain connected speech?	No
Discretionary Clinical Observation 9: Screening for Nasal Cavity Clearance (Chapter 3)	23	For examinees with perceived hyponasal resonance, does viewing the nasal cavity provide evidence of clinically relevant obstruction?	Yes

continues

Table 0–3. *continued*

Routine and Discretionary Clinical Observations		The Clinical Question	Remarkable Response
Discretionary Clinical Observation 10: Facial Dimension Estimates (Chapter 3)	24	When facial dysmorphia is noted upon superficial inspection, does evidence augment or support a specialist referral?	Yes
Discretionary Clinical Observation 11: Screening for Temporomandibular Joint Disorder (Chapter 3)	25	For individuals for whom a medical referral is planned due to reduced mandibular excursion or associated pain, does evidence augment the referral?	Yes
Discretionary Clinical Observation 12: Observations for Tongue-Thrust Swallow (Chapter 3)	26	For examinees identified to be at risk for tongue-thrust swallow, does the evidence support a diagnosis of clinically significant tongue-thrust swallow?	Yes
	27	If so, does the procedure identify the pattern as habitual or obligatory?	Either habitual or obligatory
Discretionary Clinical Observation 13: Observations for Developmental Apraxia of Speech (Chapter 3)	28	For child examinees who exhibit superficial symptoms of developmental apraxia of speech, does evidence support or rule out a diagnosis?	Yes
	29	If not, does the evidence support a referral for more in-depth testing?	Yes
Discretionary Clinical Observation 14: Observations for Acquired Apraxia of Speech (Chapter 3)	30	When routine inspection reveals symptoms that imply acquired apraxia of speech, does evidence support or rule out a diagnosis?	Yes
	31	If not, does evidence support a referral for more in-depth testing?	Yes
Discretionary Clinical Observation 15: Screening for Submucous Cleft of the Hard Palate (Chapter 3)	32	When examining individuals for whom integrity of the hard palate is questionable, who also exhibit signs of hypernasal speech or difficulty with obstruent consonants, does the evidence strengthen a medical referral?	Yes
Discretionary Clinical Observation 16: Screening for Surplus Nasal Airflow (Chapter 3)	33	For individuals who will be referred for evaluation of velar structure or function, does evidence strengthen a referral for more in-depth testing?	Yes

Table 0–3. *continued*

Routine and Discretionary Clinical Observations		The Clinical Question	Remarkable Response
Discretionary Clinical Observation 17: Observations for Dysarthria (Chapter 3)	34	When routine inspection reveals symptoms that imply dysarthria, does evidence confirm or rule out a diagnosis?	Confirm
	35	If evidence supports a diagnosis, does it provide enough data to reliably identify the type of dysarthria?	Varies
	36	If evidence does not support a diagnosis, does evidence support a referral for more in-depth testing?	Yes
Discretionary Clinical Observation 18: Speech Sound Stimulability Screening (Chapter 3)	37	For individuals with atypical speech sound production, when clinical teaching opportunities are presented, does the examinee respond by improving or changing the speaking pattern?	No
Discretionary Clinical Observation 19: Screening for Laryngeal and Respiratory Efficiency (Chapter 3)	38	For examinees who exhibit symptoms of laryngeal or respiratory inefficiency, does the S:Z ratio provide additional information that strengthens a medical referral for more in-depth testing?	Yes
Discretionary Clinical Observation 20: Gag Reflex Stimulation (Chapter 3)	39	For individuals who will be referred for neurologic or genetic evaluation, does response to gag reflex stimulation provide additional evidence to corroborate the referral?	Yes
Discretionary Clinical Observation 21: Prompt for Dysphagia Screening (Chapter 3)	40	Does evidence support the need for dysphagia screening in aging adults?	Yes
Discretionary Clinical Observation 22: Screening for Amblyopia (Chapter 4)	41	Does the young child examinee exhibit symptoms that suggest referral for amblyopia testing?	Yes
Discretionary Clinical Observation 23: Screening for Select Primitive Reflexes (Chapter 4)	42	For infants, toddlers, and some preschoolers suspected of having possible neurologic involvement, are primitive reflexes present and suppressed at developmentally appropriate ages?	No
Discretionary Clinical Observation 24: Additional Procedures for Patients Planning to Learn Esophageal Speech (Chapter 4)	43	For the laryngectomized patient who plans to learn esophageal speech, does evidence suggest candidacy for this type of alaryngeal speech?	No

Chapter 6 then focuses on formally documenting the inspection and its results. This includes principles and models for summarizing the results, noting evidence in the diagnostic and prognostic statements, and ensuring that clinicians have adequate information to respect scope of practice boundaries when making recommendations.

Appendices include a set of recording forms that are designed to facilitate gathering and interpreting evidence (Appendix A), an annotated list of materials and supplies (Appendix B), an optional rapid review of relevant anatomy and physiology (Appendix C), and summary of relevant cranial nerves (Appendix D).

Evidence-Based Practice and Oral-Facial Inspection

The American Speech-Language Hearing Association (ASHA) promotes incorporating principles of evidence-based practice whenever speech-language pathologists arrive at and implement clinical decisions (ASHA, 2005). Clearly the oral-facial inspection entails clinical decision making, calling for a foundation in evidence-based practice. Therefore, evidence-based practice principles are considered and applied throughout this inspection tool (ASHA, 2005; Lof & Camarata, 2013; Ylvisaker, 2004; Ylvisaker et al., 2002).

By way of review for most, evidence-based practice requires that clinicians and researchers alike integrate three fundamental principles whenever making decisions about clinical practice, with the definitive goal of ensuring that clinicians provide high-quality and individualized services in the best interest of every person in evaluation or treatment. The three essential elements of evidence-based practice are (1) clinical expertise/expert opinion, (2) external scientific evidence, and (3) client/patient/caregiver values.

The Dynamic Nature of Evidence-Based Practice

The three fundamentals listed above are recognized as *ever changing*. That is, optimally, a practitioner's clinical expertise and the available research-based external evidence are in a constant state of enhancement and improvement as clinicians gain experience and as more information is added to the existing available knowledge base. In addition, client attributes may evolve to some degree. Therefore, evidence-based practice is a dynamic process that requires continual reexamination on a day-to-day basis.

Although at first glance, the dynamic nature of evidence-based practice may resemble the impossibilities associated with aiming at a moving target, the practice also recognizes the continual evolutionary process of both clinical expertise and state-of-the-art research. Therefore, as evidence-based principles are applied to oral-facial inspection throughout the manual, we fully accept that new information will be added and will likely affect procedures and principles described herein.

Four Steps of Evidence-Based Practice

The four steps of evidence-based practice are (1) framing the clinical question, (2) finding the evidence, (3) assessing the evidence, and (4) making clinical decisions. The manual wraps itself around these four steps, with Chapters 2 through 4 focusing on framing the questions and finding the evidence, while Chapters 5 and 6 support the process of assessing the evidence and making clinical decisions.

Framing the Clinical Question

A clinical decision begins with a clinical question, and a successful outcome relies on appropriately framing the clinical question. To lend consistency to the process of framing answerable and relevant questions, define them according to four features: population (P), intervention or exposure (I), comparison (C), and outcome (O). These features are also known by the acronym *PICO*.

Furthermore, when working with non-treatment-oriented clinical questions, the C (i.e., comparison) element can be eliminated ordinarily; therefore, the *comparison* may not be considered entirely relevant for many oral-facial inspection-related inquiries. Dynamic measures, such as those involving response to clinical teaching, are the exception.

Oral-Facial Evaluation and Clinical Questions. The manual operatively tends to the evidence-based mandate for properly framed clinical questions by clearly stating a specific question or set of questions at the front end of each routine and discretionary clinical observation found in Chapters 2 through 4. For convenience, the full array of focused clinical questions appears in Table 0–3. These questions are intended to facilitate the evidence gathering that ultimately leads to answering the four overarching clinical questions shown in Table 0–2.

References to clinical questions appear throughout the manual. Therefore, Table 0–4 displays the four overarching questions and dissects them according to the PICO framework, ensuring that the underlying process meets standards for evidence-based practice.

Note that when stating clinical questions throughout the manual, for the sake of simplicity, certain parts of PICO are assumed to be *understood*. For example, the population (P) portion of the question is *understood* to comprise the persons who receive routine oral-facial inspection or who are identified as needing a particular discretionary clinical observation. The intervention or exposure (I) is *understood* to be either the full oral-facial inspection or the specific procedure being discussed at the time. Furthermore, the comparison (C) element is needed only for dynamic portions of the instrument, that is, when evaluating the examinee's response to clinical teaching. Therefore, for the purpose of this document clinical questions are often reduced to a simplified form that virtually converges on outcome (O).

Table 0–4. Evaluating the Four Overarching Clinical Questions According to PICO

Overarching Clinical Question	P Population	I Diagnostic Test	C[a]	O Outcome
1. Are all anatomical parts that are generally considered necessary or speech present, intact, and functioning adequately?	All persons receiving an oral-facial inspection	The oral-facial inspection	NA	Confirm or rule out that anatomical parts necessary for speech are present, intact, and functioning
2. Which parts are not present, intact, or functioning adequately?	Person whose oral-facial inspection identified an anatomical or physiological difference			Identify the specific anatomical or physiological differences
3. According to the evidence gathered, what exactly is the problem with the atypical part or parts?		Evidence gathered through oral-facial inspection compared to knowledge of normal anatomy and physiology		Identify the exact nature of the problems with regard to structure or function
4. Does evidence suggest a link between the identified anatomical and physiological differences and the idiosyncratic speaking pattern?		Consider identified anatomical or physiological difference(s) in the context of speaking pattern		Determine whether the anatomical or physiological difference(s) explain or partially explain the speaking pattern

Note: PICO = population, intervention/exposure, comparison, outcome; *NA* = not applicable.

[a]"Comparison": Only relevant for portions of the tool that involve clinical teaching; not relevant in this case.

Finding the Evidence

The act of clinical questioning mandates that, through formal observation, clinicians seek data that lead to an evidence-based clinical decision. Evidence can come from external scientific reviews or the expertise that the clinician brings to the inspection, and these should be integrated with the third type of evidence, which are the data gathered while inspecting the individual examinee.

Oral-Facial Evaluation and Finding the Evidence. Chapters 2 through 4 facilitate collecting evidence of the client-centered type. The recording forms are useful for organizing the client-centered evidence in preparation for interpretation and clinical decision making.

Then, Chapters 2 through 4 also provide limited external evidence for baseline purposes. Of course, each clinician brings professional experience to the inspection and is obliged to integrate it with the clinical observations as well as external evidence that the manual facilitates.

Assessing the Evidence

Not all evidence is relevant and applicable, and some evidence, although relevant and applicable, requires detailed analysis to determine the exact nature of its relationship to the perceptible clinical symptoms. Therefore, once the evidence is collected, the next step is to scrutinize it for relevance and clinical applicability.

Oral-Facial Evaluation and Assessing the Evidence. Interpreting the evidence is central to the oral-facial evaluation process. Yet assessing the evidence, and ultimately arriving at clinical decisions, can be the most challenging. This is particularly true when encountering less commonly seen symptom patterns. Examiners can refer to Chapter 5 for guidance in this area if it is needed.

Making Clinical Decisions

Properly framed clinical questions, when addressed through applicable and relevant evidence, lead to evidence-based clinical decisions that give rise to applicable and relevant evaluation and treatment plans. This is believed to be at the core of competent clinical service delivery.

Oral-Facial Evaluation and Clinical Decision Making. In reference to this manual, the clinical decision-making process appears most notably in Chapters 5 and 6, where implications are weighed, measured, and recorded. This includes any relevant diagnostic information, an evidence-based judgment of prognosis, and recommendations that may include referrals or other decisions that affect the plan of care.

The Art and Science of Applying Evidence-Based Practice to Oral-Facial Inspection

This may be a good time to recapture the three elements of evidence-based practice: (1) clinical expertise/expert opinion, (2) external-scientific evidence, and (3) client/patient/caregiver values. Up to this point, the primary focus has been on collecting client-centered evidence and comparing it to factual information, a scientific activity to be sure.

Yet oral-facial evaluation is also unmistakably an art. That is, the first element of evidence-based practice acknowledges that examiners rely on clinical intuition, experience, expertise, and professional opinion when determining the clinical focus for the inspection, selecting and applying discretionary clinical observations, collecting and interpreting the evidence, and documenting the findings. Box 0–1 expounds on the clinical-art metaphor.

More explicitly establishing the inspection as an art, note that a predictable pattern of one-to-one correspondence does not exist between physical anomaly and perceived speech disorder. For this reason, artful consideration is required when evaluating whether scientific evidence links the idiosyncratic-speaking pattern to organic features. Ideally, the evidence-based approach to clinical problem solving facilitates this unique blend of art and science.

Conclusion

Clearly, oral-facial inspection is a needed tool that speech-language pathologists should have at their

---

Box 0–1. Clinical-Art Metaphor

Compare the artistic angle of oral-facial inspection to the professional artist creating a collage. It is the skillful artist who gathers the pieces, has a plan for combining them in an aesthetically pleasing manner, and then does so in such a way as to create a work that catches the eye, is meaningful, and perhaps even makes an intentional, interpretable statement. On the other hand, a person with less skill, though well intentioned, may collect and arrange a similar array of attractive pieces in a collage format, yet fail to achieve the desired effect.

Similarly, the experienced clinician gathers the necessary data, is skilled at determining which pieces of data contribute meaningfully to the overall picture, and combines them in such a way that they make absolute sense to the next service provider who reads the documentation. Although many newer clinicians are typically excellent data collectors, bringing all relevant and only relevant pieces together into a meaningful whole is far more complex; this requires not only clinical intuition but also years of training and experience. Clinicians who are still in the process of developing a sense of clinical artistry are likely to find Chapters 5 and 6 exceptionally practical.

---

fingertips, not just for the purpose of inspecting the oral-facial region for the clientele they serve regularly but also to confidently serve when persons exhibit symptoms that may lead to referral or expose a need for further investigation. *Oral-Facial Evaluation for Speech-Language Pathologists* offers handy access to a wide range of tools that not only support the inspection process but also introduce newer clinicians to oral-facial evaluation procedures and outcomes.

Acknowledgments

These few paragraphs hardly seem adequate to properly recognize the many who supported my work while writing *Oral-Facial Evaluation for Speech-Language Pathologists*. Let me begin by thanking my husband, soulmate, and best friend, David Crane Root. As my partner in raising our special-needs son, he has come up to the plate many times so that this project could be completed on schedule within the context of our family life. I am indebted to him for the vision he has had for this endeavor from the beginning and for his willingness to contribute his excellent voiceover talent to the video.

It is also fitting to acknowledge Marcus Caleb Johnson-Root, the child actor who appears on the video, and my son. Although these comments may not be useful to him at the time of this writing, I trust that one day he will understand that he has been an important teacher to me and that raising him has given me the privilege of peeking into the world of a purely innocent person every day of my life.

Natalie Bell was my graduate assistant through the most work-intensive part of the project. She did excellently on assignments and performed outstandingly as the demonstration clinician on the video. Cara Scheidel also participated during video production, serving as an adult actor and providing assistance during a work-intensive period, and I recognize her for her fine work. Other graduate assistants who contributed to various degrees are Brenna Merry, Stacey Ulrich, Casey Alexander, Lauren Vollmin, and Margaret Carpenter.

Of course, the video's excellent appearance and artistic presentation could not have been done without the cinema and photography talent of Dr. Changhee Chun, Associate Professor of Media Arts, Science and Studies at Ithaca College. Dr. Chun generously donated his time and provided an excellent film crew to execute the filming process. Leading the crew was Jackson Jarvis Eagan, a recent Ithaca College graduate who worked closely with us during video planning, production, and editing.

Sara Gaechter is an industrious artist who diligently completed the artwork. I complement her for her hard work, willingness to make adjustments as needed, and the positive outcome that can be seen in the book's 68 illustrations.

I also wish to acknowledge the many clients and students throughout the years who have taught me abundantly while I was developing the materials that eventually became *Oral-Facial Evaluation for Speech-Language Pathologists*. Although they were not aware at the time, questions asked, responses to instruction, and the privilege of observing oral-facial idiosyncrasies contributed greatly to the endeavor's final outcome.

I extend a sincere thank you to Dr. Raymond Kent, who graciously reviewed the manuscript and wrote the foreword for the book. I found his editorial comments invaluable when making final revisions. More important, the constructive nature of his words had a profound impact on me personally, and I will always remember him for that. And thank you to the staff at Plural Publishing, as well as the anonymous reviewers who took the time to comment on my work. It has been a pleasure to work with Plural on this project. I sincerely appreciate the opportunity that the company gave me when they agreed to support this important project.

Finally, I cannot complete the acknowledgments without expressing intense gratitude to my creator, who gave me the skill and perseverance to complete a project of this magnitude, orchestrated a wide variety of professional and clinical experiences over a period of decades, and has blessed me with a wonderful life and family.

David

Thank you for being amused by my idiosyncrasies.
Thank you for appreciating my strengths.
Thank you for looking out for me.
Thank you for loving me.

Barb

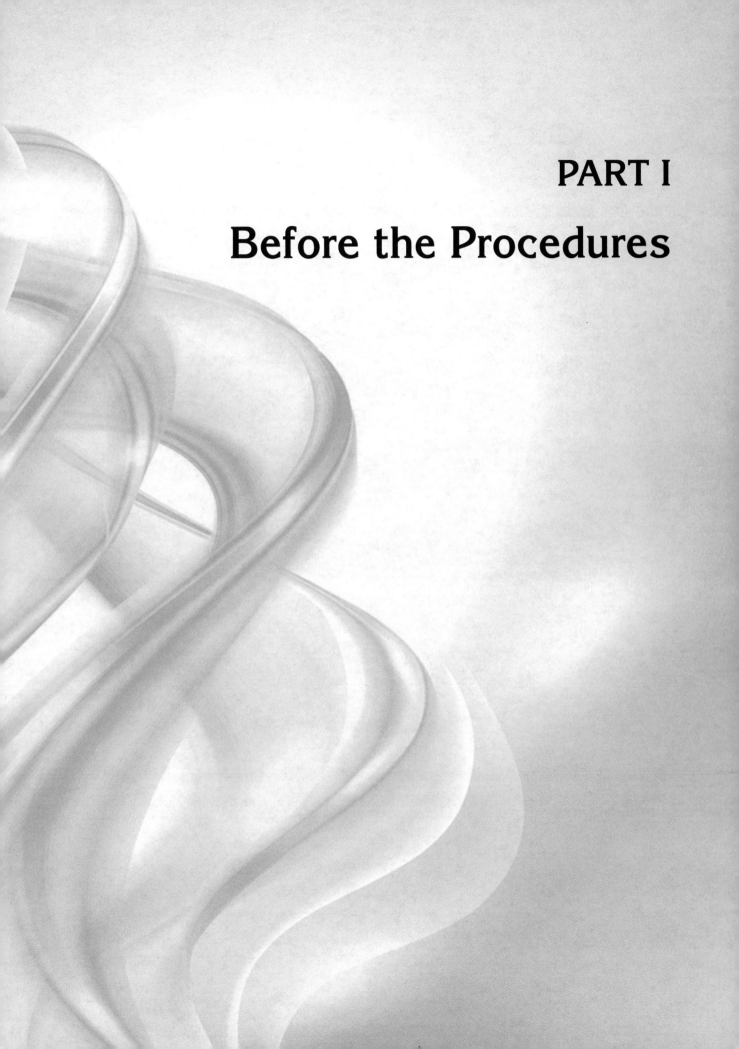

PART I

Before the Procedures

1

Getting Started

Qualifications for Examiners

Independent Inspections: Practicing Professionals and Clinical Fellows

When performing an oral-facial inspection independently, at minimum, qualified examiners are required to (1) have earned a master's degree in speech-language pathology or equivalent discipline from a program that is accredited by the Council on Academic Accreditation (CAA) or in the process of obtaining the accreditation *and* (2) either hold the American Speech-Language-Hearing Association's (ASHA's) Certificate of Clinical Competence (CCC) or are in the process of earning it. Individuals who hold the appropriate master's degree but for some reason do not maintain the ASHA CCC should at the very least maintain either a license to practice speech-language pathology in their state or a teaching certificate specific to the speech-language discipline.

Supervised Inspections: Student Clinicians

Students in clinical practicum earning clock hours in preparation for the CCC also may perform the oral-facial evaluation but only under the direct supervision of a qualified examiner who holds the ASHA CCC and meets the criteria for supervision under the guidelines of the student's accredited academic program. Furthermore, nothing prevents students who are learning about the procedures from cautiously practicing them on volunteers such as friends and relatives, provided that examinees knowledgeably consent to the inspection and the outcomes are not tendered as clinical results. In fact, practice inspections are encouraged so that students may become thoroughly familiar with the procedures and forms, while also arriving at an operative grasp of the range of normal appearances for structure and function to be encountered clinically at a later time.

Special Comments for Examiners

Newer Service Providers and Students

If you are a relatively new practitioner or a student of speech-language pathology, be assured that this manual grew out of a need expressed by individuals in your current position. The manual's structure and detail are intended to put into your hands a well-organized plan that tactically guides you through the oral-facial inspection process, so as to increase your confidence to competently evaluate a broad array of oral-facial mechanisms for structure and function.

As you grow in proficiency through experience, the need for extensive structure and detailed explanations will diminish. Yet, especially where some of the less common discretionary clinical observations and special populations are concerned, this tool is likely to continue to serve as a useful resource for years to come.

Academics and Clinical Supervisors

Preclinical Academic Teaching

Ideally, the oral-facial evaluation is introduced to students before they begin supervised clinical practice. In some programs, classroom-based exposure to oral-facial inspection is one of the first academic activities requiring students to synthesize large amounts of information learned in prerequisite coursework for the purpose of clinical decision making. Many students find this challenging, although most are relieved to at last try their hand at the practical problem solving that will eventually define their professional future.

It is at the first exposure to oral-facial inspection that full use of the manual yields the most benefit. Once a professor or supervisor lays the foundation by fully exploiting this highly structured and informative resource, students can and should practice the procedures on one another so that they become thoroughly familiar with them while also becoming acquainted with a range of normal appearances that they will inevitably view and judge later in professional practice.

Also, informal practice opportunities afford occasion to observe the few variations and anomalies that willing peers may be amenable to share, such as the occasional high palatal arch, dental misalignment or malocclusion, minor palatal fistulus, tongue-thrust swallow, or even repaired craniofacial anomaly. Although the irregularities that peers typically bring to the actual practice session are most often subclinical in nature, the opportunity to view them prior to clinical practice is invaluable.

The fundamental worth that the manual brings to your course lies in its breadth and depth. That is, the content not only scopes a wide range of possible conditions but also details procedures for identifying these idiosyncrasies, while also commenting on potential for relevance to clinical decision making.

Practicum Supervision

Supervising a student clinician's early experiences with oral-facial inspection presents many challenges. None are insurmountable, but rising above them requires supervisory vigilance as well as a generous amount of supervisory support. Less experienced clinical supervisors may find oral-facial inspection somewhat more challenging than other supervisory activities; for that reason, the comments that follow are intended to support the supervisory process on an as-needed basis.

Fundamentally, clinical supervisors serve two roles. The first and foremost is to ensure that the client receives competently delivered clinical services; the second interfaces with the first, and that is to strategically exploit teaching opportunities that benefit the student clinician. All parts of the evaluation process demand attentiveness in both of these areas, and oral-facial inspection is no exception.

With the goal of fulfilling these two intertwining supervisory roles, we strongly recommend not only being in the diagnostic room with the student and client for the entire oral-facial evaluation but also being *fully prepared* to participate in the inspection alongside the student clinician. Letting the student know in advance that this will be the case is only fair. Furthermore, expect that properly prepared students normally welcome the support since they are already cognizant that some clinical observations require more experience than they bring to the diagnostic room.

Ideally, the student performs the inspection completely and with reasonable efficiency without mediation, while you serve as a coexaminer so as to ensure a thorough and competent appraisal. To increase the likelihood of an uninterrupted procedure from start to finish, we recommend meeting with the student *prior to* the day of the clinical evaluation. The aim of the presession meeting is threefold. First, together with the student, look over the equipment and materials that the student plans to bring to the examination room, confirming that the student has amassed a full array of supplies that meet specs detailed in Appendix B. Second, give the student an opportunity to rehearse selected procedures in your presence, so that you may anticipate his or her style and even add to his or her understanding if necessary. Third, the preassessment meeting is an excellent time to help the student prepare in advance for discretionary procedures that may be anticipated based on preliminary case history intake. Taking the time to do these things prior to the session is very likely to save time during the session, while also increasing the student's confidence to perform an oral-facial evaluation on a person who has legitimate communication needs.

It is entirely possible that some clinical teaching may be needed when in the presence of the examinee. The student should be aware of this possibility so as not to feel blindsided in the event of a necessary interruption that is intended to benefit both the examinee and the student. For example, a student clinician may naïvely perform a part of the inspection in a way that is unlikely to yield the needed information; you may observe and point out a structural or functional irregularity that the student needs to see; an unanticipated discretionary clinical observation may need to be performed; or change in protocol may become evident while already engaged with the examinee in the examination room.

In anticipation of the possible need for intermediation, always let the student know in advance that the inspection should be considered a team effort, that the student is responsible to perform the procedures, that you will intervene if needed, and that you will coinspect so as to ensure that all noteworthy irregularities are noted. Go to the session prepared to work with the student as a team member. That is, wash your hands and don the gloves before the inspection begins and position yourself so as to maximize opportunity for co-observations. If it becomes necessary to demonstrate, reinstruct, or point out a feature, then politely request permission to provide input at that time thereby reducing opportunity for the student to feel undermined. Even if a student performs the activities very poorly or appears unprepared, a problem that hopefully hardly ever occurs, keep in mind that during the session, your concerns about a student's preparation or aptitude should not come across in any way so as to maintain focus on client needs and avoid potential for awkwardness.

Experienced Practitioners

As an experienced practitioner, you have most likely adopted a working set of oral-facial inspection procedures and at the very least are familiar with the process well enough to benefit from published checklists that can serve to remind you to do things that through years of practice you already know

how to do. You may have even developed your own checklist or protocol, or it is even possible that you smoothly execute the inspection from memory.

Certainly, those who specialize in a particular area do not need the amount of structure and detail provided herein, especially when evaluating cases that lie entirely within their area of expertise. Yet in deciding whether this manual is applicable to your practice, consider the benefit of having handy access to discretionary clinical observations that lie outside your area of expertise, information on serving individuals with special needs, detailed and orderly recording forms, and ready access to a well-ordered teaching tool when mentoring students and newer clinicians.

Suitable Populations

General Guidelines for Deciding Which Examinees Should Receive an Inspection

An Appropriate Activity for Most

As a general rule, if an examinee's communication goals include speech and the person is able to tolerate the procedures and follow the instructions, that person is more often than not able to participate in a meaningful inspection using the resources provided in *Oral-Facial Evaluation for Speech-Language Pathologists*. Although adaptations may be needed for selected special populations, the manual takes this into account by providing various suggestions that are applicable to a variety of exceptional groups. Be encouraged to consult Chapter 4 if necessary whenever working with persons whose needs are discussed in that section.

For the Few Who Are Not Able to Tolerate the Oral-Facial Evaluation

It is exceptionally rare to find a person who has potential to use spoken language who also is not able to participate in most of the activities shown in the manual, giving consideration to special needs and age-related limitations accounted for in Chapter 4. Yet, in some settings, the clientele may include an abundance of individuals who are not capable of participation due to reasons that may include multiple concomitant disabling conditions, serious illness, deteriorating health, profound physical or cognitive limitations, or other deleterious state. For individuals who cannot participate, whether and how to complete a meaningful inspection is a clinical decision that relies on professional judgment.

Consider the Examinees' Speech Sound System

Since the manual focuses on considering a person's capacity to produce speech, potential to form specific speech sounds enters the discussion repeatedly from start to finish. The sound system of reference throughout the manual is American English, unless denoted otherwise.

Many aspects described herein may be reasonably applied to other languages. Nonetheless, exercise caution if using this manual to inspect a person's capacity to produce specific features of a language other than American English, especially if the features of interest are not part of the American English speech sound system.

Oral-Facial Inspection for Persons Requesting Services to Address Language Difference

The scope of practice for speech-language pathologists continues to include services for individuals who choose speech therapy as a method for reducing the effect of a dialect or accent, apart from communication disorder. For the vast majority of these examinees, oral-facial inspection yields unremarkable findings. Yet, to verify that all parts are structurally and functionally sound, as well as confirm that no physical hindrance stands in the way of the person's communication goals, the routine oral-facial inspection is included in the protocol for all kinds of comprehensive communication evaluations (see Table 0–1). Of course, if remarkable findings are discovered, they should be treated as they would for any other person receiving oral-facial inspection.

Revisiting Oral-Facial Inspection for an Examinee Who Was Previously Evaluated

Most oral-facial evaluations are incorporated into the comprehensive diagnostic process that precedes decisions about plan of care. Occasionally, a clinically significant feature is missed during the preliminary inspection, and it becomes necessary to revisit oral-facial inspection as part of a therapy program even though the oral-facial region was already examined. When this happens, it is only necessary to revisit the parts of the inspection that may shed light on the problems the person experiences from a plan-of-care perspective (Box 1–1).

Amount of Time to Allow for Oral-Facial Inspection

Three principal factors strongly influence the amount of time needed to administer *Oral-Facial Evaluation for Speech-Language Pathologists*. They are examiner experience level, whether Routine Clinical Observation 1 (i.e., conversational speech sample, facial region inspection, breathing observations) is completed prior to the inspection as part of another assessment goal, and whether discretionary clinical observations are needed.

Examiner Experience Level

Undoubtedly, skilled practitioners have the advantage of immense familiarity with both oral-facial inspection practices and oral geography. Armed only with a barebones checklist and vivid internal visual and auditory models of both normal and aberrant findings, as well as having completed a conversational speech sample, facial region inspection, and breathing observations while interviewing or testing in other areas, many experienced clinicians can complete a basic routine inspection within 5 to 10 minutes under exemplary circumstances. On the other hand, students and less experienced clinicians require additional time to competently perform a simple routine inspection.

> ## Box 1–1. Clinical Examples: A Portion of Oral-Facial Inspection Was Revisited After Treatment Commenced
>
> ### Clinical Example 1
>
> The author strongly suspected serious tongue-tip immobility for a 4-year-old child who had received speech therapy for a few months with another service provider. The diagnostic report clearly stated that the oral-facial mechanism had been inspected and that all parts were structurally and functionally adequate for speech, and the therapy progress report indicated difficulty making therapy gains but gave no indication of concerns with tongue agility. Yet, the child's speech and oral posture convincingly suggested tongue immobility.
>
> As a result, a partial oral-facial inspection to evaluate tongue mobility was inserted into a treatment session, and it revealed exceptionally short lingual frenum, heart-shaped tongue tip, and failure to elevate the tongue tip beyond the cutting edge of the mandibular incisors. Once ankyloglossia was medically diagnosed and addressed, and the tongue was strengthened after a lifetime of inactivity, consistent and maintainable therapy gains began.
>
> ### Clinical Example 2
>
> An adolescent who had been a long-term recipient of speech therapy to remediate a set of consonants requiring lingual precision had worked with a few clinical service providers on a semester-by-semester basis. Gains in therapy were slow and characterized by loss of progress between sessions and considerable relapse during semester breaks.
>
> When attempting to achieve tongue position for target phonemes, the client's jaw consistently moved with the tongue, possibly interfering with ease of the lingual movements. Wondering if freedom of movement would be enhanced by relieving the burden of carrying the jaw along with the tongue for articulation, the portions of the oral-facial inspection that investigate differentiated tongue movements were performed in a diagnostic therapy session.
>
> This revealed difficulty with moving the tongue independently of the jaw for both speech and nonspeech activities, even with modeling and clinical teaching. As a result, a goal was added to explore whether treatment evidence supported the idea that increasing tongue independence would improve articulation. In this case, it did.
>
> ### Summary
>
> In these examples, only the portions of the oral-facial inspection that addressed newly emerging clinical questions were administered upon reinspection. Typically, this is an acceptable approach when taking a second look at someone whose oral-facial mechanism was already examined.

Whether Conversational Speech Sample, Facial Region Inspection, and Breathing Observations Are Completed Prior to the Inspection

Since the oral-facial inspection is usually completed at the end of an assessment session that comprises a range of procedures (see Table 0–1), many opportunities to complete these observations occur well in advance of the formal oral-facial inspection, and experienced clinicians take advantage of them. Thus, whenever this happens, the amount of time needed for oral-facial inspection can be reduced considerably.

Whether a Discretionary Clinical Observation Is Needed

The discretionary procedures are only administered on an as-needed basis. Most oral-facial inspections end with Routine Clinical Observation 8, yield unremarkable findings, and reveal no need for any discretionary procedures. For all experience levels, this type of inspection requires the least amount of time.

Discretionary procedures are clearly a wild card, however. If any are needed for an individual, the number typically does not exceed three. Some discretionary procedures can be completed in only a moment, such as stimulating the gag reflex; others may be more time-consuming, requiring as much as 3 to 5 minutes each.

Estimating Time to Allocate for Oral-Facial Evaluation

The ideal conditions for streamlining the oral-facial inspection are experienced clinician; conversational speech sample, facial region inspection, and breathing observations completed prior; and no need for any discretionary clinical observations. This oral-facial inspection can be completed in fewer than 10 minutes.

The least favorable conditions for efficient inspection are first-time examiner; conversational speech sample, facial region inspection, and breathing observations not yet completed; and a need for three or more discretionary clinical procedures. This oral-facial inspection may require as much as 30 minutes of clinical time. A lengthy inspection such as this is the exception rather than the rule.

Table 1–1 provides a framework for estimating the amount of time needed depending on the specific parameters that apply. Of course, the framework provided in the table can be used to arrive at an estimate only.

Getting Started

Before beginning an oral-facial evaluation, acquire all equipment and supplies that are listed in Table 1–2.

An annotated version of the same list appears in Appendix B.

Table 1–2 exists as a convenient reference for service providers who are familiar with the purposes and procedures associated with each item, whereas the annotated list (see Appendix B) provides additional detail that may be needed for some. We strongly suggest that newer clinicians carefully read the detailed equipment descriptions before beginning so as to be certain that the available supplies are useful for accomplishing the intended purpose.

Also, before beginning, carefully consult Chapters 2 and 3. By so doing, you will gain familiarity with the routine and discretionary clinical observations and have an understanding of the method for recording the findings. Furthermore, since an examinee may require modification, accommodation, or out-of-the-ordinary consideration due to age or special need, consult Chapter 4 if the examinee corresponds to any group whose needs are addressed therein before proceeding with the inspection.

Newer clinicians are strongly advised to practice administering the procedures as an academic activity and consult with the supervisor before proceeding with an actual case. Once you have done these things, you are ready to prepare the work area and instruct the examinee.

Prepare the Work Area for Testing

Objective

Ensure that all materials are readily accessible and that the work area and supplies are properly sterilized to protect yourself as well as the examinee.

Equipment

Gather all equipment and supplies. They are required for the setup unless otherwise indicated.

Setup Procedures

Check Batteries. So as to minimize the risk of unnecessary interruption, check batteries that supply power to any battery-operated equipment.

Table 1–1. Framework for Estimating Amount of Time to Allocate for Oral-Facial Inspection

Condition That May Influence Amount of Time Needed	Amount of Time Needed Under That Condition	Total Estimated Time in Minutes (Range)	
		Minimum Time	Maximum Time
Clinician experience	Time Needed for Routine-Clinical Observations 2–8 Expert　　　　　　　　　　Novice ◄————————————————► ≤10 minutes　　　　　　15 minutes	≤10	15
Conversational-speech sample, facial-region inspection, breathing observations not completed prior	Add 5 to 10 minutes	≤15	25
One to three discretionary-clinical observations may be needed, potentially adding 5 minutes to the inspection. The columns to the right estimate the maximum amount of time that each discretionary-clinical observation may require.	(see sub-table below)	≤16	30

Discretionary-Clinical Observation	Estimated Time in Minutes
9. Nasal Cavity Clearance	1
10. Estimating Facial Dimensions	1
11. Screening for Temporomandibular Joint Disorder	1
12. Tongue-Thrust Swallow Observations	1
13. Observations for Developmental Apraxia of Speech	3
14. Observations for Acquired Apraxia of Speech	3
15. Screening for Submucous Cleft Palate	1
16. Screening for Surplus-Nasal Airflow	1
17. Observations for Dysarthria	3
18. Speech Sound Stimulability Screening	2
19. Screening for Laryngeal and Respiratory Efficiency	2
20. Gag-Reflex Stimulation	1
21. Prompt for Dysphagia Screening	<1
22. Screening for Primitive Reflexes	3
23. Screening for Amblyopia	1
24. Checking Potential for Esophageal Speech	5

Table 1–2. Equipment and Supplies

Part of the Inspection	Item Needed	Purpose of the Item
Preparing the work area	Spare batteries	Be prepared to replace batteries before they die
	Disinfectant soap	Hand washing
	Disinfectant wipes	Disinfecting work surfaces and equipment
	Alcohol wipes	
	Tissues	In case of poor saliva management, nasal discharge, or need to manage excretions of any type
	Small plastic box	For equipment storage in some populations
During inspection	Pen and recording form	For recording responses
	Latex-free, powder-free examination gloves	Protect you and the examinee from the spread of germs
	Penlight	Illuminate the oral cavity for inspection
	Individually wrapped, disposable tongue depressor	Lip and tongue strength and mobility evaluation; oral interior inspection
	Stopwatch	Verbal diadochokinesis; vowel prolongation; laryngeal and respiratory efficiency
	Recording device	Conversational speech sample; verbal diadochokinesis; vowel prolongation; laryngeal and respiratory efficiency
	Millimeter ruler	Facial dimension estimates; temporomandibular joint screening
	Small cup of water	Tongue-thrust swallow procedure
	Small compact mirror or reflective surface	Surplus nasal airflow screening
	Extra-long cotton swab	Gag reflex; primitive reflexes
	Eye test paddle	Amblyopia screening
	Large in-room mirror	Response to clinical teaching
Interpreting data	Calculator	Facial dimension estimates; respiratory and laryngeal efficiency

Change batteries if there is any chance they may be due for replacement. Do not wait for batteries to fail before replacing them; the risk of lost data is not worth the cost of replacing a battery that may not last through the session.

Select Applicable Recording Form and Complete Identifying Information. Appendix A houses a series of recording forms, including a general form, followed by six modified forms that apply to specified populations. Choose the one that applies to your client, defaulting to the general form for most people.

Complete the identifying information section at the top of the appropriate form *before* the examinee arrives.

Sanitary Precautions. Many clinicians have inadequate training with regard to infection control. Yet precautions to avoid sharing germs are important in all settings, particularly when serving the seriously ill, the medically fragile, and individuals with infectious disease (Bankaitis, Kemp, Krival, & Bandaranayake, 2006; Kummer, 2008; Mosheim, 2005).

That is, in a hospital setting, we commonly examine persons who may be carrying contagious disease (e.g., methicillin-resistant staphylococcus aureus (MRSA), influenza, streptococcus, staph), often without knowledge of the presence of the virus or bacteria. This is especially true when the person is in the early stages of an illness or was recently exposed to a contaminated surface. For this reason, precautionary measures protect both you and the next patient who uses the same work surfaces and equipment. Likewise, every examinee deserves to know that a sanitary protocol is in place to protect from viruses and bacteria that have been left behind by other patients as well as any microorganisms that the examiner may carry at the time of the inspection.

Since bodily fluids can be hazardous and some contaminants are even capable of surviving on dry surfaces, out of consideration for the examinee and for yourself, take precautions to minimize potential for spreading germs. Suggested routine sanitary measures include the following:

- Remove and dispose of all cords, strings, and lanyards that may be attached to certain equipment before proceeding with the sterilization process (e.g., stopwatch or penlight). This is done to prevent unintended contamination of sanitized equipment resulting from proximity to porous material that characteristically resists sterilization (Chen, 2012; Lalla, Dingle, & Cheong, 2005).
- Immediately prior to beginning the inspection, wash hands and wrists thoroughly using disinfectant soap. This may require a quick hand-washing break after completing other diagnostic procedures that conceivably exposed hands to possible contaminants.
- Use a disinfectant wipe to cleanse a large area on the table surface (e.g., about twice the size of a standard placemat). The sanitized area will be used to place the equipment and supplies when working with older children and adults. For younger children and anyone else who may be distracted by the supplies or tempted to reach for them, in addition to sanitizing the table, cleanse a small plastic box (i.e., about the size of a small shoebox), so that the items may be placed in the box outside of the examinee's line of sight but handily accessible for you.
- Use a small amount of alcohol to sterilize unwrapped examination equipment (i.e., penlight, pen, mirror, millimeter ruler, recording device, stopwatch, small eye-test paddle). Wrapped items should remain in the sterile wrapping (i.e., tongue depressor, extra-long cotton swab). Some items are not wrapped and do not lend themselves to sterilization but are best kept in a handy location (i.e., tissues, cup of water, spare gloves, calculator, replacement batteries).
- Immediately after sanitizing the area and the supplies, arrange each article on the disinfected area as shown (Figure 1–1). Left-handed examiners are encouraged to move the pen and recording form to the far left for convenience, keeping all other items in the order and arrangement as shown. If using a box, place all sanitized items in the box.

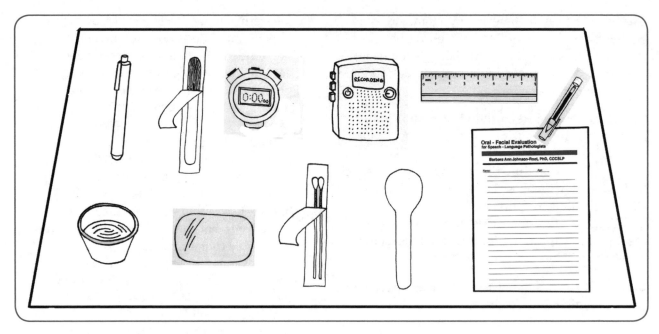

Figure 1–1. Arrangement of equipment.

- Put on the examination gloves, taking care to avoid contamination. Bare hands should only come in contact with the cuff portion of each glove. Properly sized gloves can be slipped on efficiently and hygienically. Once gloved, do not touch any surface that has not been sterilized or is not part of the sanitary procedure. That is, avoid touching hair, face, ears, clothing, furniture, books, or any other item that was not sanitized. Note that latex-free gloves are recommended to avoid allergic reaction that, in cases of latex sensitivity, can range from mild irritation to life-threatening anaphylaxis.
- Leave the gloves on throughout, changing them if ever suspecting contamination due to contact with nonsanitized surfaces. For your own safety, it is particularly important to wear gloves when coming in contact with body fluids (e.g., saliva, nasal discharge, perspiration).
- When ready to remove gloves, consider the exterior to be contaminated. Use the gloved dominant hand to slip the cuff over the nondominant hand such that the glove that was on nondominant hand becomes an inside-out wad. Enclose the wad inside the gloved fist of the dominant hand and slip the second cuff over the hand and wad. The result should be an inside-out glove with a wadded glove inside of it. Dispose. If gloves are needed after removing them, repeat the process of putting on a new pair as instructed above.

Instruct the Examinee or Guardian

Objective

Ensure that the examinee or guardian is informed about the procedures, reasonably comfortable with them, and aware of the general type of information likely to result.

Give the Instructions

Once the setup is complete, use your own words, developmentally appropriate ordinary language (i.e., no acronyms or professional jargon), and a friendly conversational tone to prepare the examinee for the inspection. Communicate the following talking points to the examinee or guardian:

- The oral-facial evaluation is a customary part of every speech-language evaluation.
- It involves inspecting all observable body parts necessary for speaking so that we may ascertain whether all parts are present, complete, and working properly.
- This is done to look into whether there is a physical explanation for the speech problem that brought you here or if there is any physical problem that we should address in order to help you.
- None of the procedures are painful or harmful.
- A few items situated on the table may not be needed.
- The oral-facial evaluation findings may lead to more detailed testing or possibly referral to another professional.
- You may ask questions before we begin or at any time. Do you have any questions now? (If *yes*, either answer briefly or diplomatically table the question for a more appropriate time. If *no*, move on.)
- Are you ready? Let's begin!

Transition From Instructions to Procedures

In transitioning from instructions to procedures, refrain from any inclination to apologize in anticipation of the inspection. Simply state what you are about to do using a pleasant and matter-of-fact tone; then proceed with a friendly yet professional demeanor.

Conclusion

Procedures associated with clinical observations appear in the next few chapters. The amount of flexibility depends on the clinician's degree of familiarity with the overall process.

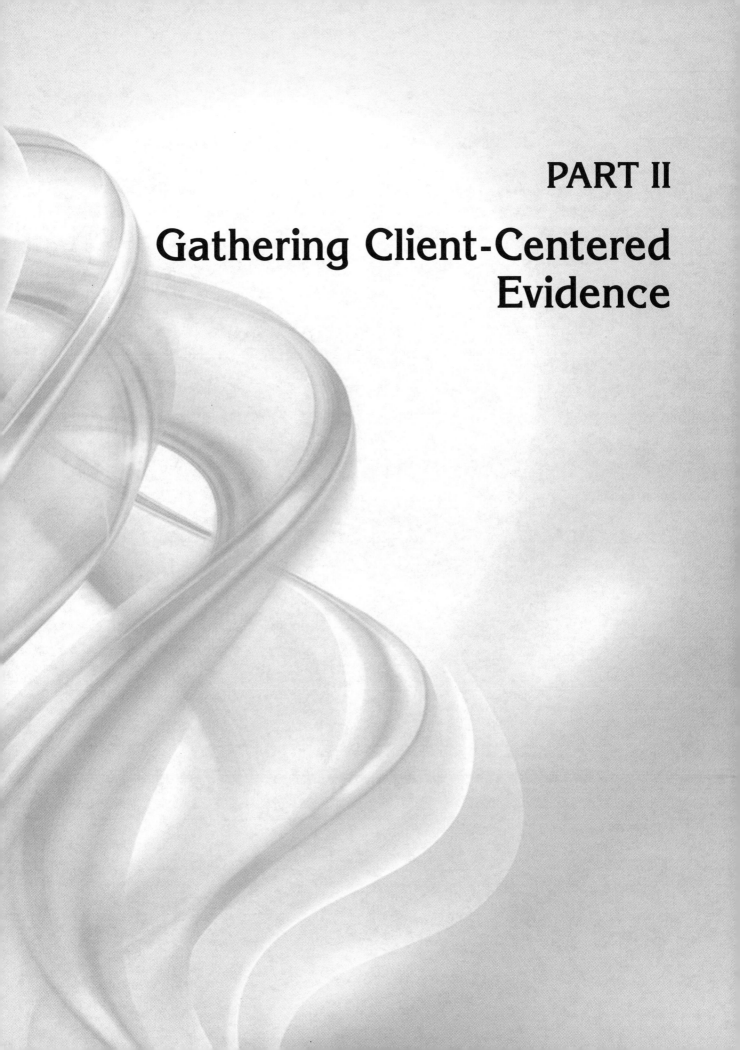

PART II
Gathering Client-Centered Evidence

2

Instructions for Routine
Oral-Facial Evaluation Procedures

Chapter 2 tactically guides a basic routine oral-facial inspection in an orderly fashion, employing a series of broadly applicable procedures that, when applied systematically, are intended to shed light on pertinent anatomic and physiologic idiosyncrasies. Findings that result from routine procedures have potential to (1) confirm that an identified communication disorder has no verifiable anatomic or physiologic basis, (2) provide physical evidence that explains or partially explains a communication disorder, (3) suggest a discretionary inspection procedure that should be performed only if routine observations expose a need, or (4) reveal the need for more in-depth testing that is beyond the scope of the oral-facial inspection.

Identify or Rule Out
Relevant Physical Anomaly

For most oral-facial inspection participants, the examiner has no prior knowledge of physical anomaly. For these individuals, the inspection is intended to rule out or expose the possibility of a physical explanation and, if a physical explanation is found, to describe the features and extrapolate with regard to their potential for relationship to the speaking pattern. Most frequently, no relevant physical evidence materializes; nevertheless, for the few whose physical symptoms are found to be definitively linked to a communication disorder, findings can significantly influence diagnosis and a plan of care.

Shed Light on a Previously
Identified Communication Disorder

Since a direct relationship cannot be established between most oral-mechanism idiosyncrasies and specific speaking patterns, the mere presence of a physical anomaly is not always clinically relevant. In some cases, however, clinical relevance is not only clearly evident but called to our attention prior to the inspection, such as in the cases of cleft palate, motor-speech disorder, or vocal pathology. Clinical relevance of physical symptoms is not particularly difficult to ascertain in these extreme cases, and certainly the oral-facial inspection can be useful for more clearly illuminating symptoms that are patently obvious.

Point to a Discretionary
Clinical Observation

Routine findings can expose the need for more information to rule out or confirm a diagnosis or to supplement evidence that supports a needed plan of action. There are times when the additional information can be obtained within the context of oral-facial evaluation, using procedures that extend beyond the scope of routine practices. The discretionary clinical observations that reside in Chapters 3 and 4 comprise the scope of discretionary procedures found in this manual.

Prompt More Thorough Testing Beyond the Scope of Oral-Facial Inspection

At times, an identified need for more information mandates testing outside the scope of oral-facial evaluation. This may refer to additional testing within the speech-language pathology discipline (e.g., dysphagia, velopharyngeal competency, or motor-speech testing). The circumstance may also denote a need for referral outside of the speech-language pathology discipline (e.g., primary care physician, genetics, otorhinolaryngologist, ophthalmologist, dentist, orthodontist, prosthodontist, oral surgeon).

Clearly, arranging for more in-depth testing within the speech-language pathology discipline can be fairly simple. For example, if anticipating a recommendation for intervention, the additional testing can be completed in the context of diagnostic therapy. Yet, whenever proposing further evaluation outside the scope of speech-language pathology, a formal referral is required and further action may be suspended until the specialist weighs in on the client's condition.

Orderly and Consistent Evidence Gathering

Each inspection procedure described in this manual follows the same sequential reasoning, ensuring systematic data collection throughout the inspection. Figure 2–1 illustrates the logic behind the process using a flowchart format. Further facilitating order, the recording forms support the process of tracking evidence.

Organization of Procedures

One goal associated with this manual is to present clear, minimally interrupted sequential instructions

for routine and discretionary oral-facial inspection. Therefore, each procedure reviews the relevant clinical question(s) (see Table 0–3), lists materials and supplies needed for that procedure, spells out the exact inspection process, describes normal and atypical findings, and ends with directions for considering discretionary procedures if they apply.

Additional details deemed relevant to the procedures but not necessarily integral to the step-by-step instructions are also interwoven throughout the chapter. These can be found in neighboring text boxes, whose purpose is to provide information that supports procedural instructions. The text box narratives are separated in this way to preserve instructions as a cohesive whole with minimal interruption to flow while still adding useful commentary.

Similarly, clinical implications are not deliberated within the context of the procedures. Instead, they are found in Chapter 5.

The Eight Routine Clinical Observation Procedures

Routine Clinical Observation 1: Conversational Speech Sample, Facial Region Inspection, and Respiration Observations

The Associated Clinical Questions

Clinical Questions 1 to 5 (see Table 0–3) can be divided into three parts. That is, the first three questions are relevant to conversational speech sample, the fourth is relevant to facial region inspection, and the fifth is relevant to breathing observations.

An answer of *yes* to any of the first five clinical questions potentially flags a remarkable finding. The procedures are useful for answering the questions *and* for describing relevant symptoms.

Clinical Questions Associated With Conversational Speech Sample. Clinical Question 1 (see Table 0–3) asks, "Does the conversational speech sample reveal a specific atypical speaking pattern that should be further explored during a later

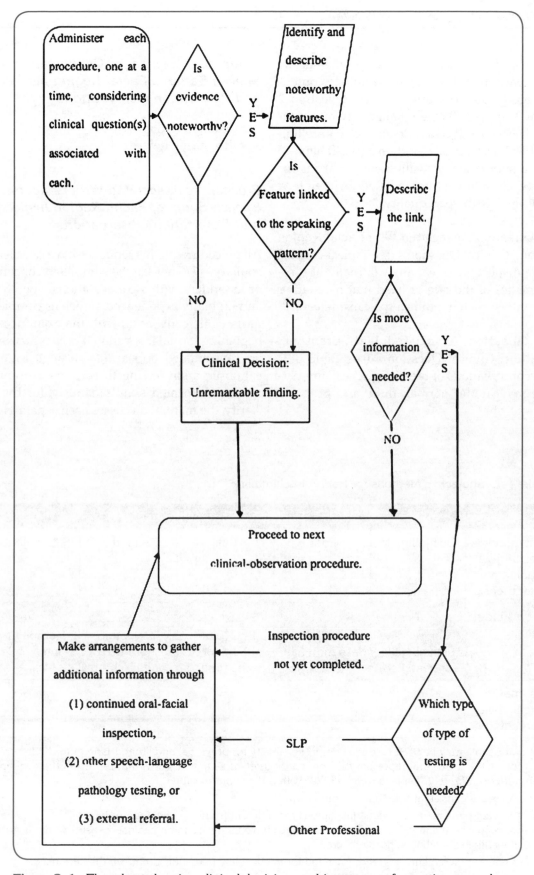

Figure 2–1. Flowchart showing clinical decision-making process for routine procedures.

part of the inspection so as to discover whether the speaking pattern has an organic etiology, potentially affecting plan-of-care?" Clinical Question 2 (see Table 0–3) asks, "Is the intelligibility rating for connected speech judged as fair, poor, or unintelligible?" (Table 2–1). Clinical Question 3 (see Table 0–3) asks, "Is a spontaneous swallow, while at rest or during speech, followed immediately by cough or noticeable change in vocal quality?"

Clinical Question Associated With Facial Region Inspection. Clinical Question 4 (see Table 0–3) asks, "Does the inspection reveal any externally observable anomalies of the face or head that may either interfere with speech or guide a specialist referral?"

Clinical Question Associated With Breathing Observation. Clinical Question 5 (see Table 0–3) asks, "Do observations of breathing reveal any pattern that may hinder normal, fluid, and properly resonant speech?"

Equipment Needed for Conversational Speech Sample, Facial Region Inspection, and Respiration Observations

- Examination gloves
- Recording device

Procedures Associated With Conversational Speech Sample, Facial Region Inspection, and Respiration Observations

All procedures in this sequence have two elements in common: (1) They can be completed concomitant to or in tandem with a conversational speech sample, and (2) many experienced clinicians complete these parts while conversing with the examinee prior to beginning formal inspection. For these reasons, they are consolidated, appearing as a single routine clinical observation having three parts. Although they can be performed simultaneously, for the sake of clarity, the manual discusses each separately.

Table 2–1. Subjective Methods for Rating Intelligibility[a]

	Subjective Rating Options				
Categories[b]: Descriptive Qualitative Judgment	Unintelligible	Poor	Fair	Good	Excellent
1–5 rating scale	1 Completely unintelligible (or nearly so)	2 Intelligible less than half of the time	3 Intelligible about half of the time	4 Intelligible more than half the time	5 Completely intelligible
Estimated intelligibility percentage[c]	0%[d] . . . . 100% →				

[a]The same table may be used to judge comprehensibility for preverbal and limited-language children. Simply replace the words that represent the concept of *intelligibility* with words that represent the concept of *comprehensibility* (e.g., replace *unintelligible* with *not comprehensible*).

[b]Categories are consistent with the recording form.

[c]An estimated percentage of overall intelligibility is different from a percentage of intelligible words based on a word count. Although word count percentages have utility for some clinical measures, that is not the type of intelligibility rating suggested here.

[d]Round-number increments are recommended for intelligibility percent estimates if they are used.

Conversational Speech Sample. The conversational speech sample is the fundamental piece. Although in most cases, the sample was taken prior to the oral-facial inspection, the information that it yields can become a useful point of reference when evaluating whether or how physical idiosyncrasies affect the reality of communication in connected speech. Therefore, if a sample was not already obtained, take time to chat with the examinee briefly before moving on, and use a recording device to preserve the sample so that further judgments can be made later.

If not certain as to exactly what is meant by *conversational speech sample*, consult Box 2–1.

One fundamental goal of the conversational speech sample is to provide a basis for *rating intelligibility*. Rating overall intelligibility is normally subjective; thus, there is no one right way to do it. A few options for subjectively rating intelligibility are shown in Table 2–1. The recording form simply asks for a categorical intelligibility rating *from unintelligible to excellent*, which is consistent with the first row of the table.

Box 2–1. What Is a Conversational Speech Sample?

A conversational speech sample is a brief informal conversation during which the clinician makes judgments concerning general aspects of language and speech. There are many ways to collect a conversational speech sample. For many, preliminary small talk combined with case history interview avails an excellent opportunity to hear and judge a habitual speaking pattern. Although a reading sample does not provide the best illustration of natural speech, it may be used with caution if a true spontaneous sample is not obtainable. Essentially, any connected speech that the examinee engages in at any time during the assessment is useful for judging conversational speaking patterns.

Conversational Starters for Older Children and Adults

Some topics may elicit conversation while also providing relevant insight into the communication concerns. These may be initiated with invitations to talk, such as the following:

- What brings you here today?
- What do you hope the communication evaluation will accomplish for you?
- Tell me about how your communication concerns affect your life.

- If there is one thing about communication that could change and make a positive difference in your life, what would that be? And how would this make a difference?

Other topics are simply small talk; they also can begin with an invitation to share. Sample topic areas may include the following:

- Weather
- Finding parking or finding the clinic
- The person's day so far
- A current event that is noteworthy and unlikely to be controversial or emotionally charged
- The person's work, if an adult
- The person's area of study or life at school, if a student
- Favorite activity during free time

Initiating Conversations With Younger Children

For younger children, the conversational speech sample is usually most efficiently elicited through play or an interactive game. For most children, these acts take place prior to the oral-facial inspection.

Intelligibility rating is a critical piece of oral-facial inspection. If physical anomaly becomes evident, and it is found to be linked to speech production, degree of impact on intelligibility has the potential to affect both diagnosis and plan of care.

Another function of the conversational speech sample is to provide a *venue for identifying possible symptom categories*, such as articulation, phonology, motor speech, voice, resonance, and fluency concerns. This enables preliminary judgments relative to specific audible symptoms that potentially affect the remainder of the inspection (Bankson, Bernthal, & Flipsen, 2009; Bauman-Waengler, 2011; Duffy, 2013; Gordon-Brannan & Weiss, 2007; Hegde & Freed, 2013; Johnson, 1996; Lowit & Kent, 2011; Yorkston, Beukelman, Strand, & Hakel, 2010).

For instance, articulatory precision, as well as number and types of articulation errors when noted in connected speech, may reveal patterns that can influence a diagnosis of articulation or phonological or motor-speech disorder. Prosodic features, such as speech rate, phrase length, and inflection patterns, may be useful for defining a motor-speech or fluency disorder. Voice quality observations may add insight into a motor-speech or voice disorder. Last, perceptible resonance irregularities can give information about a motor-speech disorder or concerns with a person's ability to control nasal-oral coupling and uncoupling during connected speech.

For convenience, Box 2–2 lists speech sound substitutions that may be noted in individuals who have difficulty controlling nasal-oral coupling and uncoupling during connected speech. If these patterns are noted, even if craniofacial anomaly or velopharyngeal insufficiency has not already been identified, the examinee is considered potentially at risk. This has potential to influence a decision to perform certain discretionary clinical observations that follow.

Furthermore, during the informal conversation, take care to observe *external structures of the face and head, along with breathing patterns both at rest and in motion;* as a result, you will be prepared to comment on the integrity of the *facial region* as well as *breathing.* Observations of this type that are made during connected speech can clarify which observations have potential for clinical relevance.

Facial Region Inspection. Because the oral-facial inspection is typically one of the last procedures performed during the comprehensive diagnostic protocol (see Table 0–1), it is likely that opportunity to consider facial features already presented itself many times before arriving at this juncture. For instance, the case history interview allows an opportunity to observe the face at rest during listening and in motion when responding to interview questions. Generally, experienced examiners make the most of these extemporaneous opportunities.

Yet, if for some reason the observations were not made prior, take the time to view the face. To survey the face at rest, ask the person to look directly at you for a moment and visually examine the features.

Box 2–2. Consonant Substitutions That May Imply Difficulty Separating the Oral and Nasal Resonating Chambers

Some consonant substitutions may be indicators of difficulty uncoupling the oral and nasal resonating chambers for pressure consonants during connected speech. That is, if someone has difficulty creating the intraoral pressure required for obstruent consonants, that person may attempt to approximate the target by creating pressure below or behind the oral resonating chamber in some other way. Some examples of substitution patterns of this type include the following:

- Glottal stops
- Pharyngeal stops
- Coarticulation of an oral and glottal stop
- Pops, clicks, and other nonspeech attempts at pressure consonants
- Pharyngeal fricatives
- Posterior nasal fricatives (i.e., nasal snorts)
- Anterior nasal fricatives (i.e., facial grimacing)

Then, so as to observe the face in motion, engage the person briefly in reasonably relevant small talk, and carefully observe facial features while the person is speaking.

Ideally, you will elicit a variety of spontaneous facial expressions. Take care to note movement and symmetry during speech, while smiling, and for any other type of expression that you may bring out.

Normally, when speaking, the face is symmetrical and moves symmetrically. Also whether at rest or during speech, the face should be free of scarring or malformation.

Facial region inspection can also be a pivotal procedure with regard to noticing the *potential for genetic or otorhinolaryngologic symptoms*. Craniofacial irregularities may or may not be relevant from a speech-language pathology perspective, but all should be noted given that some judgments are not formalized until additional information is in. Furthermore, because externally observable traits can suggest the possibility of a syndrome or craniofacial anomaly, even if speech-language pathology indicators are not readily observed, physical features potentially call attention to the need for a genetic or otorhinolaryngology referral.

There are literally thousands of features that, when occurring in a cluster, may be of interest to a genetic specialist. Individual books that are devoted to describing genetic disorders do not have the capacity to house a complete set of symptoms or symptom clusters associated with *all* possibilities, and many syndromic patterns are still not yet clearly defined (Robin, 2008; Shprintzen, 1997). Therefore, a comprehensive list of symptoms associated with syndromes cannot be part of this manual.

For this reason, if observing any feature listed in Table 2–2, consider it noteworthy and mark your observation on the recording form. Because the list provided in the table is not exhaustive, consider that dysmorphia of any kind, even if the description does not appear in the table, has potential for relevance to genetic and otorhinolaryngology professionals.

Some facial-region observations *may suggest neurologic involvement*. Facial asymmetry either at rest or in motion, ptosis of any feature, a jaw that seems to hang open at rest, asymmetrical angles of the mouth at rest or during speech, fasciculations in the perioral region, unequal elevation of the mouth angles during a spontaneous emotional smile, and poor saliva management are some examples (Duffy,

Table 2–2. Some Observable Features That May Imply Need for Genetic Consult

Eye Features	Nose Features	Ear Features	Lip Features	Jaw Features	Other Features of Face/Head/Body
Hypertelorism	Flat nasal bridge	Malformed ears	Thin or short upper lip	Micrognathia	Hypoplastic midface
Hypotelorism	Low nasal bridge	Hypoplasia of pinna	Lip pits (i.e., on interior surface of lower lip)	Macrognathia	Elongated face
Long or short palpebral fissures	Bulbous nasal tip	Absence of pinna	Flat philtrum	Retrognathism	Cranial asymmetry
Epicanthal folds in non-Asian subject	Depressed nasal tip	Low-set ears		Prognathism	Prominent forehead
Eyelid ptosis					Microcephaly
Marcus Gunn jaw wink					Macrocephaly
Strabismus					Atypical stature
Wandering eye					Any dysmorphic feature

2013; Hegde & Freed, 2013; Lowit & Kent, 2011; Yorkston et al., 2010).

Some externally observable features may suggest *possible nasal airflow obstruction* if associated with hyponasality. These may include small or obstructed nares, flat nasal bridge, and nasal asymmetry (Gordon-Brannan & Weiss, 2007; Kummer, 2008).

Some observable features may testify to a *history of oral-facial surgeries secondary to cleft palate or other craniofacial anomaly*. These may include flat nasal tip, scarring of cupid's bow, or flat zygomas (Kummer, 2008).

Open-mouth posture, if noted, is remarkable, especially if accompanied by symptoms of voice disorder, congestion, or poor saliva management. This trait may bear witness to any number of potential concerns, including problems with nasal cavity clearance, malocclusion, poor facial-muscle tone, oral-motor dysfunction, allergies, chronic congestion, vocal-fold attrition, changes in skull growth, high palatal arch, and elongated retrognathic face. Furthermore, when accompanied by forward-tongue posturing, open-mouth posture can turn out to be one of many indicators to consider when deciding whether to screen for tongue-thrust swallow (Bresolin et al., 1984; Hanson & Mason, 2003; Kummer, 2008; Schlenker, Jennings, Jeiroudi, & Caruso, 2000; Sivasankar & Fisher, 2003).

When observing the facial region, take note as to whether the examinee's *overall posture* seems conducive or disadvantageous to efficient speech production, especially for those with evidence of respiratory or laryngeal tension. Normally, the head and neck should be held erect, the back should be straight, and shoulders should be positioned toward the back (i.e., not bent in a forward direction). A natural, relaxed, and comfortable appearance is desirable.

Evidence of muscle tension, which may manifest as stiffness or tightness in the neck, jaw, shoulders, or even the scapula, is remarkable, as are any indicators of habitual shoulder elevation or unnatural bend in the shoulder or back structure. Postural symptoms may coincide with voice disorder and can contribute to observations relative to respiration, which are discussed below (Courtney, 2013; Perri & Halford, 2004; Schneider & Sataloff, 2007).

Breathing Observations. Observe breathing both at rest and during speech. Normally, breathing is virtually inaudible and accomplished with the mouth closed. Shoulder movement, upper thoracic movement, audible symptoms, and struggle are not part of the normal respiratory pattern.

Whenever breathing calls attention to itself in any way, use the recording form to document remarkable observations. Timing of air exchange, depth of air intake, and opening used for taking in and letting air out should all be considered.

When observing the *timing of air exchange*, notice duration of inhalation and exhalation cycle both at rest and during speech. At rest, the amount of time required for inhalation should correspond *approximately* to the amount of time required for exhalation, although exhalation may be somewhat longer. However, during speech, exhalation requires considerably more time as compared to inhalation, depending on the type of speaking activity. If the person displays a breath-timing pattern other than the one described in this paragraph, the observations are noteworthy (Bauman-Waengler, 2011; Boone, McFarlane, Von Berg, & Zraick, 2010; Seikel, King, & Drumright, 2010).

Also observe *depth of air intake* both at rest and during speech. Bear in mind that *diaphragmatic breathing* is most advantageous and categorically necessary for the vocal projection associated with public speaking and singing. Furthermore, diaphragmatic breathing optimally balances muscle effort for both inspiration and expiration, allows exchange of larger airflow volumes, and reduces potential for tension in the neck and shoulder muscles (Iwarsson, 2001; Schneider & Sataloff, 2007).

When individuals use a diaphragmatic breathing pattern, breathing calls virtually no attention to itself. The only observable motion may be a slight expansion and contraction in the abdominal region.

Thoracic breathing is shallower. There are two types: lower-thoracic and upper-thoracic breathing (Courtney, 2013; Schneider & Sataloff, 2007).

Lower-thoracic breathing is common and possibly even standard for the vast majority of people. This pattern is generally acceptable for conversation but not when speaking conditions require vocal projection such as public speaking, acting, and singing. It is also not acceptable if punctuated by gasps or periods of stopping the airflow. Lower-thoracic breathing may be slightly noticeable and is characterized by expansion and contraction of the lower thorax (Boone et al., 2010; Courtney, 2013; Schneider & Sataloff, 2007).

On the other hand, *upper-thoracic breathing* is an undesirable pattern as the airflow does not descend sufficiently to support voice projection. The obvious observable feature includes expansion of the upper thorax in the absence of notable shoulder movement (Courtney, 2013; Schneider & Sataloff, 2007).

An even shallower type, *clavicular breathing*, is too shallow for clear phonation, balanced resonance, and normal phrasing in connected speech. Clavicular breathing calls conspicuous attention to itself by observable up-and-down rhythmic shoulder movement that corresponds to each breathing cycle (Boone et al., 2010). Consider clavicular breathing remarkable, particularly for individuals with voice disorders, resonance disorders, difficulty projecting the voice adequately for comfortable conversation, or frequent breaths that interrupt speech flow.

If suspecting a problem with breath support but not noting any of the above symptoms, be on the lookout for the possibility of an attempt to speak on minimal airflow or in the absence of it. Some examples include attempting to speak on *residual air* or even during the *inspiratory phase* of breathing. These can be recognized by audible stridor and glottal fry (Schneider & Sataloff, 2007).

Orifice used for inhalation and exhalation can also be identified while observing respiration. Breathing observations should also pinpoint which opening the person uses habitually to take in and let out air (i.e., nasal or oral). *Nasal breathing* is desirable and is characterized by mouth-closed posture at rest, although the lips may be parted.

Oral breathing, on the other hand, is not desirable and is characterized by mouth-open posture and dropped mandible when at rest. Mouth breathing may be an indicator of congestion or nasal obstruction, or it may simply result from a lingering habit secondary to resolved temporary obstruction. More concerns with mouth breathing are discussed in a previous section that discussed open-mouth posture.

Some other types of breathing that may call attention to themselves include *cortical breathing* and *oppositional breathing*. Cortical breathing can be recognized when the person exerts excessive muscular force while attempting to breathe for speech. Oppositional breathing is noted if the thorax and diaphragm seem to oppose each other in the act of breathing for speech, resulting in discernible struggle (Nicolosi, Harryman, & Kresheck, 2004). Although these are not common, due to their potential for interference with speech flow or vocal efficiency, they are considered clinically relevant if observed.

As a rule, any breathing pattern that calls attention to itself has potential for clinical relevance and is remarkable.

Managing Evidence From Conversational Speech Sample, Facial Region Inspection, and Breathing Observations

This set of observations enables clinicians to comment cogently with regard to the following:

- Speech production patterns noticed in connected speech, including articulation, voice, and resonance
- Subjective rating of overall intelligibility in conversational speech
- Whether a swallow, during speech or at rest, is followed immediately by a cough or change in vocal quality that may imply a need for dysphagia screening
- Externally observable anomalies of the face or head that may either interfere with speech or guide a specialist referral
- Whether respiratory pattern is adequate for normal, fluid, and properly resonant speech

Discretionary Clinical Observations to Perform or Rule Out After Conversational Speech Sample, Facial Region Inspection, and Breathing Observations

At this juncture, a decision can be made as to whether the client should participate in two discretionary clinical observations. Although detailed in Chapter 3, both are named below and followed by a bulleted list of indicators that suggest a need for the discretionary procedure.

- Consider nasal cavity clearance screening (i.e., Discretionary Clinical Observation 9) if noting the following:
  o Hyponasality during any speech or nonspeech activity
  o Nasal asymmetry
  o Visible or audible symptom of congestion
- Consider facial dimension estimates (i.e., Discretionary Clinical Observation 10) if noting the following:
  o Disproportionate facial features

Discretionary Clinical Observations to Consider if Supported by Additional Data

If detecting any symptoms that, with benefit of additional data, could lead to one or more of the remaining discretionary clinical observations, make note on the recording form. Observations that potentially lead to a discretionary procedure decision appear in Table 2–3.

Routine Clinical Observation 2: Assess Lips and Tongue for Mobility and Strength

Clinical Question Associated With Assessing Lips and Tongue for Mobility and Strength

Clinical Question 6 (see Table 0–3) asks, "When inspecting lips and tongue for strength and mobility, does the examinee exhibit any irregularities that potentially explain articulatory errors noted during speech?" An answer of *yes* to the clinical question potentially flags remarkable implications. The procedures that follow are useful for answering the clinical question *and* for identifying the nature and impact of any irregularities.

Clearly Differentiated Lip and Tongue Movements

Procedures provide an opportunity to observe lips and tongue during motion. During these activities, take care to note whether the articulators move freely

and independently, without assistance from other moveable parts. See Box 2–3 for more information.

Equipment Needed for Assessing Lip and Tongue Strength and Mobility

- Examination gloves
- Tongue depressor
- Penlight
- Large in-room mirror

Procedures Associated With Assessing Lip and Tongue Strength and Mobility

Lip Mobility Activities. Ask the examinee to *pucker the lips* (e.g., purse or protrude lips). Demonstrate if needed. The normal response is a symmetrical and fully rounded pucker that occurs effortlessly, without delay, and involves lip movement only. Any response other than this is remarkable.

Box 2–3. Differentiated Lip and Tongue Movements

The goal for most lip and tongue activities is to achieve a clearly differentiated and independent movement that involves only the one articulator (i.e., lips or tongue). For example, if instructions are to move the tongue in a particular direction, expect the tongue to move independently without simultaneous assistance from the neck or jaw.

To maximize the likelihood of success when attempting to elicit clearly differentiated independent movements, (1) instruct plainly, (2) carefully observe so as to detect neck or jaw movement, and (3) reinstruct with demonstration if necessary, so as to give the person an opportunity to exhibit a clearly differentiated response. If differentiated movements are not achieved for either the lips or tongue, this has potential for clinical relevance, particularly for individuals with imprecise speech involving that articulator.

Table 2–3. Conversational Speech Sample, Facial Region Inspection, or Breathing Observations That Suggest Discretionary Observations After Additional Data Are Gathered

Symptom	Possible Discretionary Clinical Observation to Consider	Routine Clinical Observations That May Contribute to Decision
Limited mandibular excursion during conversation	Temporomandibular joint disorder screening (i.e., Discretionary Clinical Observation 9)	1 5
Interdental lisp during conversation, or forward-tongue posturing either during conversation or at rest	Tongue-thrust swallow procedure (i.e., Discretionary Clinical Observation 12)	1 2 3 5
Sound transpositions, difficulty with multisyllabic words or words of increased length and complexity, perseveration across word boundaries, dysfluency, or choppiness	Observations for developmental apraxia of speech (i.e., Discretionary Clinical Observation 13) in children	1 2 7
	Observations for acquired apraxia of speech (i.e., Discretionary Clinical Observation 14) in people whose symptoms emerged postlingually	
Hypernasal resonance or difficulty with obstruents (i.e., with regard to obstruents, some substitution patterns may denote difficulty with separating the oral and nasal cavities for speech. Examples are listed in Box 2–2.)	Screening for submucous cleft (i.e., Discretionary Clinical Observation 15)	1 5 7 8
	Screening for surplus-nasal airflow during speech (i.e., Discretionary Clinical Observation 16)	1 3 8
In individuals who have experienced a neurologic episode: a jaw that seems to hang open at rest, asymmetrical angles of the mouth at rest, fasciculations in the perioral region, unequal elevation of the mouth angles during a spontaneous emotional smile, or any kind of facial asymmetry either at rest or in motion	Observations for dysarthria (i.e., Discretionary Clinical Observation 17)	1 2 5 6 7 8
Voice quality that indicates possible inefficient use of the larynx	Observations for dysarthria (i.e., Discretionary Clinical Observation 17)	1 7 8
	Screening for laryngeal efficiency (i.e., Discretionary Clinical Observation 19)	
Any symptom that suggests a possible neurologic etiology	Gag-reflex stimulation (i.e., Discretionary Clinical Observation 20)	1 6 7 8
Cough or voice change after swallow Recent neurologic incident, neurologic disease, or laryngectomy	Prompt for dysphagia screening (i.e., Discretionary Clinical Observation 21)	1 7 8 14 20

Be alert that some examinees, if asked to demonstrate kissing, may smack their lips without puckering if lip rounding is difficult. If this happens, although the response is noteworthy, the next activity may provide additional insight.

Ask the examinee to sustain an exaggerated /u/ sound. Demonstrate by saying /u/, using an excessive amount of lip rounding. The response should be fully rounded, symmetrical lips in the absence of extraneous facial movements or struggle. A weak, latent, shaky, asymmetrical, distorted, or effortful response is remarkable.

Ask the person to *spread the lips*. Demonstrate if needed. The normal response is an immediate, symmetrical, smoothly executed smile. A weak, latent, shaky, or asymmetrical response is remarkable, as is any evidence of struggle. Beware that a spontaneous social smile, if elicited, is not adequate to demonstrate ability to spread the lips voluntarily on command. Therefore, avoid relying on telling a joke, showing a funny picture, pretending to use a camera, modeling, or showing a picture of a person smiling.

Instruct the examinee to rapidly produce a *short series of bilabial consonant repetitions* (i.e., /p/ or /b/). Watch and listen carefully. Normally, expect efficiently executed bilabial consonant repetitions, where the lips fully approximate, stop the airflow, and release it. Imprecise or weak approximation is remarkable, as is any evidence of struggle.

Similarly, ask the examinee to *smack the lips*. This action requires creating and releasing a strong labial seal on command. Normally, lips should approximate and release, creating an audible smacking sound. Movements should be smooth, symmetrical, and without delay. A weak, asymmetrical, or effortful response is remarkable.

Lip Strength and Symmetry. Check *labial seal*. Instruct the person to take a breath, and use the air to puff out the cheeks, not allowing air to escape. Modeling is acceptable, even desirable.

Then, let the person know that you will poke the cheek with one finger to test lip seal. Once the person's cheeks are filled with air, using a gloved finger, gently poke the person's puffed cheek on one side so as to increase intraoral pressure. Normally, the labial seal remains intact and the cheeks

remain puffed, even when poked. An easily broken seal or air seepage either unilaterally or bilaterally is remarkable (Shipley & McAfee, 2008). Posterior or superior egress of air should also be noted if it occurs (Box 2–4). Reinstruct and repeat if results seem questionable.

Check *lip resistance*. Instruct the person to close the lips lightly and naturally. Then, place the flat side of a tongue depressor firmly but gently against the external surface of the person's closed lips (Figure 2–2). Instruct the client to use lip protrusion to push the tongue depressor away. Demonstration is encouraged, using a different tongue depressor, of course.

Normally, gentle pressure of the lips pressing against the tongue depressor is detectable. If this does not occur, for individuals with imprecise articulation of bilabial stop and plosive consonants, the finding is remarkable. Furthermore, forward lip movement should be accomplished independently, without participation or assistance from the mandible or neck. Because independent and differentiated lip movement is the goal, if any other moveable part comes forward when the examinee is attempting to use lips to push the tongue depressor away, take the time to evaluate whether the ancillary movements can be brought under purposeful control.

Box 2–4. In the Event of Posterior or Superior Egress of Air

If the captured air seems to escape without breaking the labial seal, then it is possible that either the velar seal may be inadequate for intraoral pressure or the hard palate may lack integrity. This is particularly noteworthy for clients with compromised obstruent consonants or imbalanced resonance. Bear in mind, however, that the ability to hold air within the oral cavity does not definitively rule out difficulty with uncoupling the nasal and oral cavities since some examinees may close off a posterior or superior oral egress by creating a seal between the tongue blade and the velum or palate.

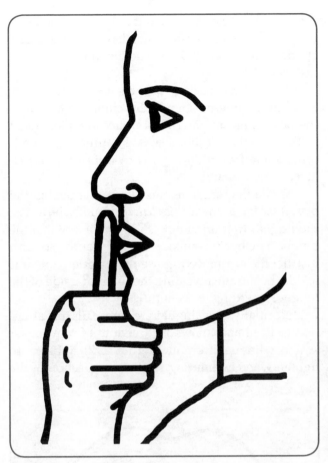

Figure 2–2. Tongue depressor position for testing lip and tongue strength.

One way to do that might be to reinstruct in a way that does not call obvious attention to the error. For instance, you may say, "Great! Now, let's try it *another* way. This time, use your lips only; so try not to move your jaw or neck when pushing the tongue depressor away." If the mandible and neck continue to participate in the lip movement activity even with these instructions, it may be worthwhile to provide a mirror and try again. Since it has already been established that differentiated lip movements are challenging for the examinee, this would be done to judge the extent to which the lips depend on other body parts to assist in simple movement and whether differentiated movements can be accomplished with the benefit of visual feedback.

Tongue Mobility. Several tongue movement exercises follow, and noteworthy symptoms are similar

for each. Therefore, Box 2–5 summarizes the normal and remarkable symptoms as they apply to all tongue mobility tasks.

Check *tongue protrusion*. Ask the person to stick the tongue straight out. Demonstrate if needed. For adolescents and adults, eliciting tongue protrusion in this way requires little explanation but may be more complicated when giving instructions to children (Box 2–6).

If the tongue tip seems to drop when protruded, although this may be a sign of weakness, it may be

---

Box 2–5. Clinically Significant Symptoms for Tongue-Movement Activities

Normally, tongue movements are smooth, coordinated, and even. Extraneous, jerking, writhing, poorly differentiated, involuntary, incomplete, and effortful movements are all noteworthy. Similarly, preference for the right or left side, reduced speed or range of motion, and weakness or flaccidity should be recorded if noticed (Bauman-Waengler, 2011; Duffy, 2013; Dworkin & Culatta, 1996; Gordon-Brannan & Weiss, 2007; Yorkston et al., 2010).

Box 2–6. Eliciting Tongue Protrusion in Children

One excellent way to elicit tongue protrusion in young children is to ask the child to point the tongue at a particular object that is obvious but not within reach, such as a colorful child-friendly picture on the wall, a door knob, a toy on a shelf, or the clinician's raised hand. Always refrain from suggesting any method for tongue protrusion that may prompt parental disapproval (e.g., do not correlate tongue protrusion with an act that is associated with disdain toward a friend or sibling).

that the person's tongue inadvertently succumbed to gravity. For this reason, it is worthwhile to reinstruct, emphasizing the idea of sticking the tongue *straight out* without allowing the tip to drop.

Normally, tongue protrusion occurs symmetrically, on a horizontal plane (i.e., not downward or upward), without extraneous movements, and should be of adequate excursion to accomplish the consonants /θ/ and /ð/. Any other response is remarkable. Box 2–5 lists symptoms that can be useful in identifying clinically significant symptoms.

This is an expedient time to take note of the *tongue-tip shape*, which should be slightly and symmetrically rounded (Figure 2–3), not angular (Figure 2–4), flat (Figure 2–5), or heart shaped (Figure 2–6). If an unusually shaped tongue tip accompanies imprecise articulation, consider this finding remarkable.

Inspecting *tongue elevation* includes two parts. First, judge whether the examinee demonstrates the ability to intentionally elevate the tongue tip when instructed to do so; then inspect the lingual frenum.

Ask the person to stick out the tongue and point it upward. Demonstrate if needed. If evaluating a child, refer to Box 2–7 for suggestions on how to instruct.

Normally, expect upward excursion that is adequate for tongue-tip sounds. Touching the tongue to the nose is not required, but noticeable movement in the direction of the nose is. Failure to elevate is remarkable for individuals with imprecise lingua-alveolar consonants.

While the tongue is raised, use the penlight to *inspect the lingual frenum for length.* Usually, however, the lingual frenum is not readily visible when the tongue is elevated outside of the mouth. So, also instruct the examinee to raise the tongue while it is inside the mouth, revealing the full underside of the tongue, including its frenum.

Normally, the lingual frenum calls no attention to itself and allows for freedom of movement. A short lingual frenum (Figure 2–7) appears to tighten when attempting to allow inspection of the

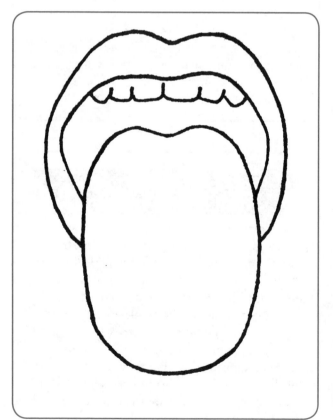

Figure 2–3. Rounded tongue tip.

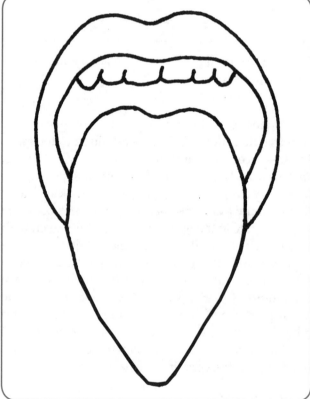

Figure 2–4. Angular tongue tip.

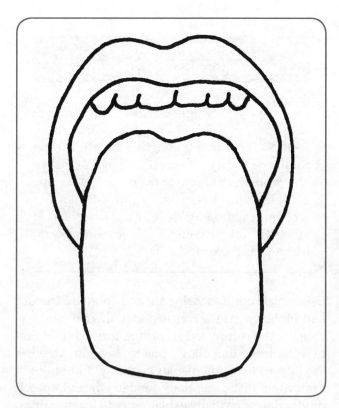

Figure 2–5. Flat-shaped tongue tip.

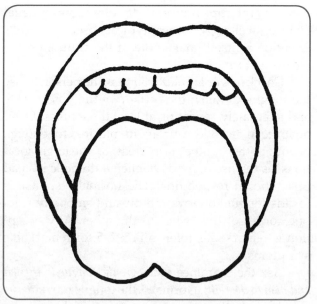

Figure 2–6. Heart-shaped tongue tip.

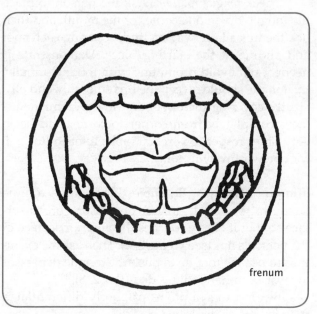

Figure 2–7. Short lingual frenum.

Box 2–7. Suggestions for Instructing Tongue Elevation

Some examinees may contend that they are unable to accomplish tongue elevation if they believe the goal is to touch the nose with the tongue. If this happens, encourage the person to use the tongue to point at the ceiling without tilting the head back.

Also, with some children, the instruction, "stick out your tongue and touch your nose," may result in the child sticking out the tongue and touching the nose with a finger. Be careful to avoid this and other confusing word sequences when instructing.

tongue's underside and seems to hinder upward lingual movement. Another notable feature of a short frenum is a heart-shaped tongue tip (see Figure 2–6).

A short lingual frenum *may be* clinically relevant for individuals with difficulty producing the tongue-tip sounds (Bankson et al., 2009; Gordon-Brannan & Weiss, 2007; Shipley & McAfee, 2008).

Furthermore, when inspecting the underside of the tongue, take note of its texture, coloration, and general appearance. If discoloration, unusual texture, swelling, or other atypical observation calls attention to itself, make note of the feature on the recording form.

Check *tongue lateralization.* Ask the person to use the tongue to touch the corners of the lips quickly and alternately, repeating at least three times. Demonstrate if needed, but avoid placing food (e.g., peanut butter or other tasty treat) on the target locations, as the use of food *can* elicit automatic instead of volitional responding. The normal response is for the tongue to move rapidly and smoothly from one corner of the orifice to the other. Any exception is remarkable; refer to Box 2–5 for remarkable symptoms.

Ask the examinee to *wiggle the tongue to the left and then to the right.* Normally, the tongue movements should be rhythmic, as well as of perceivably normal rate and excursion. Any other response is remarkable; refer to Box 2–5 for noteworthy symptoms.

Check *tongue rotation.* Ask the person to place the tongue tip on one corner of the mouth and then lick the lips all the way around, covering each spot and ending at the starting place. Demonstrate if needed, but avoid prompting with food. Normally, the tongue should sweep the lips smoothly and efficiently, covering the upper and lower stomian surfaces completely from corner to corner and back. Any other response is remarkable; refer to Box 2–5 for noteworthy symptoms.

Tongue Strength. To subjectively judge tongue strength, position the tongue depressor's broad surface so that it barely touches the anterior surface of the person's lips (see Figure 2–2). Then ask the examinee to use the tongue to push the tongue depressor away. Use imitation if needed (Box 2–8).

Be alert to symptoms of poorly differentiated movements as described earlier (e.g., forward neck or jaw movement). Poorly differentiated movements are remarkable. If noted, reinstruct (i.e., as directed in the section on evaluating lip strength).

Normally, the action is gentle pressure resulting from the tongue pushing against the tongue depressor. The response should be immediate and symmetrical, and movements should involve the tongue only. Any other finding is remarkable and should be recorded.

Box 2–8. Subjectively Judging Tongue Strength

Subjectively judging tongue strength through resistance is a widely used and acceptable method for *screening* tongue strength during routine oral-facial inspection. Because instrumentation is available to measure this feature, concerns with tongue strength can lead to a recommendation for more scientifically based strength measurements (Solomon, Clark, Makashay, & Newman, 2008).

Evidence From Assessing Lip and Tongue Strength and Mobility. At the conclusion of this set of observations, the completed recording form should display evidence that allows one to ascertain whether the lips and tongue display mobility and strength symptoms that potentially hinder efficient speech production or partially explain speech irregularities.

Discretionary Clinical Observations to Consider if Supported by Additional Data. Although lip and tongue strength and mobility observations do not lead directly to a decision about a discretionary clinical observation, some data can contribute to a decision for discretionary procedures after more data are collected. Refer to Table 2–4 for more information.

Routine Clinical Observation 3: Assess Dental Alignment and Bite

Clinical Question Associated With Assessing Dental Alignment and Bite

Clinical Question 7 (see Table 0–3) asks, "Does a systematic inspection of dentition reveal bite or alignment irregularities that potentially influence an identified atypical speaking pattern or imply a need for specialist referral?" An answer of *yes* potentially has remarkable implications. Dental alignment and bite inspection is useful for answering the question *and* for identifying the nature and impact of any irregularities.

Table 2–4. Lip and Tongue Strength and Mobility Screening Results May Suggest Discretionary Observations After Additional Data Are Gathered

Symptom	Possible Discretionary Clinical Observation to Consider	Routine Clinical Observations That May Contribute to Decision
When checking labial seal, the oral cavity deflates without breaking the labial seal	Screening for submucous cleft (i.e., Discretionary Clinical Observation 15)	1 2 5 7 8
	Screening for surplus-nasal airflow during speech (i.e., Discretionary Clinical Observation 16)	1 2 7 8
	Observations for dysarthria (i.e., Discretionary Clinical Observation 17)	1 2 5 6 7 8
When checking labial seal, lips part either unilaterally or bilaterally, causing air to escape	Observations for dysarthria (i.e., Discretionary Clinical Observation 17)	1 2 5 6 7 8
Difficulty with volitional tongue or lip movements in the absence of difficulty with moving the same structures automatically	Observations for developmental apraxia of speech (i.e., Discretionary Clinical Observation 13)	1 2 7
	Observations for acquired apraxia of speech (i.e., Discretionary Clinical Observation 14)	
Any discoordination, asymmetry, atrophy, fasciculation, tremor, extraneous movements, inadequate range of movement, or atypical rate or rhythm of movement	Observations for dysarthria (i.e., Discretionary Clinical Observation 17)	1 2 5 6 7 8
Any neurologic symptom, including those that lead to screening for apraxia or dysarthria	Stimulate gag reflex (i.e., Discretionary Clinical Observation 20)	1 2 6 7 8
	Prompt for dysphagia screening (i.e., Discretionary Clinical Observation 21)	1 2 7 8 14 20

Clinical Relevance of Dental Bite and Alignment

Dental bite and alignment are two distinct but overlapping concepts. Dental bite is ascertained by examining the relationship between the maxillary and mandibular incisors, whereas dental alignment is determined by examining the arrangement of each tooth independently.

Normal and atypical bite and alignment are defined and illustrated (Box 2–9 and Figures 2–8 through 2–15; Box 2–10 and Figures 2–16 through 2–25). Any findings other than standard bite and alignment are potentially remarkable; however, many individuals compensate well for differences in dental bite and alignment. Therefore, findings relative to clinical observations in this area are clinically relevant *only if* differences seem to partially or fully explain concomitant atypical consonant production *or if* they imply the need for genetic consultation.

Box 2–9. Normal and Atypical Dental Bite

Normal Bite

As a rule, maxillary incisors reside barely anterior to mandibular incisors and cover one third to two thirds of the mandibular incisors' anterior surface. There should be little or no space between the anterior surface of the mandibular incisors and the posterior surface of the maxillary incisors.

Common Atypical Bite Patterns

Labels for common dental arrangements that do not meet the above-stated criteria for normal bite include the following:

- *Closed bite*—Maxillary-central incisors cover more than two thirds of or completely cover the anterior surface of mandibular-central incisors; also called *overbite, excessive maxillary-incisor supraversion,* or *deep overbite* (see Figure 2–9).
- *Open bite*—Anterior mandibular and maxillary teeth fail to occlude. There are two basic types.

  o A *central open bite* requires an opening between the mandibular and maxillary incisors (see Figure 2–10A).
  o A lateral open bite may be noted when the lateral incisors or cuspids are infraverted at all four quadrants, leaving lateral openings (see Figure 2–10B).
- *Flared bite*—Maxillary and mandibular incisors flare outward, toward the lips (see Figure 2–11).
- *Cross bite*—Central-mandibular incisors are positioned to the right or left as compared to central-maxillary incisors (see Figure 2–12).
- *Edge-to-edge bite*—Biting surface of maxillary incisors meets biting surface of mandibular incisors (see Figure 2–13).
- *Overjet*—Maxillary incisors are tilted forward such that the maxillary lower edge is significantly anterior to the superior edge of mandibular incisors (see Figure 2–14).
- *Underbite*—Mandibular incisors are positioned anterior to maxillary incisors (see Figure 2–15).

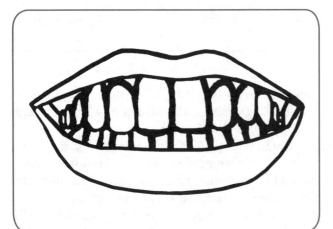

Figure 2–8. Normal bite.

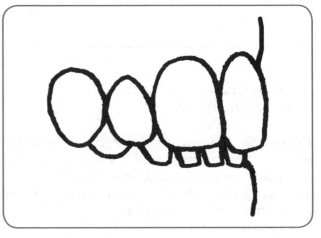

Figure 2–9. Closed bite.

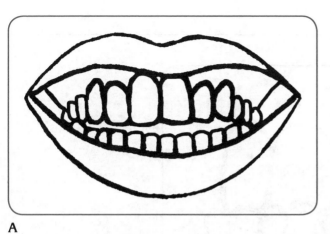

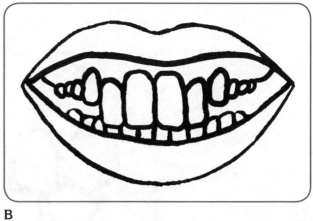

A

B

Figure 2–10. **A.** Open bite, central. **B.** Open bite, lateral.

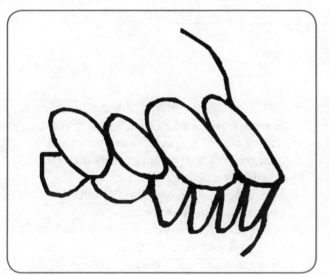

Figure 2–11. Flared bite.

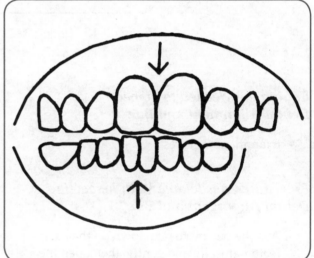

Figure 2–12. Cross bite.

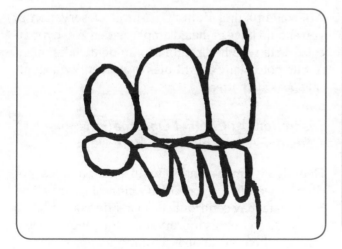

Figure 2–13. Edge-to-edge bite.

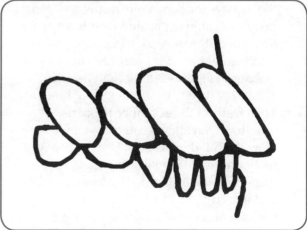

Figure 2–14. Overjet.

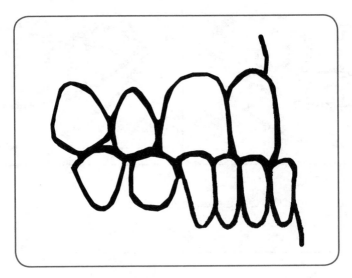

Figure 2–15. Underbite.

Equipment Needed to Inspect Dental Alignment and Bite

- Examination gloves

Procedures Associated With Inspecting Dental Alignment and Bite

- Ask the person to bite down on the back teeth naturally and gently; then open the lips so that the front teeth can be viewed. Demonstration is encouraged. If parting the lips manually seems necessary, use gloved fingers to open the lips and view the incisors for dental bite inspection. Most people are able to position their teeth and lips without manual assistance.
  - Carefully view the incisor relationship. Refer to Figures 2–8 through 2–15 and Box 2–9 when classifying dental bite.
- Then instruct the examinee to open the mouth, which allows you to systematically view the full dental array. Use the penlight to view dental layout by quadrant, inspecting the teeth for alignment, number, and integrity.
- Classify alignment concerns if any are noted, paying particular attention to any that have the potential to affect speech, such as teeth positioned in such a way that they reduce available space for tongue mobility, or anterior dental arrangements that negatively influence airflow.
- The presence of decay or poor dental hygiene is also noteworthy.
- Alignment definitions are detailed in Box 2–10, and illustrations appear in Figures 2–16 through Figure 2–25.

Consider Evidence Resulting From Inspecting Dental Alignment and Bite

After completing Routine Clinical Observation 3, you should have gathered ample evidence to hypothesize as to whether irregularity in dental alignment or bite potentially contributes to an identified atypical speaking pattern.

Discretionary Clinical Observations to Consider After Collecting More Data

Dental alignment and bite inspection does not directly lead to a discretionary clinical observation. Some data may contribute to a later decision relative to the discretionary observation for tongue-thrust swallow. Refer to Table 2–5 for more information.

Box 2–10. Normal and Atypical Dental Alignment

Normal Dental Alignment

Incisors should be juxtaposed to one another and arranged in an even line that is slightly curved toward the back of the mouth (see Figure 2–16). The maxillary dental arch is generally longer and wider than the mandibular arch (Bankson et al., 2009).

Number and Alignment of Teeth

To report clinically relevant results, the examiner should know the names of the teeth, including quadrant designation. There is variability according to age for this information.

Young Children

For young children who have a full set of deciduous dentition, each quadrant has five teeth: central incisor, lateral incisor, bicuspid, and two molars. Figure 2–16A names deciduous teeth and provides ages of both eruption and shedding.

School-Age Children

Numbers of teeth vary depending on stage of shedding deciduous dentition and eruption of permanent dentition. Figures 2–16A and 2–16B should be helpful if used together, along with knowledge of the child's chronological age.

Adolescents and Adults

Each quadrant has seven or eight teeth: central incisor, lateral incisor, cuspid, two bicuspids, and two or three molars. Figure 2–16B displays permanent teeth, with the approximate ages of eruption.

Dental Misalignment

Most misalignment configurations are only potentially useful to explain speech errors when the dental arrangement alters the airflow, provides evidence of tongue thrust, implies a particular syndrome or craniofacial anomaly, or interferes with tongue mobility; otherwise, they are typically unremarkable. Common misalignment configurations include the following.

Axioversion. *Axioversion* is a general term used to describe a tooth that is slanted or tipped on an improper axis. There are two basic types: distoversion and mesioversion.

A *distoversion* (see Figure 2–17) is an axioversion that is slanted or tipped away from the middle of the dental arch, also called *facioversion* because the tooth leans in the direction of the face. There are two basic types of distoversion: *labioversion* and *buccoversion*. A labioversion is a distoversion that leans toward the lips, usually involving incisors and cuspids; labioversion includes *flared bite* and *overjet* (see Figures 2–11 and 2–14). A buccoversion is a variation on distoversion that leans toward the cheeks. This classification usually involves premolars (also called bicuspids) or molars (see Figures 2–16A and 2–16B).

A *mesioversion* is an axioversion that is slanted or tipped toward the midline or tongue. It may also be called *linguaversion* (see Figure 2–18).

Torsioversion. A torsioversion is a tooth that is rotated along the vertical axis, upright but twisted (see Figure 2–19).

Transversion. In the event of transversion, the teeth are present but in wrong sequential order (see Figure 2–20). This arrangement is not common, may be noteworthy if making a genetic referral, but is rarely clinically relevant from a speech-language pathology perspective.

Infraversion. The tooth has not emerged completely enough to reach the line of occlusion (also described as a short tooth) (see Figure 2–21A). Although this *may* apply to teeth in the process of erupting, the configuration is more likely to be noteworthy for fully erupted permanent teeth that do not reach the occlusal edge. In fact, it is best to refer to a partially erupted tooth as partially erupted, not as an infraversion, since the configuration is most likely temporary.

Supraversion. A tooth's biting surface extends beyond that of adjacent teeth; the tooth may appear too long in comparison to neighboring teeth (see Figure 2–21B).

Jumbling. Teeth overlap or are massed together; synonym: *crowding* (see Figure 2–22).

Supernumary Tooth. A supernumary tooth is an extra tooth. In some cases, an extra tooth may insert itself within the dental arch, as shown in Figure 2–23A. In other cases, a supernumary tooth may grow in a surprising location such as behind the dental arch (see Figure 2–23B) or even in the hard palate (see Figure 2–23C). Supernumary teeth may interfere with tongue movement for articulation in some cases.

Edentulous Space. An edentulous space is a gap resulting from a missing tooth (see Figure 2–24). In order for space to qualify as an edentulous space, it must occur in the location that typically accommodates dentition that is not present.

If all teeth are missing, the person's mouth is said to be edentulous. Missing teeth are only relevant if they are useful for explaining an atypical speech pattern.

Interdental Space. An interdental space is a gap between sequential teeth, not resulting from missing teeth (see Figures 2–25A and 2–25B); this may also be called *diastema*.

Dental Decay

Dental decay is remarkable, from a hygiene perspective.

Dental Appliances

Some older adults may wear dental appliances, such as dentures or partial plates. There is no need to ask the person to remove the dental appliance to inspect the hard palate, since one can assume that palatal integrity is not a concern with the adult examinee. Furthermore, there is no need to count teeth or consider dental misalignment because the prosthodontist who fitted the appliance would have taken these concerns under consideration when fitting the device. However, if the examinee reports pain associated with the appliance, if the appliance seems to move about during speech, or if imprecise speech seems to result from a poorly fitted dental appliance, these features are remarkable.

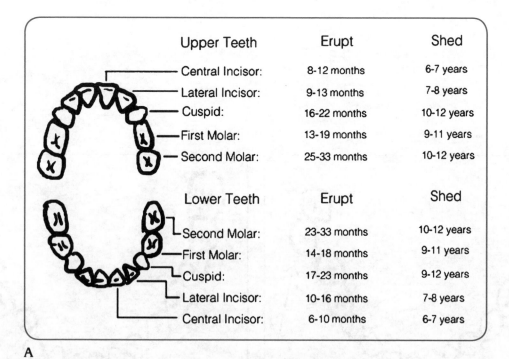

Upper Teeth	Erupt	Shed
Central Incisor:	8-12 months	6-7 years
Lateral Incisor:	9-13 months	7-8 years
Cuspid:	16-22 months	10-12 years
First Molar:	13-19 months	9-11 years
Second Molar:	25-33 months	10-12 years

Lower Teeth	Erupt	Shed
Second Molar:	23-33 months	10-12 years
First Molar:	14-18 months	9-11 years
Cuspid:	17-23 months	9-12 years
Lateral Incisor:	10-16 months	7-8 years
Central Incisor:	6-10 months	6-7 years

A

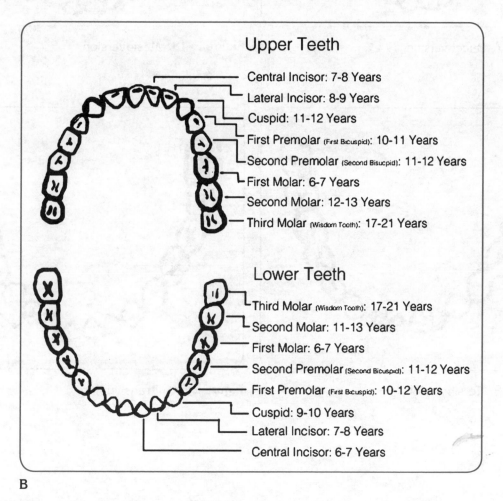

Upper Teeth

Central Incisor: 7-8 Years
Lateral Incisor: 8-9 Years
Cuspid: 11-12 Years
First Premolar (First Bicuspid): 10-11 Years
Second Premolar (Second Bisucpid): 11-12 Years
First Molar: 6-7 Years
Second Molar: 12-13 Years
Third Molar (Wisdom Tooth): 17-21 Years

Lower Teeth

Third Molar (Wisdom Tooth): 17-21 Years
Second Molar: 11-13 Years
First Molar: 6-7 Years
Second Premolar (Second Bicuspid): 11-12 Years
First Premolar (First Bicuspid): 10-12 Years
Cuspid: 9-10 Years
Lateral Incisor: 7-8 Years
Central Incisor: 6-7 Years

B

Figure 2–16. A. Deciduous teeth, with ages of eruption and ages of shedding. **B.** Permanent teeth, with ages of eruption.

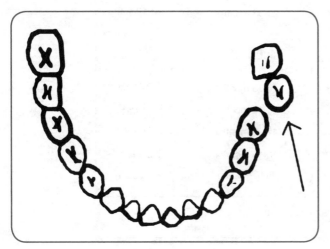

Figure 2–17. Buccoversion.

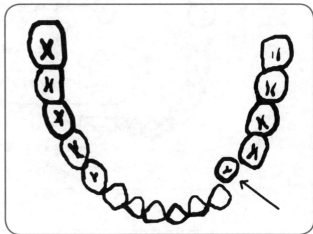

Figure 2–18. Mesioversion.

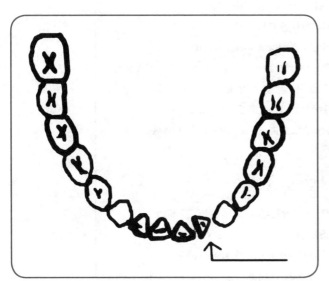

Figure 2–19. Torsioversion.

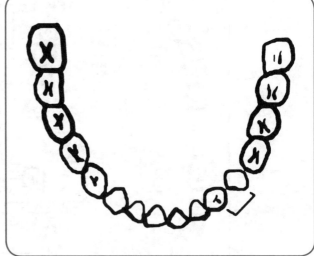

Figure 2–20. Transversion.

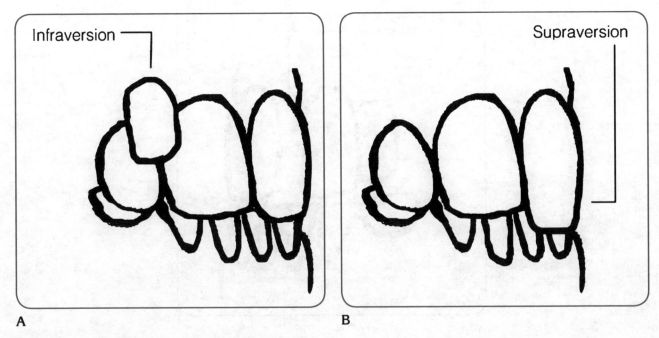

Figure 2–21. **A.** Infraversion. **B.** Supraversion.

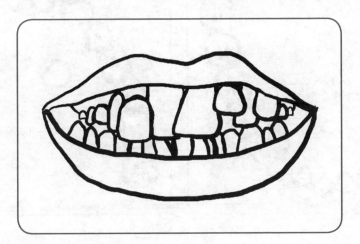

Figure 2–22. Jumbling.

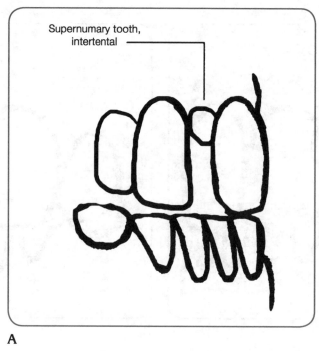

A

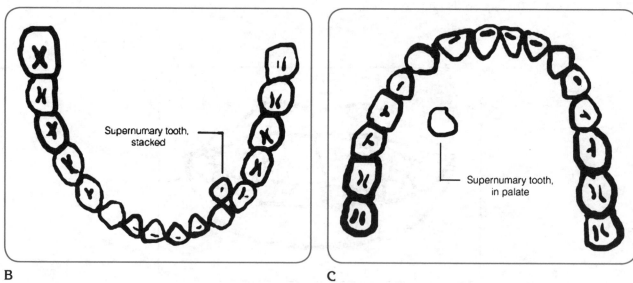

B

C

Figure 2–23. **A.** Supernumary tooth, interdental. **B.** Supernumary tooth, stacked. **C.** Supernumary tooth, in palate.

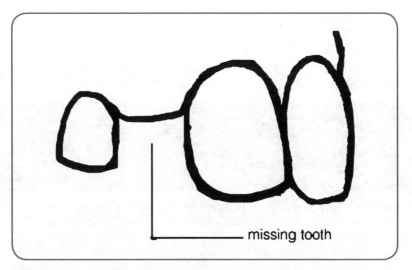

Figure 2–24. Edentulous space.

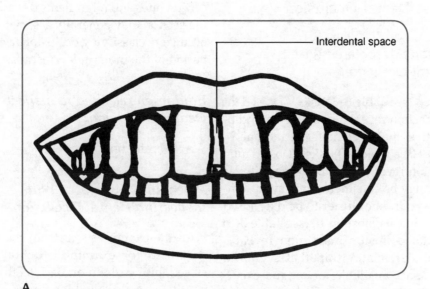

A

B

Figure 2–25. **A.** Interdental space. **B.** Interdental spaces.

Table 2–5. Dental Alignment and Bite Inspection Results May Suggest Discretionary Observation After Additional Data Are Gathered

Symptom	Possible Discretionary Clinical Observation to Consider	Routine Clinical Observations That May Contribute to Decision
Open or flared bite, overjet, deep overbite	Tongue-thrust swallow procedure (i.e., Discretionary Clinical Observation 12)	1 2 3 5

Routine Clinical Observation 4: Assess Dental Occlusion

Clinical Questions Associated With Assessing Dental Occlusion

Clinical Question 8 (see Table 0–3) asks, "Does dental occlusion inspection reveal a maxillary-mandibular relationship that implies craniofacial anomaly?" Clinical Question 9 (see Table 0–3) asks, "Does dental occlusion inspection reveal a maxillary-mandibular relationship that may be considered one symptomatic element of a syndromic cluster to be diagnosed by a specialist?" Clinical Question 10 (see Table 0–3) asks, "Does dental occlusion inspection reveal a maxillary-mandibular relationship that seems to reduce intraoral space available for tongue excursion?" Clinical Question 11 (see Table 0–3) asks, "Does dental occlusion inspection reveal a maxillary-mandibular relationship that seems to result in improper alignment between the tongue and palatal surface, potentially affecting articulatory precision?"

An answer of *yes* to any of these clinical questions has the potential for noteworthy implications. Inspecting dental occlusion is useful for answering the four questions *and* for identifying the nature and impact of any irregularities noted.

What Is Dental Occlusion?

Dental occlusion refers to the relationship between the first maxillary molar and the first mandibular molar. Occlusion classifications are defined in Box 2–11 and illustrated in Figure 2–26. Although certain bites and alignments described in the preceding section may generally associate with a particular occlusion, classifying occlusion *requires* direct examination of the molar relationship.

Equipment Needed to Inspect Dental Occlusion

- Examination gloves

Procedure Associated With Inspecting Dental Occlusion

With the examinee's teeth in the same position as described for examining dental bite above (i.e., closed, biting down on back teeth) and lips relaxed, gently use a gloved index finger and thumb to open the lips on one side so as to view the molar relationship. Classify the person's occlusion according to criteria defined and illustrated in Box 2–11 and Figure 2–26.

Evidence From Inspecting Dental Occlusion

After inspecting dental occlusion, you have evidence to determine whether a Class II or III malocclusion is present and, if so, whether the occlusal relationship potentially contributes to an identified speaking pattern. Findings are only clinically relevant if they seem to explain or partially explain atypical speech or imply craniofacial concerns if combined with other symptoms.

Box 2–11. Normal and Atypical Dental Occlusion Classifications

Because occlusion refers to the mandibular-maxillary molar relationship, it can only be confirmed by examining the relationship between these teeth. Therefore, even when perceived jaw size or positioning seems to imply a particular occlusion, and even though jaw size and positioning can coincide with a particular occlusion, the relationship between first maxillary molar and first mandibular molar must be ascertained to classify occlusion.

Neutroclusion

The first maxillary molar rests above the first mandibular molar, with the center of the maxillary molar slightly behind. Neutroclusion is the normal anterior-posterior relationship between mandible and maxillary palatal arches (see Figure 2–26A). If accompanied by dental misalignment, it may be classified as Angle's Class I Malocclusion.

Neutroclusion is typically unremarkable in and of itself. However, it may be accompanied by concerns with dentition that are marked as remarkable after evaluating dental alignment and bite.

Distoclusion

The first maxillary molar rests above the first mandibular molar with the center of the maxillary molar slightly in front. Although distoclusion may co-occur with overbite, retrognathic jaw, or micrognathia, this is not always the case. Distoclusion is also called Angle's Class II Malocclusion (see Figure 2–26B).

Whenever distoclusion is identified, it is remarkable. However, distoclusion has clinical significance only if it provides evidence relative to the clinical questions shown above.

Mesioclusion

The first maxillary molar rests above the first mandibular molar with the center of the maxillary molar considerably behind. Mesioclusion may be associated with underbite or prognathic jaw but not always. Mesioclusion is also called Angle's Class III Malocclusion (see Figure 2–26C).

Whenever mesioclusion is identified, it is remarkable. However, mesioclusion has clinical significance only if it provides evidence relative to the clinical questions shown above.

Routine Clinical Observation 5: Assess Oral Interior

Clinical Questions Associated With Assessing Oral Interior

Clinical Question 12 (see Table 0–3) asks, "When asked to lower the jaw, does the examinee's mandible move with adequate excursion to allow for viewing the oral cavity?" Clinical Question 13 (see Table 0–3) asks, "When lowering and raising the jaw while the examiner manually applies resistance, does the examinee exert adequate strength to overcome the resistance symmetrically?" Clinical Question 14 (see Table 0–3) asks, "Does inspecting the oral interior expose any structural irregularities, such as missing, damaged, or malfunctioning parts, that may potentially explain or partially explain the examinee's idiosyncratic speaking pattern?"

An answer of *no* to Clinical Questions 12 and 13 has potential for clinical implications, as also does an answer of *yes* to Clinical Question 14. These clinical questions are useful for identifying muscular weakness, temporomandibular joint dysfunction, and the nature and impact of any internal oral irregularities.

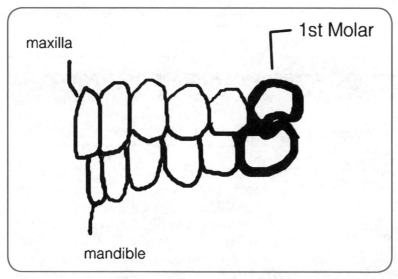

A

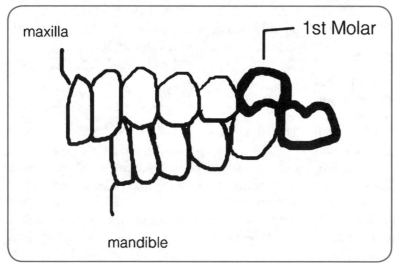

B

Figure 2–26. **A.** Neutroclusion.
B. Distoclusion. **C.** Mesioclusion.

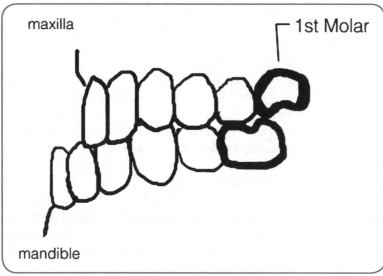

C

Equipment Needed for Inspecting Oral Interior

- Examination gloves
- Tongue depressor
- Penlight

Procedures Associated With Inspecting Oral Interior

Instruct the person to open the mouth for viewing. Unless otherwise indicated, avoid tilting the head back as this may displace certain moveable structures, yielding potentially incorrect results (Bankson et al., 2009). Box 2–12 provides additional suggestions to facilitate the oral interior inspection.

Box 2–12. Notice for Inspecting Oral Interior

The client needs to assume an open-mouth posture at least once to allow for intraoral viewing. So as to avoid requesting that the person open the mouth repeatedly or hold it open for an extensive period, the clinician does well to have a working knowledge of the oral geography, the recording form, labels for common aberrations, and the objectives for performing each movement.

The best way to become familiar with oral geography is to perform the oral-facial evaluation on many individuals until fully acquainted with what to expect. Everyone is encouraged to take opportunities to do this if not yet comfortable enough to identify irregularities with relative ease. In addition, a rapid functional review of oral-facial anatomy and physiology appears in Appendix C, and *if needed*, take the time to study it.

Experienced clinicians who are intimately familiar with oral geography may complete all of Routine-Clinical Observation 5 quickly and efficiently. Newer clinicians may require more time and perhaps several looks to accomplish the same goal.

Observe Mandibular Movement and Strength. Oral interior inspection begins by asking the person to open the mouth. Before viewing the interior, however, notice whether the person's mouth opens freely, adequately, symmetrically, and without extraneous movement.

Then, let the examinee know that you will make an attempt to close the jaw when it is open, that you will similarly make an attempt to open it when it is closed, and that the examinee should resist your efforts to change the jaw position. Then proceed to evaluate jaw strength by requiring the examinee to resist your courteously executed attempts to thwart jaw movements.

A normal response is smooth, symmetrical jaw movement with full excursion and competent resistance to the examiner's attempts at changing jaw position. If any of the following is noted, the symptom is remarkable: restricted mandibular movement, asymmetrical movement, difficulty resisting pressure, or extraneous motion.

Oral Interior Inspection. View the oral interior, illuminating it with a penlight. Individually examine each feature listed below.

Color of the oral interior should be healthy shades of pink, consistent with the person's pigmentation. Any gross irregularities in coloration are remarkable.

Inspect the tongue for *surface, size, and shape*. Normally, the *tongue's surface texture* is relatively smooth. Papillae (i.e., sensory end organs, or taste buds) should be small in size and visible. The tongue should be free of bumps, grooves, or atypical texture. Furthermore, shriveled appearance or deep crevices are considered atypical. Any anomaly noted in this paragraph is remarkable.

Tongue width and length ideally correspond to the size and shape of the oral interior. A small tongue may be associated with atrophy. On the other hand, large tongue size can restrict freedom of lingual movement within the cavity or even change oral structure to accommodate. Whether small or large, unusual tongue size is only clinically relevant if concomitant to imprecise articulation or structural changes.

The *tongue should be symmetrical*, with left side resembling the right, and the *tip should be gently rounded*. Asymmetry under any condition is remarkable, as is any tongue-tip shape other than gently rounded.

Other noteworthy observations may include fasciculations, intention or resting tremor, any kind of extraneous movement, or scar tissue. Any abnormality noted is remarkable if it has potential for relevance to the communication concern.

Inspect the *hard palate*, which is the bony structure that comprises the roof of the oral cavity. Hard palate features that that are of potential interest include the alveolar ridge, palatal arch, median palatal raphe, posterior nasal spine, foveae palati, mucosal membrane, and coloration.

To *view the hard palate*, ask the person to tilt the head back as far as possible. Then shine the penlight on the roof of the mouth.

The *alveolar ridge* (Figure 2–27), located on the anterior hard palate, is easily recognized as a fairly symmetrical pattern of bumps (i.e., rugae) resembling a small inverted mountain range immediately posterior to the maxillary incisors. The normal alveolar ridge is free of gross irregularities, which if present may suggest possible cleft (Figure 2–28A), fistulus (Figure 2–28B), or submucous cleft. In relation to the tongue, the alveolar ridge normally lies directly superior to the tongue tip. Any asymmetry, evidence of incompleteness, other structural irregularity, or indication of atypical alignment with the tongue tip is remarkable.

The *palatal arch* (see Figure 2–27) should be complete and free of clefts, fissures, or fistulae (see Figure 2–28). Normally, the shape of the palate is gently arched, neither shallow nor severely vaulted. The shape and depth of the palatal arch, and whether the structure is irregular or asymmetrical, is noteworthy if concomitant to a corresponding atypical speaking pattern.

The *median palatal raphe* (see Figure 2–27) is a noticeable palatal midline seam (i.e., slight indentation) that under normal circumstances separates right and left sides of the hard palate into equal parts. Deviation in its configuration is remarkable.

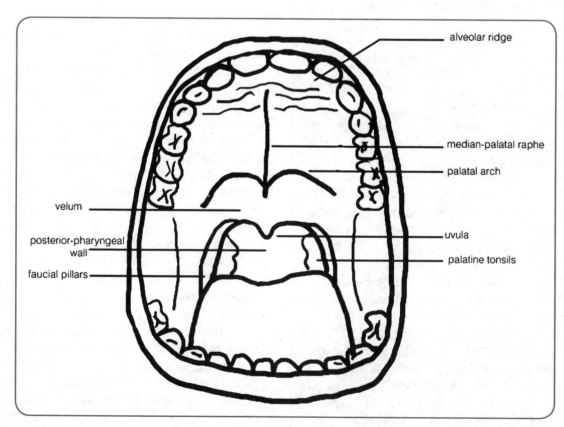

Figure 2–27. Oral interior: alveolar ridge, palatal arch, median-palatal raphe, velum, uvula, faucial pillars, palatine tonsils, and posterior-pharyngeal wall.

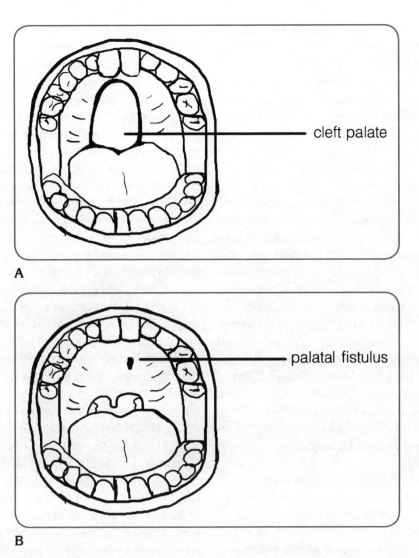

Figure 2–28. **A.** Palatal cleft. **B.** Palatal fistulus.

The *posterior nasal spine* is a small angular landmark that resides at midline on the posterior border of the hard palate. Although this landmark may be observable through visual inspection, it may not be. Therefore, if it is not noticed and concerns about palatal integrity exist, make note and then plan to examine this feature through palpation when screening for submucous palatal cleft.

Foveae palati are a pair of small bilateral depressions at the juncture of the hard palate and velum, and they may be observable for some examinees. They serve as openings for salivary glands (Kummer, 2008). In many cases, foveae palati are not noticeable; therefore, their discernible presence or absence is not remarkable. Palatal foveae are mentioned to prevent unnecessary reporting of a concern when they are noted.

The *palatal mucous membrane* is normally opaque, smooth, and consistent with oral interior shading. Slight symmetrical shading consistent with contour is expected. Asymmetry, dark or bluish shading, translucency, symptoms of inflammation, and irregular configuration are remarkable.

The mere presence of *scar tissue* does not characteristically interfere with speech. However, scar tissue may divulge evidence of a previous surgery or injury with clinical implications. For this reason, the presence of scar tissue is remarkable for the person with a perceptible communication disorder that may be explained or partially explained by the location or extent of the visible scar.

The *coloring of the palate* should be uniform and consistent with the overall oral interior. Bluish coloration at any palatal location should be noted, especially if associated with hypernasal resonance or difficult obstruent production. Bluish coloring near or at midline is especially noteworthy.

Observe the *velum* with a mouth-open posture, the neck erect, and the head not tilted toward the back. The velum (see Figure 2–27), also called the soft palate, should be symmetrical, complete, and of adequate length to presumably reach the posterior pharyngeal wall for velopharyngeal closure. No rhythmic or arrhythmic involuntary movements of the velum should be observed when at rest or in motion.

The velum is capable of being raised, lowered, and tensed. However, inspecting velar movement is the subject of Routine Clinical Observation 6 that follows. While still addressing Routine Clinical Observation 5, the focus is limited to ascertaining the integrity of the physical structure while *at rest*. Remarkable velar features include asymmetry, irregularity in size or shape, involuntary movements, or discoloration.

For the sake of efficiency, experienced clinicians may prefer to insert Routine Clinical Observation 6 (i.e., assessing velar movement) at this juncture since the mouth is already open and the velum is in full view. For more detail, refer to procedures and expectations that appear under that heading.

Inspect the *uvula*. Typically, the uvula is a single structure that hangs from the center of the posterior velar margin (see Figure 2–27). The shape, size, configuration, location, or absence of the uvula may be but is not always noteworthy. Common differences in uvular symmetry and formation are defined in Box 2–13 and illustrated in Figures 2–29 and 2–30.

Inspect the *faucial pillars* (see Figure 2–27). These soft structures flank the pharyngeal opening as inferior extensions of the lateral velum. They are useful as landmarks and should be symmetrical. As a rule, faucial asymmetry corresponds to velar asymmetry and may therefore be remarkable if associated with hypernasality, difficulty with pressure consonants, or neurologic episode.

Look for and inspect the *palatine tonsils* (see Figure 2–27). If present, they typically come in a pair and should be somewhat wrinkled in texture, slightly visible, posterior to the faucial pillars, and immediately anterior to the posterior pharyngeal wall. Normally, in prepubescent children, palatine tonsils tend to be somewhat large even when not inflamed, atrophy during puberty, and later become quite small in size for many adults. Potentially noteworthy tonsillar conditions are described in Box 2–14, and an example appears in Figure 2–31.

Inspect the *posterior pharyngeal wall*. Similarly, the posterior pharyngeal wall (see Figure 2–27) should be consistent with the oral interior in color and texture. Size of the pharyngeal cavity should be adequate to serve as an unobstructed nasal egress. Note any aberrations in color, texture, or relationship to the posterior oral cavity boundaries.

Evidence From Oral Interior Inspection. After oral interior inspection (i.e., Routine Clinical Observation 5), response form data bear witness to whether all structural parts of the oral interior are present and intact. If any physical anomaly is noted, a decision is made as to whether it likely contributes to an idiosyncratic speaking pattern.

Discretionary Clinical Observations to Perform or Rule Out. At this juncture, enough evidence has been amassed to make an informed decision about whether to proceed with two discretionary procedures. They are named below, followed by a list of indicators that suggest their need.

- Consider screening for temporomandibular joint disorder (i.e., Discretionary Clinical Observation 11) if noting the following:
  - Limited mandibular excursion during speech or nonspeech activities (i.e., as noted in Routine Clinical Observations 1 and 5)
  - Reported sensation of localized or referred pain when moving the jaw (i.e., as noted in Routine Clinical Observation 5)
- Consider observation for tongue-thrust swallow (i.e., Discretionary Clinical Observation 12) if noting the following:

Box 2–13. Atypical Uvular Configurations

Uvular Asymmetry

A uvula that *hangs to the right or left* when at rest may be associated with velar asymmetry (see Figure 2–29). This is remarkable if concomitant to hypernasal resonance or difficult obstruent consonants.

Dysmorphic Uvula

A *bifid*, *stubby*, or *notched* uvula (see Figures 2–30A, 2–30B, and 2–30C, respectively) may be associated with submucous cleft or velar insufficiency. These formations are noteworthy if concomitant to hypernasal resonance or difficulty with obstruent consonants (Bankson et al., 2009; Bauman-Waengler, 2011; Dworkin, Marunik, & Krouse, 2004; Reiter, Brosch, Wefel, Schlömer, & Hasse, 2011; Shprintzen, Schwartz, Daniller, & Hoch, 1985).

Bifid Uvula

A bifid uvula characteristically has two tags instead of one. However, the two parts can stick together, making it difficult to identify bifid uvula. If in doubt, you may separate the two tags by gently flipping the uvula with the tongue depressor, if the examinee tolerates.

Stubby Uvula

A stubby uvula has a short and boxy appearance and may also be described as hypoplastic. Although not bifid or notched, its presence similarly is noteworthy for examinees with hypernasal speech, difficulty with obstruents, or feature clusters associated that imply a syndrome.

Notched Uvula

A notched uvula has an incomplete inferior separation between the two halves. In cases where the notch is very small, it may appear as a dimple at the base of the uvula. Notched or dimpled uvula is remarkable.

Absent Uvula

Some individuals present without a uvula. If this structural difference is observed, it may be remarkable from a genetic or otorhinolaryngology perspective.

- Age-inappropriate oral habits, bruxism, sleep apnea, allergies pica (i.e., as noted during case history intake)
- Interdental lisp, forward tongue posturing, mouth-open posture, habitual oral breathing, chronic chapped lips, unilateral lip or cheek biting, tongue sucking, tongue or lip resting posture idiosyncrasies, poor saliva management, or deviated septum (i.e., as noted during Routine Clinical Observation 1)
- Restricted upper lip movement (i.e., as noted during Routine Clinical Observation 2)
- Open bite, flared bite, cross bite, or deep overbite (i.e., as noted during Routine Clinical Observation 3)
- Any of the following if associated with forward tongue posture: extra-large palatine tonsils, small pharyngeal orifice, shallow or vaulted hard palate, incomplete eruption of anterior dentition, restricted lingual frenum, palatal asymmetry, or suspected temporomandibular joint disorder (i.e., as noted during Routine Clinical Observation 5)

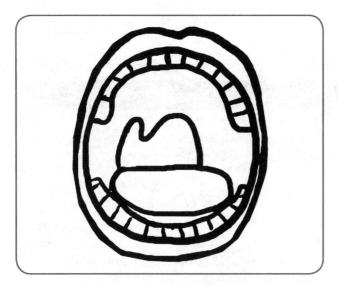

Figure 2–29. Deviating uvula, velar asymmetry.

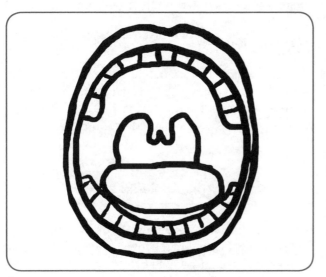

A

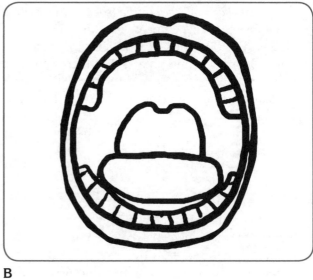

B

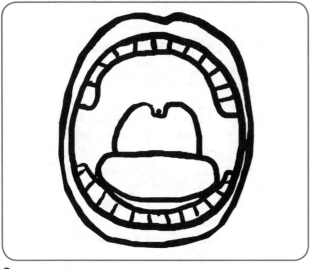

C

Figure 2–30. **A.** Bifid uvula. **B.** Stubby uvula. **C.** Notched uvula.

Box 2–14. Potentially Noteworthy Palatine Tonsil Observations

Inflamed, Enlarged, or Discolored Palatine Tonsils

Palatine tonsils that appear to be inflamed or red, of a color not consistent with the overall oral interior, of smooth texture, enlarged, or *kissing tonsils* (see Figure 2–31) are potentially noteworthy. Enlarged palatine tonsils can influence resonance.

Unequally Sized Palatine Tonsils

If palatine tonsils are conspicuously of unequal size, this is noteworthy. Unequally sized palatine tonsils can influence resonance.

Absent Palatine Tonsils

The absence of palatine tonsils bilaterally is not usually remarkable. However, the absence of only one tonsil may be worthy of investigation; therefore, it is remarkable.

Surgically Removed Palatine Tonsils, Concomitant to Hypernasal Speech

If palatine tonsils have been removed surgically, and if hypernasal speech is detected, it is a good idea to find out whether the tonsillectomy included adenoidectomy. Tonsillectomy with adenoidectomy is the typical standard of care for individuals with chronic tonsillitis or multiply replaced myringotomy tubes. For the few individuals who rely on adenoidal tissue to complete velopharyngeal closure, the removal can affect resonance as well as the ability to achieve intraoral pressure. Therefore, the finding is significant.

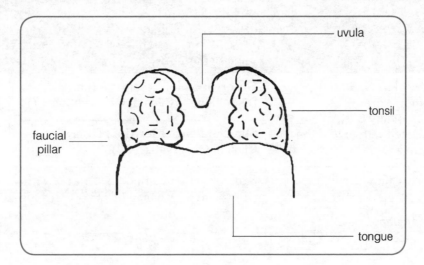

Figure 2–31. Enlarged palatine tonsils.

Discretionary Clinical Observations to Consider if Supported by Additional Data. Even if the oral interior inspection uncovers no direct reason to explore additional discretionary procedures, some of the information gathered through this process has potential to strengthen a decision to perform a discretionary clinical observation to be decided later in the sequence. Refer to Table 2–6 for more information.

Routine Clinical Observation 6: Assess Velar Movement

Clinical Questions Associated With Assessing Velar Movement

Clinical Question 15 (see Table 0–3) asks, "When prompting velar movement through /ɑ/ phonation, does the velum appear to move symmetrically and with adequate excursion?" Clinical Question 16 (see Table 0–3) asks, "Is the velar dimple observed to be properly located during /ɑ/ phonation?"

If the answer to either clinical question is *no*, findings may be remarkable. The procedures that follow are useful for answering the questions *and*

for identifying the nature and relevance of any irregularity.

Velar Movement

To accomplish most speech sounds of American English and many other languages, speakers approximate the velum and posterior pharyngeal wall using a sphincter-like action, creating a barrier that separates the nasal and oral cavities, preventing nasal airflow emissions or excessive nasal resonance. Figure 2–32 shows a sagittal view of the velopharyngeal port in the closed and open positions. Box 2–15 briefly addresses velopharyngeal closure's relevance to speech.

Velopharyngeal closure, although essential to both articulation and resonance, cannot be observed directly through the oral orifice. Evidence of movement and symmetry can be noted using the procedures described herein, but nasopharyngoscopy is required to evaluate closure and valve competence.

Table 2–6. Oral Interior Inspection Results May Suggest Discretionary Observations After Additional Data Are Gathered

Symptom	Possible Discretionary Clinical Observation to Consider	Routine Clinical Observations That May Contribute to Decision
Any evidence of weakness, atrophy, fasciculation, tremor, extraneous involuntary motion of any part, or asymmetry associated with any of the above-named features	Observation for dysarthria (i.e., Discretionary Clinical Observation 17)	1 2 5 6 7 8
	Stimulate gag reflex (i.e., Discretionary Clinical Observation 20)	1 5 6 7 8
Any evidence of structural irregularity or scar tissue of any part	Screening for submucous cleft (i.e., Discretionary Clinical Observation 15)	1 5 7 8
Bluish shading of the hard palate near the median raphe, translucency of hard palate		
Absent or deformed uvula		
Nasal spine not palpable		
Asymmetry if associated with any of the structural differences noted above		

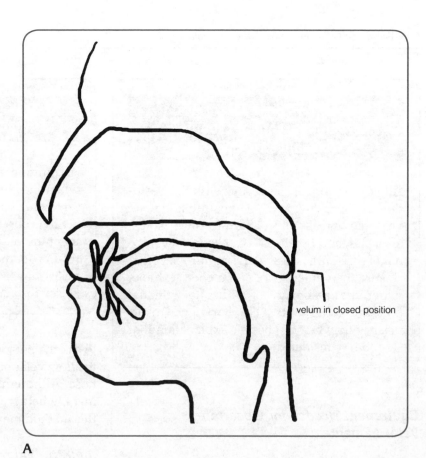

velum in closed position

A

Figure 2–32. **A.** Velum in closed position, sagittal view. **B.** Velum in open position, sagittal view.

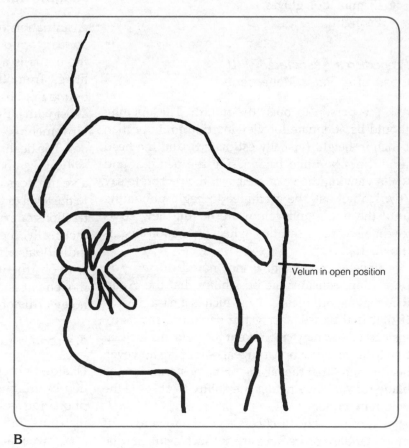

Velum in open position

B

55

Box 2–15. Brief Description of Velopharyngeal Closure's Relevance to Speech

All vowels and all consonants with the exception of /m/, /n/, and /ŋ/ require adequate velopharyngeal closure. Stop-plosives, stops, affricates, and fricatives (i.e., obstruent consonants, pressure consonants) require stronger closure than other sounds. If a client exhibits hypernasal resonance or difficulty with the pressure consonants, velopharyngeal insufficiency may be one possible explanation that should be considered.

Box 2–16. Suggestion for Viewing Velar Movement

A common and easily avoided error occurs when the clinician instructs the person to say /ɑ/ *before* having the velum in full view. The result is observing the velum *after* velar movement instead of at the onset of it. This mistake results in missing the opportunity to view velar movement and therefore places results at risk for inaccuracy.

Equipment Needed for Observing Velar Movement

- Examination gloves
- Penlight

Procedures Associated With Observing Velar Movement

Ask the person to open the mouth. The opening should be adequate for viewing but no more than 1 inch in height (visually estimated), and the head should not be tilted back. Using the penlight and while viewing the velar area, ask the person to say /ɑ/. Do not ask the examinee to begin phonating until the uvula and velum are in full view so as to enable careful scrutiny when phonation begins (Box 2–16).

If velar movement is not noted during /ɑ/ phonation, consider the possibility that the examinee may be producing /ɑ̃/, which is a nasal vowel. If that is the case, asking the person to say /kɑ/ instead of /ɑ/ may circumvent the person's inclination to leave the velopharyngeal port open; however, bear in mind that the raising of the posterior tongue blade for /k/ may hinder the ability to observe the velum in motion.

Another way to observe velar movement, if more standard procedures are not successful, may be

to ask the person to open the mouth widely enough to allow velar observation, then breathe through the nose. Although this elicits nonspeech velar movement, whether velar movement is possible through this method may provide useful insight (Riski, n.d.).

Judging Velar Movement

At initiation of /ɑ/ phonation, the velum should appear to move up and back symmetrically. Since the uvula is a relatively prominent landmark that hangs from the center of the velum's posterior boundary, observing it during /ɑ/ phonation can assist with judging excursion and symmetry of velar movement.

The healthy velum typically elevates symmetrically and smoothly to the level of the hard palate. If a velum does not move noticeably, does not elevate to the level of the hard palate, exhibits localized contractions or extraneous movements, or moves asymmetrically, these features should be recorded. For individuals with hypernasal resonance or difficulty with obstruent consonants, atypical or absent velar movement is clinically relevant. Some examples of noteworthy observations are listed in Box 2–17.

Managing Evidence From Velar Observation

Unaided observations of velar movement are limited in utility since most velar activity during /ɑ/ phonation is impossible to view directly without instrumentation. Occult manifestations of velopharyngeal action include whether closure occurs,

Box 2–17. Noteworthy Velar Observations

Asymmetrical Velar Movement

Asymmetrical velar movement is easy to recognize in that on /ɑ/ phonation, the uvula deviates to the unaffected side and drooping is evident on the affected side. If this occurs, it is noteworthy.

Misplaced Velar Dimple

During /ɑ/ phonation, the velar dimple should be visible and in proximity to the uvula. That is, about two thirds to four fifths of the soft palate should be anterior to the dimple, and about one fifth to one third of the soft palate should be between the dimple and the uvula. A velar dimple that is positioned too far forward or too far backward is remarkable.

Poor Velar Movement and Hyponasal Speech

In some cases, velar movement may be lacking for individuals with hyponasal resonance. This may result from a variety of explanations and is remarkable.

whether the valve is competent, pattern of closure, size of the nasopharynx, and size and participation of the pharyngeal tonsil.

Yet observing elicited velar movement during oral-facial inspection yields enough information to superficially judge the following:

- Features of the velum and hard palate at rest
- Symmetry of velar movement
- Excursion and height of velar movement
- Whether the velar dimple is properly positioned to allow for velopharyngeal seal

Discretionary Clinical Observations to Consider if Supported by Additional Data

Although velar movement observations do not lead directly to a discretionary procedure, they can uncover evidence that supports a discretionary clinical observation to be completed after collecting more data. See Table 2–7 for more information.

Routine Clinical Observation 7: Assess Verbal Diadochokinesis

Clinical Questions Associated With Verbal Diadochokinesis

Clinical Question 17 (see Table 0–3) asks, "For speech-alternating motion, are the verbal diadochokinetic syllables produced with steady rate and articulatory precision?" Clinical Question 18 (see

Table 2–7. Velar Movement Observations May Suggest Discretionary Observations After Additional Data Are Gathered

Symptom	Possible Discretionary Clinical Observation to Consider	Routine Clinical Observations That May Contribute to Decision
Inadequate velar movement on /ɑ/ phonation	Observations for dysarthria (i.e., Discretionary Clinical Observation 17)	1 2 5 6 7 8
	Gag-reflex stimulation (i.e., Discretionary Clinical Observation 20)	1 6 7 8

Table 0–3) asks, "For speech-sequential motion, are the three distinctly different syllables produced accurately, rapidly, and in sequence?" Clinical Question 19 (see Table 0–3) asks, "For speech-alternating motion and speech-sequential motion, are the syllables produced with rate, volume, and precision that do not deteriorate?" Clinical Question 20 (see Table 0–3) asks, "For speech-alternating motion and speech-sequential motion, are five or six syllables produced per second?"

An answer of *no* to any of the four clinical questions potentially implies noteworthy findings. The procedures that follow are useful for answering the clinical questions *and* for identifying irregular features with relevance to speech.

Equipment Needed for Evaluating Verbal Diadochokinesis

- Stopwatch
- Recording device

Procedures Associated With Verbal Diadochokinesis Activity

A general definition for verbal diadochokinesis appears in Box 2–18. The two types of verbal diadochokinesis that are part of this inspection include speech-alternating motion and speech-sequential motion exercises. For both, precision and rate data are collected; however, the precision data take precedence over the rate data with regard to clinical utility (Bankson et al., 2009; Duffy, 2013; Kummer, 2008; Mason & Wickwire, 1978).

Box 2–18. Verbal Diadochokinesis Defined

Verbal diadochokinesisis is the term used to describe rapid alternating and rapid sequential articulatory movements, using syllables of equal stress. Two types of verbal diadochokinetic data are collected: speech-alternating motion and speech-sequential motion.

Speech-Alternating Motion. Speech-alternating motion requires an examinee to repeat the same CV syllable rapidly, at an even rate, and using a single breath. Since achieving evenly spaced syllables of equal stress can present difficulty for speakers of any stress-timed language, including American English (Box 2–19), demonstration and practice are encouraged.

Before making formal observations or taking any rate measurements, practice each syllable pattern until confident that the examinee knows exactly what to do. When ready, instruct the examinee to take a deep breath, and repeat /pə pə pə pə/ as quickly and evenly as possible for 5 seconds. Use a recording device to capture the data so that you may listen carefully at a later time to judge rhythm, precision, range of motion, and rate for each syllable group. Then repeat the same instructions and data collection procedures for syllables /tə/ and /kə/.

Speech-Sequential Motion. Speech-sequential motion requires that one rapidly repeat a sequence of articulatory movements. This is done to assess proficiency for programming and executing a series of speech movements both rapidly and sequentially.

The syllable sequence for this activity is /pə tə kə/. As with speech-alternating motion, demonstration and practice are encouraged before making formal observations. When practicing, begin with slow rates so that the examinee will be confident of the sequence before being required to reproduce it rapidly. Again, use a recording device to capture the data so that you may listen at a later time, and when listening, focus on the examinee's capacity to sequence the sounds accurately.

Procedural Adjustments for Children. Verbal diadochokinetic testing with children can require procedural adjustments. Suggestions appear in Box 2–20.

Subjective Judgments Made During the Procedure

Although most judgments pertaining to speech-alternating motion and speech-sequential motion are confirmed while listening to the recording after

Box 2–19. Achieving Syllables of Equal Stress

Since English is a stress-timed language, most native English speakers naturally produce multisyllable sequences with an unequal stress pattern. Therefore, modeling and practice are usually needed before an even syllable rate can be achieved.

Stress Timing's Influence on Prosody

One critical feature of stress-timed language is equal timing between stressed syllables. For instance, consider the sentence, "A ca*ta*strophe *happ*ened *yes*terday." Although there are a variable number of syllables between the stressed syllables (i.e., cat, hap, and yes), the three stressed syllables are equally spaced in time, with the unstressed syllables worked into the available time in between.

Native speakers of stress-timed languages rely on the *understood* rule that stressed syllables are interspersed throughout the language when pronouncing words, phrases, and other syllable sequences. Therefore, it is easier for native American English speakers to say /ˈpʌ pə pə ˈpʌ pə pə/ than to say /pə pə pə pə pə pə/. This becomes even more true when varying the onset, such that /ˈpʌ tə kə/ is far easier to say than /pə tə kə/ for American English speakers.

Nevertheless, the target for verbal diadochokinesis is steady rate and equal stress (e.g., /pə pə pə pə pə pə/, /pə tə kə/). To accomplish this, practice is needed, first for the clinician and then for the examinee.

Box 2–20. Age Considerations for Verbal Diadochokinesis

Measuring the verbal diadochokinetic rate in children younger than 6 years may not be appropriate because rate data do not typically apply to young children. However, the verbal diadochokinesis exercise may be useful because performance symptoms such as articulatory precision, rhythm, and syllable sequence may provide clues as to the nature and etiology of the child's speech production concerns (Bankson et al., 2009; Mason & Wickwire, 1978).

When testing the very young or when having difficulty achieving client participation, it is acceptable to substitute multisyllabic words with a similar phonological pattern for the traditional syllables. For example, *butter*, *pucker*, *buttercup*, and *pat-a-cake* may be appropriate for some. When using words, however, consider that because the words do not lend themselves to being produced with an equal syllable stress pattern, and because they are cognitively associated with linguistic meaning, the activity should be noted as having been altered in this way.

Nevertheless, the act of producing multisyllabic words that require rapid, alternating articulatory movements can reveal much clinically useful data. Note any performance irregularities on the recording form.

the session, some data are lost unless purposefully witnessed in the examinee's presence. Therefore, intentionally observe coordination and range of motion for the various movable articulators (i.e., lips, mandible, and tongue) while still in face-to-face contact with the examinee.

Formally Evaluating the Data After the Session

After the session but within 24 hours of it, listen carefully to the recorded data. Instructions for subjective judgments as well as rate measurements follow.

Subjective Evaluation of Recorded Data. Evaluate performance on both alternating and sequential syllables subjectively first, as subjective observations may be more useful than formal rate measurements in many cases (Bankson et al., 2009; Duffy, 2013; Kummer, 2008; Mason & Wickwire, 1978). For speech-alternating motion, focus on listening for steadiness of rhythm and articulatory precision. On the other hand, for speech-sequential motion, concentrate on whether the speaker accurately and rapidly sequences the three distinctively different syllables in succession. Moreover, for both sets of data, if rate, volume, or precision decreases over time, this is remarkable and may indicate fatigue.

Syllable Rate for Speech-Alternating Motion. For the speech-alternating motion activity, count the number of syllables produced in 5 seconds. Then divide by 5. Normally, adults produce approximately five or six syllables per second (Duffy, 2013).

Evidence From Routine Clinical Observation 7

Having completed the verbal diadochokinesis activities, you have access to subjective information that addresses whether rapid alternating articulatory movements are subject to sound transpositions, perseveration across syllable boundaries, sequencing difficulties, fatigue, or decreasing rate. You also have syllable rates per second compared with general expectations. Verbal diadochokinesis can contribute valuable data when estimating a person's neuromuscular status for speech and that ultimately may contribute to a diagnosis of motor-speech disorder (Duffy, 2013; Hanson & Mason, 2003; Hegde & Freed, 2013; Yorkston et al., 2010).

Discretionary Clinical Observations to Perform or Rule Out

Performance irregularities during verbal diadochokinesis can be an indicator of a motor-speech disorder because verbal diadochokinesis testing is especially sensitive to symptoms of both developmental and acquired apraxia of speech. The discretionary procedures that explore symptoms of apraxia are named below and followed by a list of indicators that suggest a need for testing in that area.

- Consider observation for developmental apraxia of speech (i.e., Discretionary Clinical Observation 13) if noting the following in a child examinee:
  - History of speech production problems in family, history of speech treatment in family, delayed speech development, or absence of canonical babbling between the ages of 5 and 10 months (i.e., as learned via case history intake)
  - Persisting unintelligible speech, not explained by phonological disorder or organic pathology, difficulty with multisyllabic words, sound transpositions, perseveration across word boundaries, apparent disfluency, or choppiness not consistent with fluency disorder (i.e., as noted during Routine Clinical Observation 1)
  - Difficulty with volitional tongue or lip movements in the absence of difficulty with automatic tongue or lip movements—that is, symptoms of oral apraxia (i.e., as noted during Routine Clinical Observation 2)
  - Difficulty with sequencing movements for volitional speech during verbal diadochokinesis (i.e., as noted during Routine Clinical Observation 7)
- Consider observation for acquired apraxia of speech (i.e., Discretionary Clinical Observation 14) if noting the following in an adult examinee or a person who has a history of brain injury:
  - Difficulty with words with multiple syllables or words of increased length and complexity, sound transpositions, perseveration across word boundaries, apparent disfluency, or choppiness not consistent with fluency disorder

(i.e., as noted during Routine Clinical Observation 1)

- ○ Difficulty with volitional tongue or lip movements in the absence of difficulty with automatic tongue or lip movements—that is, symptoms of oral apraxia (i.e., as noted during Routine Clinical Observation 2)
- ○ Difficulty with sequencing movements for volitional speech during verbal diadochokinesis (i.e., as noted during Routine Clinical Observation 7)

Discretionary Clinical Observations to Consider if Supported by Additional Data

Performance on verbal diadochokinesis is also likely to expose symptoms of other neurogenic speech disorders (i.e., a dysarthria), or it may be useful to support a decision as to whether audible symptoms of submucous cleft are apparent. Refer to Table 2–8 for more information on whether evidence suggests a possible need for discretionary procedures that examine these areas.

Routine Clinical Observation 8: Assess Vowel Prolongation

Clinical Questions Associated With Assessing Vowel Prolongation

Clinical Question 21 (see Table 0–3) asks, "When sustaining a vowel, does the examinee's voice exhibit pitch, quality, loudness, and evenness that are perceived to be within normal limits?" Clinical Question 22 (see Table 0–3) asks, "When sustaining a vowel, do duration and loudness suggest breath support that is adequate to sustain connected speech?"

An answer of *no* to either clinical question can imply remarkable findings. The procedures that follow are useful for answering the two clinical questions *and* for identifying features as well as relevance when irregularities are found.

Equipment Needed for Vowel Prolongation Exercise

- Stopwatch
- Recording device

Table 2–8. Verbal Diadochokinesis Results May Suggest Discretionary Observations After Additional Data Are Gathered

Symptom	Possible Discretionary Clinical Observation to Consider	Routine Clinical Observations That May Contribute to Decision
Reduced range of movement, slowness, consonant imprecision, evidence of fatigue (i.e., decreasing rate, volume, precision)	Observations for dysarthria (i.e., Discretionary Clinical Observation 17)	1 2 5 6 7 8
Any symptom that leads to observations for acquired apraxia of speech (i.e., Discretionary Clinical Observation 14) or observations for dysarthria (i.e., Discretionary Clinical Observation 17)	Gag-reflex stimulation (i.e., Discretionary Clinical Observation 20)	1 6 7 8
	Prompt for dysphagia screening (i.e., Discretionary Clinical Observation 21)	1 7 8 14 20
Any evidence of hypernasality or difficulty with obstruents	Screening for submucous cleft palate (i.e., Discretionary Clinical Observation 15)	1 5 7 8

Procedures Associated With Vowel Prolongation Exercise

Ask the person to take the deepest breath possible, then use it to say /ɑ/ for as long as possible, using a steady tone, holding on to the sound until completely out of air. Without demonstration, many examinees either take a shallow breath or stop phonating before running out of air. For that reason, demonstration, even a little competition, is encouraged to facilitate accurate results.

Allow three trials. Use a recording device to preserve all three, thus making it possible to check data objectively at a later time. The official rate measurement is the best of the three trials. Duration that approximates 20 seconds or more is desirable for adults and 10 seconds or more for children. Sustaining the vowel for less time is noteworthy.

Note perceived vocal quality, pitch, loudness characteristics, and effort. Any aberration in these is noteworthy, as is deterioration of any kind with consecutive trials.

Evidence Resulting From Vowel Prolongation Exercise

Having completed the vowel prolongation exercise, you now have enough information to comment on whether breath support seems adequate for speech. Furthermore, you will have made subjective judgments with regard to laryngeal function.

Discretionary Clinical Observations to Perform or Rule Out

It is after Routine Clinical Observation 8 that you have enough information to decide whether to perform the remaining Chapter 3 discretionary clinical observations. Each is named and followed by a list of indicators that suggest the need for the procedure.

- Consider screening for submucous cleft (i.e., Discretionary Clinical Observation 15) if noting the following:
  - History of middle ear effusion and reflux (i.e., as learned during case history intake)
  - Hypernasal resonance or difficulty with pressure consonants, particularly of the voiceless variety (i.e., as noted during Routine Clinical Observation 1)
  - Posterior or superior leakage of air during labial seal activity (i.e., as noted during Routine Clinical Observation 2)
  - Palatal asymmetry, dark or bluish shading at palatal midline, palatal translucency, bifid uvula, or anterior or posterior placement of the velar dimple (i.e., as noted during Routine Clinical Observation 5)
  - Hypernasal resonance or difficulty with pressure consonants during verbal diadochokinesis (i.e., as noted during Routine Clinical Observation 7)
  - Hypernasal resonance during vowel prolongation (i.e., as noted during Routine Clinical Observation 8)
- Consider surplus nasal airflow screening (i.e., Discretionary Clinical Observation 16) if noting the following:
  - Hypernasal resonance or audible nasal airflow during speech or nonspeech activities, short utterance length, difficulty with obstruent consonants with or without hypernasality, atypical resonance, or compensatory articulatory substitutions for obstruents (i.e., as noted during Routine Clinical Observation 1)
  - Posterior or superior leakage of air during labial seal activity (i.e., as noted during Routine Clinical Observation 2)
  - Velar movement on /ɑ/ phonation is asymmetrical, weak, or absent (i.e., as noted during Routine Clinical Observation 6)
  - Difficulty with obstruent consonants during verbal diadochokinesis (i.e., as noted during Routine Clinical Observation 7)
  - Hypernasal resonance noted during vowel prolongation (i.e., as noted during Routine Clinical Observation 8)
- Consider observations for dysarthria (i.e., Discretionary Clinical Observation 17) if noting the following:
  - Jaw hangs in open position when at rest, mandible deviates to right or left at rest

or in motion, oral asymmetry at rest or in motion, or fasciculations in the perioral area (i.e., as noted during Routine Clinical Observation 1)

- ○ Labial asymmetry at rest or in motion, or unilateral or bilateral labial seal weakness (i.e., as noted during Routine Clinical Observation 2)
- ○ Tongue: extraneous movements at rest or in motion, deviation at rest or in motion, weakness, imprecise movements, reduced range of motion, or fatigue (i.e., as noted during Routine Clinical Observation 2)
- ○ Mandible: deviates to right or left when lowered, weak resistance, or extraneous movements (i.e., as noted during Routine Clinical Observation 5)
- ○ Tongue: asymmetry, deviation, signs of atrophy, fasciculations, or extraneous movements at rest or in motion (i.e., as noted during Routine Clinical Observation 5)
- ○ Velum: asymmetry at rest or in motion, rhythmic or arrhythmic movements at rest or in motion, or unilateral or bilateral weakness (i.e., as noted during Routine Clinical Observation 5)
- ○ Weak or asymmetrical velar movement on /ɑ/ phonation (i.e., as noted during Routine Clinical Observation 6)
- ○ Verbal diadochokinesis: imprecise articulation, reduced range of motion for articulators, decreasing rate, slow rate, or evidence of fatigue (i.e., as noted during Routine Clinical Observation 7)
- ○ Evidence of hypernasality or fatigue during sustained vowel (i.e., as noted during Routine Clinical Observation 8)
- Consider speech sound stimulability screening (i.e., Discretionary Clinical Observation 18) if noting speech sound errors not fully attributable to organic anomaly, or stimulability test not completed prior (i.e., as noted during any routine clinical observation)
- Consider laryngeal and respiratory efficiency screening (i.e., Discretionary Clinical Observation 19) if noting the following:

- ○ Voice quality that indicates possible inefficient use of larynx (i.e., as noted during Routine Clinical Observation 1)
- ○ Failure to sustain the vowel for at least 20 seconds for adults or 10 seconds for children (i.e., as noted during Routine Clinical Observation 8)
- Consider gag reflex stimulation (i.e., Discretionary Clinical Observation 20) if noting the following:
- ○ Hypernasal resonance during speech, difficulty with obstruents, or craniofacial symptoms leading to genetic referral (i.e., as noted during Routine Clinical Observation 1)
- ○ Suspected inadequate velar movement (i.e., as noted during Routine Clinical Observation 6)
- ○ Any symptom leading to observations for developmental or acquired apraxia of speech (i.e., as noted during Routine Clinical Observation 7)
- ○ Hypernasal resonance during sustained vowel or any symptoms leading to observations for dysarthria (i.e., as noted during Routine Clinical Observation 8)
- ○ Any symptom suggesting a need for neurologic or genetic referral (i.e., as noted during any routine clinical observation)
- Consider prompt for dysphagia screening (i.e., Discretionary Clinical Observation 21) if noting the following:
- ○ Recent history of cerebrovascular accident, neurologic episode, or laryngectomy (i.e., as learned during case history intake)
- ○ Voice change or cough immediately after swallow (i.e., as noted during Routine Clinical Observation 1)
- ○ Flagged for apraxia or dysarthria observations (i.e., as noted during Routine Clinical Observations 7 and 8)
- ○ Abnormal volitional cough (i.e., as noted in Discretionary Clinical Observation 14)
- ○ Abnormal gag reflex (i.e., as noted during Routine Clinical Observation 20)

Concluding an Oral-Facial Evaluation

The discussion on concluding the oral-facial evaluation is inserted here for practical reasons. However, bear in mind that when discretionary clinical observations shown in Chapter 3 or 4 are to be performed, they should be completed before bringing the inspection to a close.

What the Oral-Facial Inspection Accomplishes

Having completed the inspection, you have collected concrete evidence to support a statement that either (1) dismisses organic etiology from consideration or (2) identifies specific aberrant structures or functions that are believed to potentially contribute to the identified speech production pattern. In addition, the inspection may result in recommendations and referrals that should be addressed. (See Chapter 5 for more information on how to interpret the data.)

Transition From Oral-Facial Evaluation to the Next Activity

After completing all procedures, including any necessary discretionary clinical observations, begin the transition from the oral-facial inspection to the next activity on the assessment plan. The next activity is often the closing interview or a short break that precedes the closing interview. This is because the oral-facial evaluation is often the last procedure completed during an evaluation, due to its potentially invasive nature, which can interfere with rapport needed for other procedures.

When ready to move on, using a friendly tone as well as age-appropriate verbiage, state that the person has successfully completed the oral-facial evaluation part of testing. Congratulate or otherwise encourage the person appropriately according to age and disposition. Comments should emphasize participation, perseverance, or whatever positive quality seems fitting to the client's response to the inspection protocol.

For children, a reward (e.g., sticker or token toy) for participation may be an effective way to acknowledge participation. Although some children may request, avoid dispensing clinical supplies such as flavored tongue depressors or examination gloves as they may pose liability if injury results.

Also, circumvent questions about findings until ready to discuss clinical implications at the closing interview. If questions about oral-facial evaluation results come up spontaneously before the closing interview, commend the person for having a great question, write the question down, and affirm that you will respond in a few moments when discussing results of the full battery of tests.

This concludes instructions for basic oral-facial inspection procedures. The next chapter gives instructions on how to administer 13 of the discretionary clinical observations when they are deemed necessary.

3

Instructions for Discretionary Clinical Observations

At times, routine procedures evoke awareness of a need for a closer look so that the clinician can focus on a particular aspect of oral structure or function. For that reason, Chapter 3 adds a series of discretionary clinical observations that, when appropriately and strategically applied, can strengthen a diagnosis, referral, or recommendation or can simply provide additional information that complements routine findings.

How and When to Insert the Discretionary Clinical Observations

When considering whether to add a discretionary clinical observation, there is only one recommended guideline: Before proceeding, complete the corresponding checklist that is shown on the recording form, or at least give consideration to the criteria highlighted therein.

Although discretionary observations appear on the recording forms after the full set of routine procedures, experienced clinicians can assume a comfortable degree of latitude when deciding how and when to insert a discretionary observation since there is no intention to restrict experienced clinicians from using professional judgment with regard to sequencing. Less experienced clinicians, however, are encouraged to defer discretionary testing until after completing routine data collection following the sequence provided until fully confident.

Orderly Data Collection

As with routine procedures that appear in Chapter 2, each discretionary clinical observation follows a consistent and orderly sequence. That is, each begins by explaining when to consider the particular procedure. Instructions then proceed by presenting a clinical question or series of clinical questions, list of equipment and supplies, and guidelines for performing the procedures, including information on normal and aberrant findings.

As is also true for routine procedures, when commentary is deemed necessary but not contiguous with the instructions, text boxes are inserted so as to minimize interruption to flow. Furthermore, details relevant to interpretation are located in Chapter 5.

The Discretionary Clinical Observations

Thirteen discretionary clinical observations are housed in this chapter. Three additional discretionary procedures are associated with special populations and can be found in Chapter 4, which addresses inspection procedures for individuals with special needs.

When adding the discretionary observations to the manual, a decision was made with regard to numbering the procedures. Since routine procedures are numbered 1 through 8 (Chapter 2), discretionary procedures begin with the number 9 and proceed through the number 24. By continuing with the numbering sequence, instead of beginning a new sequence, all procedures in the manual have a unique number that does not depend on prefix or home-chapter heading. The 13 discretionary procedures associated with Chapter 3 are as follows:

- Screening for nasal cavity clearance
- Facial dimension estimates
- Screening for temporomandibular joint disorder
- Observations for tongue-thrust swallow
- Observations for developmental apraxia of speech
- Observations for acquired apraxia of speech
- Screening for submucous cleft
- Screening for surplus nasal airflow during speech
- Observations for dysarthria
- Speech sound stimulability screening
- Screening for laryngeal and respiratory efficiency
- Gag reflex stimulation
- Prompt for dysphagia screening

Discretionary Clinical Observation 9: Screening for Nasal Cavity Clearance

Narratives provided by Bankson, Bernthal, and Flipsen (2009), Gordon-Brannan and Weiss (2007), Hanson and Mason (2003), Kummer (2008), Paskay (2012), and Riski (n.d.) were consulted and integrated with clinical experience when developing the nasal cavity clearance screening sequence.

When to Consider Nasal Cavity Clearance Screening

One should consider screening for nasal cavity clearance if noting any symptom flagged in the corresponding decision box on the recording form. Yet, take into account that if the examinee manifests symptoms of cold, flu, or allergy concomitant to hyponasal resonance, the condition may be temporary; therefore, the decision to perform the screening can be tabled until transitory symptoms resolve.

Clinical Question Associated With Screening for Nasal Cavity Clearance

Clinical Question 23 (see Table 0–3) asks, "For examinees with perceived hyponasal resonance, does viewing the nasal cavity provide evidence of clinically relevant obstruction?" An answer of *yes* suggests potential for clinically significant findings relative to nasal cavity clearance. Procedures that follow are useful for answering the question *and* for defining perceptible features and relevance of any anomaly observed.

Bear in mind that only superficial features of the nasal passages can be viewed using the procedures described herein and that size and condition of the posterior nasal chambers, nasopharynx, and pharyngeal tonsil (i.e., adenoid) cannot be seen through the nasal orifice. Therefore, if no obstruction is noted during nasal cavity-clearance screening, this does not rule out the possibility of occult obstruction.

Consequently, if perceiving hyponasal resonance and if this superficial screening fails to reveal evidence of obstruction or malfunction, instrumentation is required to more fully account for hyponasality. This type of testing goes beyond the scope of oral-facial evaluation and therefore results in a recommendation or referral.

Equipment Needed for Nasal Cavity-Clearance Screening

- Examination gloves
- Penlight
- Tissues (may be needed)

Procedures for Screening Nasal Cavity Clearance

- Don examination gloves if you have already removed them for some reason. Use gloving and ungloving procedures outlined in Chapter 1.
- Using the penlight, examine nasal passages bilaterally for symmetry and bilateral clearance. Any perceived obstructions due to mucosal swelling, deviated septum, growths, hypertrophied conchae, or excess mucus are all remarkable.
- Instruct the examinee to close the mouth and inhale deeply through the nose and

then expel the inhaled air, also via the nose. Be advised that mucus emission may necessitate the handy access to tissues. If risk of nasal discharge is evident, one may either opt to table this exercise until another session when symptoms have resolved or offer the opportunity to release nasal discharge prior to beginning.

- ○ Repeat the procedure for up to 20 breath cycles. Any difficulty admitting or discharging air via the nasal passages is remarkable.
- ○ While the examinee is exhaling nasally, use a gloved finger to alternately occlude each naris, one at a time. Difficulty expelling air through either or both nares is remarkable.
- • Instruct the examinee to close the lips and say /m →/ for 5 seconds. Difficulty with prolonging the nasal phoneme /m/ is remarkable.

Discretionary Clinical Observation 10: Facial Dimension Estimates

Narratives provided by Bergman (1999), Hanson and Mason (2003), Kummer (2008), and Prendergast (2012) were consulted and integrated with experience when developing procedures for estimating facial dimensions. Furthermore, we applied the measurements described herein to more than 30 faces representing a variety of ages, genders, and races to confirm the procedure as well as criteria for judging dimensions.

When to Consider Facial Dimension Estimates

In some cases, a person's facial dimensions seem disproportionate upon superficial viewing. Informal judgments of this sort are generally based on an examiner's experience with viewing thousands of faces throughout a lifetime of personal and, in many cases, clinical experience.

Whenever routine findings raise suspicions of facial dysmorphia that may be a part of a genetic syndrome or may interfere with the freedom or accu-

racy of tongue mobility or resonance, it is appropriate to proceed to this section so that facial dimension estimates can more specifically define the features observed. Refer to the corresponding decision box on the recording form when deciding whether to estimate facial dimensions.

Clinical Question for Estimating Facial Dimensions

Clinical Question 24 (see Table 0–3) asks, "When facial dysmorphia is noted upon superficial inspection, does evidence augment or support a specialist referral?" An answer of *yes* implies a potentially significant finding. The procedures that follow are useful for answering the clinical question *and* for surmising the nature of the anomaly when dysmorphia seems to affect overall facial dimensions, lower-third facial dimension, size and spacing of the eyes, facial angle, or Frankfurt horizontal plane. Diagnosing any conditions as a result of this screening is outside of the scope of practice for speech-language pathologists.

Equipment Needed for Facial Dimension Estimates

- • Examination gloves
- • Millimeter ruler
- • Calculator (may be needed)

About Facial Landmarks

Identifying key facial landmarks is fundamental to estimating facial dimensions. Therefore, the landmarks used as points of reference for this screening are listed and briefly described in Table 3–1. For clarity, the same landmarks are shown on frontal view of a human face (Figure 3–1A) and a similar profile view (Figure 3–1B).

Obviously, differences exist among individuals with regard to facial dimensions. Box 3–1 provides clarification.

Procedures for Estimating Facial Dimensions

General Notes. Calculations may be needed when estimated findings seem questionable and possibly relevant to communication or health. So as to focus

Table 3–1. Facial Landmarks Relevant to Facial Dimension Estimates

Landmark	Location and Description
Glabella	Most prominent point of the midline between the eyebrows
Subnasale	Horizontal line segment where the base of the nose meets the upper-most boundary of the philtrum
Menton	Most inferior point on the chin
Stomian	Line segment denoting where the upper and lower lips meet
Supramentale	Crease between the lower lip and the chin
Pogonion	Most anterior point of the chin
Palpebral fissures	Eye slits
Tragion	Superior-most point on the tragus, which is the cartilaginous projection in the auricle that is directly anterior to the external auditory canal
Lid-cheek junction	Inferior-most point of the zygomatic arch

on the procedures that involve the examinee while in the examination room, executing the math can be postponed until after the session.

Before beginning, slip on the examination gloves if you have taken them off for any reason. Refer to gloving and ungloving procedures described in Chapter 1.

Estimating Overall Facial Dimension. Instruct the examinee to look straight ahead, with the lips in a closed position. It may be helpful to suggest fixing both eyes on an object that is either at eye level or slightly above. Once the person's gaze and facial expression are appropriately fixed, estimate overall facial dimension using either profile or face-to-face point of view:

- Visually estimate the distance between the examinee's hairline (i.e., estimated hairline if absent or receded) and glabella, between glabella and subnasle, and between subnasale and pogonion, as shown in Figure 3–1C.
- Each of these three segments should occupy approximately one third (i.e., 33%) of the examinee's facial height.
- Exact equity is not the standard. However, if the thirds of the face are judged to be grossly uneven, use the millimeter ruler

to measure the segments, and after the session, use the calculator to compute the percentage that each segment occupies so that you may include the disparity in your documentation and in your communication with the referral recipient.

- Judge the area of concern according to whether the jaw, forehead, or midface is perceived as oversized or undersized.
- Consider grossly uneven facial segments as remarkable, especially if co-occurring in a symptom cluster implying possible syndrome or if the disparity potentially sheds light on an identified communication disorder.

Estimating Lower-Third Facial Dimension. Again, instruct the examinee to look straight ahead, fix the eyes on a stationary object at or slightly above eye level, and assume a closed-mouth position. Once the person has assumed the proper facial posture, estimate the dimensions for the lower third of the face:

- Visually estimate the distance between the subnasale and stomian, between the stomian and supramentale, and between supramentale and pogonion, as shown in Figure 3–1D.
- Each of the three segments should occupy approximately one third (i.e., 33%) of the

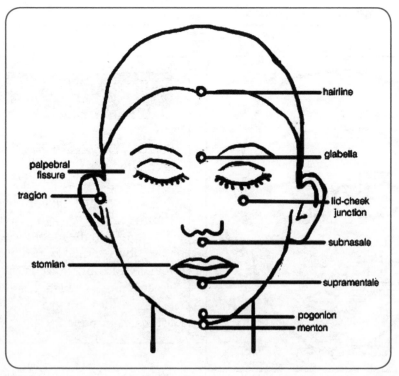

A

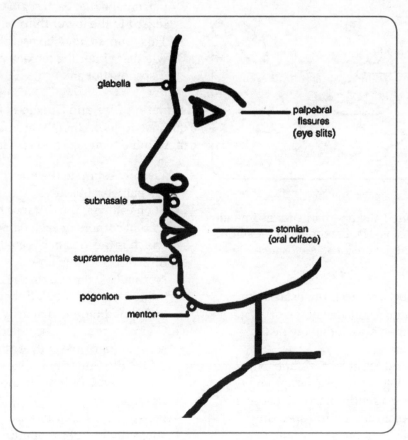

B

Figure 3–1. **A.** Facial landmarks, frontal view. **B.** Facial landmarks, profile view. *continues*

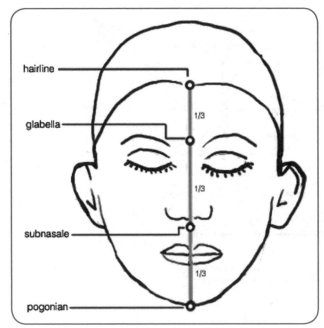

C

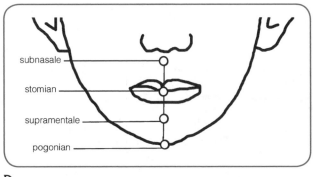

D

Figure 3–1. *continued* **C.** Landmarks for estimating overall facial dimensions. **D.** Landmarks for estimating lower-third facial dimensions. *continues*

total distance between the subnasale and pogonion. Again, results are noteworthy only if the segments are judged to be exceptionally uneven.

- If judging the three segments as uneven, and if this finding occurs in a symptom cluster implying a syndrome, or if it seems to partially explain an atypical speaking pattern, this observation is remarkable.
- If the three segments are judged as uneven, use the millimeter ruler to measure the height of the three lower-face segments.

Some variations in facial structure may be accounted for by race, heredity, or maturation; furthermore, a wide variety of idiosyncratic facial structures have no known relationship to any syndrome and have no discernable impact on tongue mobility or precision. Therefore, unless otherwise indicated, findings are remarkable only if appearing to affect speech, if occurring in cluster implying syndrome, or if dimensions are grossly dissimilar from the estimates provided.

Later, use the calculator to compute the percentage that each segment occupies with regard to the lower third of the face.

- This estimate may be useful in pinpointing whether either the maxilla or mandible is disproportionate.

Estimating Size and Spacing of Eyes. Instruct the examinee to look directly at your eyes so that you can examine their size and spacing:

- Visually estimate the horizontal width of the palpebral fissures.
- Then estimate the distance between the medial corners of each palpebral fissure, which is the area between the eyes that is directly above the nose.
- Normally, the three distances are approximately equal. If they are grossly different, then the disparity is noteworthy.
- Concerns that may be noted include wide-set eyes, narrow-set eyes, small or large orbits, dissimilarity in size when comparing the two eyes, or long or short palpebral fissures.
- For some, a disparity may be noted subjectively, but pinpointing the exact feature that is disproportionate may not be obvious. If this happens, report the proportions only and leave further

descriptive information up to the genetic specialist or otorhinolaryngologist who will evaluate next.

Estimating Facial Angle. Instruct the examinee to look straight ahead, eyes fixed on a selected stationary object, and mouth closed. Prepare to estimate the facial angle; a profile perspective is desirable:

- Use the straightedge to connect the glabella with the pogonion, as shown in Figure 3–1E.
- Normally, when connecting the glabella and pogonion in this way, the straightedge naturally arrives at an approximate vertical placement, perpendicular to the horizontal plane.
- The straightedge, placed in this manner, should intersect the subnasale plane.
- Findings are remarkable only if the line deviates grossly from a vertical position or if the subnasale plane is missed completely. Although it would be possible to use a protractor to measure the facial angle, if it

is estimated to be greater than or less than 90°, anticipate that exact dimensions will be taken during more in-depth testing that will result from medical referral.

- Judging facial angle as appreciably different from 90° can be helpful to the next service provider when suspecting atypical size or position of the jaw.

Estimating Frankfurt Horizontal Plane. Again instruct the examinee to look straight ahead, fixing both eyes on a stationary object that is at or slightly above eye level. Once the correct posture has been assumed, visually estimate the Frankfurt horizontal plane, which has value for estimating the height of the ears and eyes in relationship to one another:

- Use the straightedge to assist while you create an imaginary line between the tragion and the ipsilateral lid-cheek junction. These two landmarks, when connected, normally form a horizontal line (Figure 3–1F).

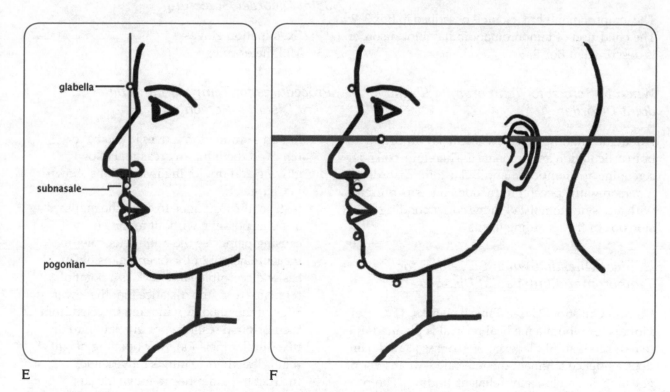

E   F

Figure 3–1. *continued* **E.** Landmarks for estimating facial angle. **F.** Landmarks for estimating Frankfurt horizontal plane.

- If the line that results deviates considerably from a horizontal plane, then this finding is remarkable. The concern in this case is that the positioning of the ears or eyes may be improper, which can be associated with a syndrome when occurring in a symptom cluster.

Discretionary Clinical Observation 11: Screening for Temporomandibular Joint Disorder

In preparing the temporomandibular joint screening, the following resources were consulted and integrated with clinical experience: Farina et al. (2009), Gordon-Brannan and Weiss (2007), Hanson and Mason (2003), Paskay (2012), Schmitter et al. (2008), Shipley and McAfee (2008), Stern and Greenberg (2013), and Wright and North (2009).

The Temporomandibular Joint and Temporomandibular Joint Disorder

The temporomandibular joint is described in Box 3–2. The condition of temporomandibular joint disorder is described in Box 3–3.

When to Screen for Temporomandibular Joint Disorder

Adequate mandibular movement is important to both articulation and resonance. Therefore, consider screening for temporomandibular joint disorder if a person with speech production concerns presents with any symptom listed in the corresponding decision box of the recording form.

Clinical Question When Screening for Temporomandibular Joint Disorder

Clinical Question 25 (see Table 0–3) asks, "For individuals for whom a medical referral is planned due to reduced mandibular excursion or associated pain, does evidence augment the referral?" An answer of *yes* suggests a clinically relevant finding. The procedures that follow are useful for answering the question *and* for pinpointing the extent to which the

---

Box 3–2. The Temporomandibular Joint

The temporomandibular joint is dissimilar from most joints in the human body in that it is not a simple hinge but instead is a compound joint. The primary function of the temporomandibular joint is to raise and lower the jaw for articulation, resonance, and eating.

To locate the temporomandibular joint on yourself, place two fingers on your own face in front of either ear at the level of the ear canal. Then raise and lower your jaw. By so doing, you will feel the jaw move, and thereby locate the joint location.

---

concern affects communication as well as other daily living activities, such as eating.

Equipment for Temporomandibular Joint Disorder Screening

- Examination gloves
- Millimeter ruler

Procedures for Temporomandibular Joint Disorder Screening

- Put on examination gloves if you have removed them for any reason. Follow gloving and ungloving instructions shown in Chapter 1.
- Instruct the examinee to open the mouth as far as possible without forcing or causing pain. Use the millimeter ruler to measure height of the opening, using an easily discernible landmark as a point of reference (e.g., the distance that the lower edge of the maxillary incisors traveled from their original resting spot in relation to the mandibular incisors). Any opening height that is less than 40 mm is remarkable.
- Instruct the examinee to move the jaw from side to side as far as possible without forcing or causing pain. Measure range of

Box 3–3. Temporomandibular Joint Disorder

As a rule, temporomandibular joint disorder, which is also known as *temporomandibular joint dysfunction*, is a repetitive-motion disorder of the jaw, most often resulting from either subluxation (i.e., partial dislocation) or luxation (i.e., complete dislocation) of the temporomandibular joint (described in Box 3–2).

Etiology of Temporomandibular Joint Disorder

Muscle spasms and pain can result when the levator muscles are forced to maintain the jaw's malposition under the circumstances of luxation or subluxation. Less common etiologies for temporomandibular joint disorder may also include infection, tumor, blow to the jaw, disk displacement, edema, effusion, or joint inflammation secondary to arthritis.

Incidence of Temporomandibular Joint Disorder

Persons with temporomandibular joint disorder usually first notice symptoms between 20 and 40 years of age. Although up to 30% of the population experience at least one symptom during their lifetime, only 6% to 7% experience symptoms severe enough to necessitate seeking relief through medical intervention.

Symptoms of Temporomandibular Joint Disorder

In addition to severe pain, reduced range of motion, stiffness, catching, and locking, temporo-mandibular joint disorder can also result in atypical sounds associated with jaw movement. That is, a less severe condition may result in clicking, snapping, or popping sounds. A sound that indicates a more severe condition is the sound that resembles footsteps on loose gravel, also called *crepitus*. Crepitus is the sound of bone rubbing against bone.

Temporomandibular joint disorder pain can be extreme. Most typically, the pain is localized in the regions associated with the masseter muscle, in the anterior temporalis, or in the preauricular area. Although most often the pain is dull and achy or associated with the feeling of pressure, the sensation can also resemble burning, stabbing, or throbbing.

Pain associated with temporomandibular joint disorder may or may not be at the exact joint location and in fact may refer to an ipsilateral-lower molar or the ear. Similarly, an earache or toothache may be perceived in the ipsilateral temporomandibular joint as opposed to the actual site of inflammation.

Temporomandibular Joint Disorder's Relevance to Speech-Language Pathology

Because temporomandibular joint disorder can limit mandibular excursion, it can result in indistinct articulation as well as reduced size of the oral chamber for resonance and airflow egress during speech. It can also cause mandibular tongue thrust, associating it with a type of tongue-thrust swallow that involves mandibular as well as tongue protrusion.

motion, again using an easily discernible landmark as a point of reference. For instance, in most cases, the dividing line between the two maxillary incisors is a clear line that can be found easily, as is the dividing line between the two mandibular incisors, and unless there is cross bite, the two dividing lines are continuous with one another. Thus, measuring the distance that represents lateral jaw excursion can be facilitated by measuring the distance between the two dental midlines when the examinee has lateralized the jaw as much a possible. Any measurement less than 7 mm is remarkable.

- Instruct the examinee to protrude the jaw as far as possible without forcing or causing pain. Measure range of motion, again using natural incisor position as the landmark. Any measurement less than 6 mm is remarkable.
- Instruct the person to open and close the mouth rapidly:
  - Touch the joint so as to judge whether popping, clicking, or grinding during jaw movement is palpable. Any sensation of these is remarkable.
  - Ask the person to report whether the opening and closing of the mouth results in a sensation of popping, snapping, or grinding. Any report of these is remarkable.
  - Ask whether the examinee experiences pain in the jaw, ear, or lower molar. If pain is reported, ask the person to subjectively rate pain severity on a 5-point scale, where 1 represents *no pain* and 5 represents *maximum pain*. Any 2 to 5 rating is remarkable.
- Instruct the examinee to move the mandible from side to side rapidly. Ask the person to report any sensation of pain, popping, clicking, snapping, or grinding and to subjectively rate pain using the 5-point scale described above. Any testimony of audible or felt symptoms is remarkable, as is the numeric pain rating if pain is reported.

Discretionary Clinical Observation 12: Tongue-Thrust Swallow Procedure

In assembling procedures for identifying tongue-thrust swallow, resources that were consulted include Andrianopoulos and Hanson (1987); de Felicio and Ferreira (2008); de Felicio, Folha, Ferreira,

and Medeiros (2010); Flipsen, Bankson, and Bernthal (2009); Fraser (2006); Hanson and Mason (2003); Karacay, Akin, Ortakoglu, and Bengi (2006); Knösel, Klein, Bleckmann, and Engelke (2012); Lebrun (1985); Marasa (2007a, 2007b, 2008); Mason (1988); Paskay (2012); Peng, Jost-Brinkmann, Yoshido, Chou, and Lin (2004); Singh, Prerna, Dua, and Jain (2011); Smithpeter and Covell (2010); and Wadsworth, Maul, and Stevens (1998). These reports were integrated with experience in diagnosing and treating the condition in clinical practice and supervision.

The Controversy About Tongue-Thrust Swallow

Controversy surrounds the diagnosis and clinical relevance of tongue-thrust swallow. Box 3–4 sheds light on the diagnostic perspective and comments on how the procedures offered herein may be useful for identifying individuals with the condition. The other side of the controversy concerns clinical relevance to speech-language pathology. Box 3–5 speaks to this issue.

Clinical Questions Associated With the Tongue-Thrust Swallow Procedure

Clinical Question 26 (see Table 0–3) asks, "For examinees identified to be at risk for tongue-thrust swallow, does evidence support a diagnosis of clinically significant tongue-thrust swallow?" An answer of *yes* indicates the possibility of a noteworthy result, leading to Clinical Question 27, which asks, "If so, does the procedure identify the pattern as habitual or obligatory?" The procedures that follow are useful for both identifying tongue-thrust swallow *and* distinguishing between habitual and obligatory varieties.

When to Perform Tongue-Thrust Swallow Inspection

Check for tongue-thrust swallow in any person with relevant speech production disorder, age 12 years or older, who displays symptoms listed in the corresponding decision box on the recording form. Also, when evaluating children between 5 and 12 years of age, if tongue-thrust swallow symptoms are noted,

Box 3–4. Diagnosing Tongue-Thrust Swallow: A Controversial Topic

Considerable effort was made to create a set of clinically useful procedures that take a range of perspectives into consideration. However, one cannot ignore the noteworthy disagreement concerning whether tongue-thrust swallow can be identified reliably without instrumentation. Since speech-language pathologists are qualified to diagnose and treat the condition, we leave this judgment up to the individual clinician. That is, if symptoms of tongue-thrust swallow are definitively exhibited using the procedures described herein, the speech-language pathologist should make a professional decision as to whether to order ultrasonography for the purpose of confirming the diagnosis. Obviously, whenever the findings are questionable and potentially relevant to speech, the referral for more in-depth testing should be made.

To make meaningful observations relative to tongue-thrust swallow, the examiner should first understand salient features of tongue-thrust swallow and distinguish them from features of the more typically occurring standard swallow. Likewise, in the event that a tongue-thrust swallow pattern is identified, clinicians should be prepared to distinguish between two types so as to provide an appropriate plan of care. The two types of tongue-thrust swallow to be considered are habitual and obligatory.

Box 3–5. Clinical Relevance of Tongue-Thrust Swallow

Tongue-thrust swallow is an atypical swallow pattern that can not only be associated with an easily recognized articulation error pattern but also can co-occur with oral-structural anomalies that necessitate compensatory strategies when attempting to produce standard phonemes of the language. Although many individuals are capable of compensating, because the pattern can be changed through therapy and changing the pattern can eliminate the need for energy-sapping compensatory movements, some maintain that early identification and treatment can make a difference to many.

emptive measures that address the swallow as part of a plan of care.

To more effectively identify candidates for tongue-thrust swallow observations, it is helpful to first understand the differences between the typical swallow pattern and the tongue-thrust swallow pattern. Box 3–6 distinguishes between these two.

Equipment Needed for Tongue-Thrust Swallow Procedure

- Examination gloves
- Cup of water
- Penlight (may be needed)

Procedures for Identifying Tongue-Thrust Swallow

Tongue-thrust swallow is generally considered easy to identify manually both during speech and during swallowing, yet a few have expressed concern that inspection procedures can disturb the lip muscles enough to operably interfere with findings. Our experience leans toward agreeing with those who find the condition to be easily identifiable without resorting to expensive testing for most examinees, although exceptions can occur.

you may use clinical judgment to determine whether the swallow pattern should be evaluated as a possible contributor to a speech production problem. If tongue-thrust swallow coincides with speech characteristics common to that pattern, even younger than age 12 years, it may be expedient to take pre-

Box 3–6. Tongue-Thrust Swallow Contrasted to Typical Swallow Pattern

The term *tongue-thrust swallow* is the preferred label for the swallow pattern described in this section and has been intentionally selected from an assortment of terms that may be associated with the phenomenon. Other terms include *reverse swallow*, *deviate swallow*, *infantile swallow*, and *immature swallow*; they are not used in this manual because they are considered potentially misleading. Also, the term *oral-facial myofunctional disorder* may be used to describe some swallowing disorders, including tongue-thrust swallow, but it was not chosen since the term encompasses a broader spectrum of swallowing patterns than the specific pattern discussed under this heading.

Even the term *tongue-thrust swallow* may be somewhat misleading because the word *thrust* implies a forceful forward action of the tongue, but in actuality, the swallow pattern of interest may be more accurately described as having a difference in the tongue's direction during the swallow, with less emphasis on a difference in the amount of force applied during the swallow.

Typical Swallow

Normally, the adult swallow involves gently closing the jaw, followed by upward and backward motion of the tongue with the tongue blade forcing a seal with the hard palate. This action is used to push the contents of the mouth toward the pharyngeal orifice, where it exits the oral cavity and proceeds downward toward the esophagus.

Tongue-Thrust Swallow

In the case of tongue-thrust swallow, however, the mandibular and maxillary teeth do not occlude during the swallow. Also, the tongue moves in a forward direction at the onset of the swallow, proceeds to insert itself between the maxillary and mandibular incisors, and makes contact with the lower lip. A strong anterior seal involving the lip and cheek muscles is characteristically associated with tongue-thrust swallow, as contrasted to the superior lingua-palatal seal required for the so-called normal swallow.

The tongue-thrust swallow pattern can be associated with forward tongue posture during speech and at rest, malocclusion, altered facial development, open bite, overjet, and problems with articulation, specifically dentalization of the alveolar consonants and overexaggeration of the interdental consonants. Tongue-thrust swallow can also co-occur with mastication and deglutination problems, habitual oral breathing, habitual open-mouth posture, incomplete eruption of anterior teeth, restricted upper-lip movement, restricted lingua-frenum, temporomandibular joint disorder, age-inappropriate oral habits (e.g., thumb sucking, bottle feeding, pacifier use beyond infancy, or pica), bruxism, biting or resting objects between the teeth (e.g., pencils), chronically chapped lips, unilateral lip or cheek biting resulting in palatal arch asymmetry, tongue sucking, tongue or lip resting-posture idiosyncrasies, poor saliva management, adaptive sleep apnea, and extraordinarily large tonsils. Tongue-thrust swallow may also occur secondary to allergies, enlarged pharyngeal tonsil, swollen nasal membrane, deviated septum, high-palatal arch, cross bite, or vertical dental crowding due to deep overbite.

Normal Suppression of Tongue-Thrust Swallow During Development

The tongue-thrust swallow is characteristically common to all infants since the large size of the infant tongue in relation to the oral cavity necessitates sealing the anterior cavity during the swallow. As the child's oral cavity grows, a superior (i.e., lingua-palatal) seal usually replaces or suppresses the earlier anterior (i.e., bilabial) seal.

Experts disagree as to the exact age when tongue-thrust swallow is naturally suppressed in most children. A reasonably accepted age of suppression is during the years when deciduous teeth fall out and permanent teeth erupt, or roughly between 5 and 12 years of age.

Therefore, when tongue-thrust swallow is observed before the child acquires a full complement of permanent teeth (i.e., before 10 or 12 years of age), many consider this to be a developmental condition that is likely to disappear with maturation. Similarly, if the pattern is noted after this dental milestone, it can be regarded as chronic.

Consequently, it stands to reason that some individuals who display features of developmental tongue-thrust swallow do not outgrow it. Given this information, one may conclude that there is room for conjecture when considering the needs of individuals with tongue-thrust swallow during the teeth-shedding years (i.e., between the ages of 5 and 12 years).

Furthermore, it is important to note that for some people, the tongue-thrust swallow pattern is never suppressed even after age 12 years, having no negative impact on adult speech production or oral structure. In these cases, the persistent tongue-thrust swallow pattern, although potentially noteworthy for documentation purposes, is usually clinically irrelevant.

Recognizing that occasionally inspection procedures may yield tentative results, we acknowledge that ultrasonography is beneficial to confirm a diagnosis when manually attained findings are unclear. Whenever in doubt, do not hesitate to request ultrasonography. Otherwise, however, the procedures offered herein are generally accepted as reliable.

Instruct the examinee as follows:

- Take a sip of water and hold the water in the mouth for a moment.
- Close the jaw and hold it closed, while using the thumb and index finger to hold the lips open on both sides (Figure 3–2). Note: Since many tongue thrusters habitually swallow with a teeth-open position, it is essential that you instruct the person to keep the back teeth closed, preventing the water from spilling out. You may even demonstrate. Depending on age and ability to perform, some examinees may use their own fingers to hold their lips open; however if an examinee needs your assistance, gloves are required.
- Swallow, keeping the lips open and the back teeth together.

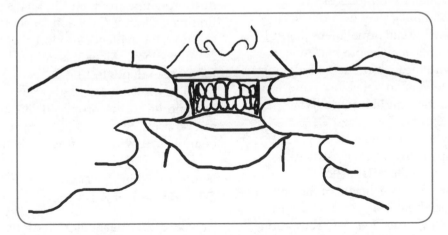

Figure 3–2. Facial position for tongue-thrust swallow observation.

Observe. Carefully observe the teeth and lips during the swallow. Tongue-thrust swallow pattern is identified if either or both of the following occurs while swallowing: (1) the tongue visibly protrudes between the incisors, involuntarily and forcefully, or (2) the lips close and either seal or attempt to seal involuntarily and forcefully. The swallow procedure may be repeated to verify results.

Habitual Versus Obligatory Tongue-Thrust Swallow. If a tongue-thrust swallow seems apparent, ascertain whether the pattern is habitual or obligatory. In the case of habitual tongue-thrust swallow, the pattern occurs in the absence of any noticeable anatomic or physiologic obstacle.

Obligatory tongue-thrust swallow, however, coincides with structural differences that seem to obstruct or prevent the normal swallow pattern. Nasal obstruction, high palatal vault, mouth breathing, open bite, and temporomandibular joint disorder are examples of some observations that have potential to interfere with a person's ability to use a standard swallow pattern.

Therefore, to determine whether the pattern is habitual or obligatory:

- Review findings noted during facial region inspection, with focus on nasal observations, breathing, and resonance (i.e., Routine Clinical Observation 1). If in doubt, reinspect; a penlight may be needed. Any physical aberration potentially suggests an obligatory pattern.
- Consider whether symptoms of temporomandibular joint disorder, such as reduced mandibular motion or painful jaw movements, may be present. Any concerns with the temporomandibular joint may point toward an obligatory pattern, especially if the mandible juts outward during the observed swallow.
- Review any notes on the recording form that speak to oral-cavity structure, including size of the palatine tonsils, size of the pharyngeal orifice, height of the palatal vault, or open bite. Reinspect if in doubt; a penlight may be needed. Any aberration may point toward an obligatory pattern.

Discretionary Clinical Observation 13: Observations for Developmental Apraxia of Speech

In building the procedures for this section, many resources were consulted and combined with clinical experiences. They include ASHA (2007a, 2007b); Buder, Chorna, Oller, and Robinson (2006); Duffy (2013); Duffy, Waumbaugh, Fredrickson, and Haley (2013); Hall (2007a, 2007b, 2007c); Kamhi (2006); Oller (1980, 2000); Oller, Buder, et al. (2013); Oller, Warlaumont, et al. (2013); Overby and Caspari (2013); Strand (2011); Strand, McCauley, Weigand, Stoeckel, and Baas (2012); and Yorkston, Beukelman, Strand, and Hakel (2010).

Clinical Questions Associated With Observations for Developmental Apraxia of Speech

Clinical Question 28 (see Table 0–3) asks, "For child examinees who exhibit superficial symptoms of developmental apraxia of speech, does evidence suggest or rule out a diagnosis?" If the answer suggests a diagnosis, this implies potentially clinically relevant findings that may indicate developmental apraxia of speech.

Yet, for some, the evidence may not clearly support or rule out a diagnosis. This is especially true when the examiner does not routinely work in the area of childhood motor-speech disorders, but can also be the case for more experienced clinicians when the child exhibits an assortment of speech production symptoms. For individuals with ambiguous findings, Clinical Question 29 should be asked: "If not, does the evidence support a referral for more in-depth testing?" A response of *yes* leads to a referral for more in-depth testing.

The procedures that follow are useful for responding to the proposed questions. Also, they can be useful when identifying specific symptoms of apraxia, if evidence supports a diagnosis.

When to Consider Observations for Developmental Apraxia of Speech

Consider this particular discretionary procedure whenever a child presents with any combination of the symptoms listed in the corresponding decision box of the recording form. A description of developmental apraxia of speech can also be found in Box 3–7.

Although symptoms associated with developmental apraxia of speech characteristically emerge in toddlers and preschoolers, it is our experience that some children with the condition receive a generic *late talker* or *unintelligible speech* diagnosis, receive therapy at a young age that does not specifically target apractic symptoms, make slow progress in therapy continuing through the school-age years, and may even be subject to repeated re-evaluations well beyond the time that would have been excellent for an initial diagnosis. So as to prevent missing a latent identification opportunity, the procedures to observe

for developmental apraxia of speech are offered in this section.

Because many children with developmental apraxia of speech are seen for their first assessment as toddlers, this is an area of testing that more frequently applies to children in the 3- to 5-year age group. Therefore, consult adaptations for younger children in the appropriate section of Chapter 4 for more information.

Objective When Observing for Developmental Apraxia of Speech

Ideally, the procedure suggests or rules out a diagnosis of developmental apraxia of speech. Less

---

Box 3–7. Developmental Apraxia of Speech Described

Developmental apraxia of speech, also called by many other names, including childhood apraxia of speech, is a speech disorder that manifests in early childhood. Fundamentally, developmental apraxia of speech is characterized by a set of symptoms that suggest challenges with regulating volitional movements and sequences of movements required for speech. It is considered a disorder of speech-motor control and often occurs concomitantly with other conditions that may include but are not limited to language disorder, academic disability, gross and fine motor irregularities, difficulty with role-playing sequences of daily routines, and feeding concerns.

Developmental apraxia of speech presents as a symptom cluster, where a number of symptoms are associated with the condition, but no one symptom is yet considered the cardinal feature, and not all associated symptoms are required to make the diagnosis. Therefore, diagnosing the condition can be seriously challenging to clinicians who do not work with the population on a regular basis or do not specialize in diagnosing and treating the disorder. Having established that the cluster of symptoms can only loosely guide a diagnosis, it is also important to recognize that oral-facial inspection is sensitive to the symp-

toms and, if interpreted accurately, can provide evidence that substantially contributes when confirming or ruling out developmental apraxia of speech.

One important developmental feature of the disorder is the absence of canonical babbling during the appropriate stage. Canonical babbling is the repetitive sequencing of consonant-vowel syllables and is a common act of vocal expression in normally developing children between the ages of 7 and 10 months.

Another important developmental characteristic is a significantly delayed onset of verbal language, with first words emerging well into the second or even the third year of life for some. In fact, many children with developmental apraxia of speech do not use spoken language consistently until they are 4 or 5 years of age.

Some parents may bring their child with developmental apraxia of speech for speech-language evaluation as a young toddler or in the preschool years, but a small number of children may receive evaluation or reevaluation upon entering school or even later. Regardless of when the child is seen, it is of utmost importance that the condition be accurately diagnosed as early as possible so that appropriate treatment can ensue.

frequently, it may expose concrete evidence that leads to a recommendation or referral for more in-depth testing. Since some examiners may encounter childhood apraxia on occasion, lacking regular exposure to the condition, the observations can also provide structure for examiners who may not feel confident making a diagnosis or substantiating a referral to a specialist who is qualified to make the diagnosis.

Equipment Needed When Observing for Symptoms of Developmental Apraxia of Speech

Observations for developmental apraxia of speech require no special equipment.

Procedures for Developmental Apraxia of Speech Observations

Developmental Apraxia of Speech Observations for Preverbal and Limited-Language Children

- Return to the case history intake form or ask the parent to verify the following:
  - Did the child babble? Specifically, did the child use canonical babbling between the ages of 5 and 10 months? If the answer to either of these questions is *no*, then the finding is remarkable.
  - Would you consider the child to have been an unusually quiet baby? If the answer is *yes*, the finding is remarkable.
  - If the child is preverbal and older than 18 months, does the child prefer to communicate using gestures? If the answer is *yes*, the finding is remarkable.
- Return to the recorded social interaction gathered during Routine Clinical Observation 1 or request that the parents provide recorded evidence of the child interacting socially during play. Note the following:
  - Do single-word utterances dominate, and are they frequently holophrastic? If the child is older than age 18 months, an answer of *yes* is remarkable.
  - Does the child communicate more effectively using gestures than speech?

If the child is older than age 18 months, an answer of *yes* is remarkable.
  - Does the child frequently supplement unintelligible speech with gestures and environmental sounds (e.g., /bɝd/ → /bud/ supplemented by making a chirping sound, or /ˈdɑ dɪ/ is used to express the words *daddy* and *doggy*, and the child communicates the intended message by supplementing the homonym with a learned American Sign Language [ASL] sign)? If the answer is *yes*, the finding is remarkable.
  - Does the child make unusual speech sound production errors (e.g., vowel distortions, consonant insertions, voicing confusions, metathetic errors, perseveration across word boundaries, nonspeech sounds)? If so, the presence of unusual speech sound production errors is remarkable.
- If the child uses simple multiword utterances, then proceed to observations for developmental apraxia of speech in verbal children, and complete the procedures to the extent that the child tolerates.

Observation Procedures for Developmental Apraxia of Speech in Verbal Children

- In an effort to challenge the child's ability to plan and sequence motor movements for speech, ask the child to repeat the multisyllabic words shown on the recording form. Watch for manner-type substitution errors (e.g., fricative → stop), speech sound additions, prolongations, repetitions, nonphonemic productions (e.g., pops, clicks), voicing and nasality errors, vowel and diphthong errors, difficulty with sequencing phonemes in syllables, inconsistent errors, silent or audible articulatory groping, silent posturing of articulators, unusual prosodic patterns, and dysfluency or choppiness. If noting any of these features, the finding is remarkable.

- For children who have demonstrated the ability to speak in sentences, instruct to repeat the silly sentences shown on the recording form, similarly challenging the ability to plan and sequence motor movements for speech at a more complex level. Watch for the same types of error patterns. If noticing any of the error patterns listed in the paragraph above, the finding is remarkable.

Discretionary Clinical Observation 14: Observations for Acquired Apraxia of Speech

In developing this section, the following authorities were consulted and combined with clinical experience: Duffy (2006, 2011, 2013); Duffy and Josephs (2012); Duffy et al. (2013); Haley, Jacks, de Riesthal, Abou-Khalil, and Roth (2012); McCullough et al. (2005); Waumbaugh (2006); Waumbaugh, Duffy, McNeil, Robin, and Rogers (2006); Waumbaugh, Nessler, Cameron, and Mauszycki (2013); Yorkston et al. (2010); and Ziegler, Aichert, and Staiger (2012).

When to Check for Acquired Apraxia of Speech in an Adult Examinee

Acquired apraxia of speech is described in Box 3–8. Routine procedures described in Chapter 2 purposefully call attention to differences between automatic and volitional responses for both speech and non-speech activities. Consider the apraxia of speech procedure if noting evidence of a person having acquired any symptom flagged in the corresponding decision box on the recording form. Pay particular attention to individuals for whom the onset of symptoms is associated with cerebrovascular accident, traumatic brain injury, or neurogenic disease.

Clinical Questions Associated With Acquired Apraxia of Speech Procedure

Clinical Question 30 (see Table 0–3) asks, "When routine inspection reveals symptoms that imply acquired apraxia of speech, does evidence support or rule out a diagnosis?" If the answer supports a diagnosis, this suggests clinically relevant findings with regard to apraxia of speech.

For some, the evidence may not clearly support or rule out a diagnosis. This is most often the case

---

Box 3–8. Acquired Apraxia of Speech Described

Primarily, acquired apraxia of speech manifests as an impaired capacity to plan or program movements necessary for speech. Although there may be differences in symptoms based on etiology, primary symptoms include speech sound errors, increased errors as utterance length and complexity increase, audible and silent articulatory groping, false starts and restarts, slow rate of speech, increased time needed for speech sound or syllable transitions, distorted substitutions and additions, syllable segmentation, and disordered prosody.

Adults with apraxia of speech may be able to perform certain speaking activities well when an automatic response is required but not well, or even not at all, when attempting to say the same word or words with deliberate intent. For exam-

ple, a person with apraxia of speech may fluently say the days of the week in sequence when asked to recite them but struggle to name a particular day in response to a question, "What day is today?" or "On what day did your son visit?"

Although apraxia of speech can be the predominant or only speech disorder associated with certain neurologically based communication disorders, in many cases, it co-occurs with a dysarthria, aphasia, or other type of apraxia (e.g., oral or limb apraxia). Therefore, under conditions of concomitant speech disorder, newer clinicians or clinicians who do not regularly practice in this area may experience challenges and should refer to or collaborate with an experienced practitioner until confident.

when the examining clinician lacks experience with diagnosing and treating apraxia. For examinees with this result, Clinical Question 31 should be asked: "If not, does evidence support a referral for more in-depth testing?" An affirmative response leads to a referral.

The procedures that follow are useful for responding to the proposed questions. They are also useful for identifying specific symptoms of apraxia if evidence supports a diagnosis.

Clinical Intent of the Acquired Apraxia of Speech Procedure

The procedure provides structure that is intended to support clinicians who have limited experience in this important area of diagnosis and treatment so as to corroborate a proper diagnosis, recommendation, or even referral.

Equipment Needed for Acquired Apraxia of Speech Procedure

No special equipment is needed for apraxia of speech screening.

Procedures for Acquired Apraxia of Speech Observations

- First, screen for oral apraxia to confirm or rule out whether it potentially contributes to the noted symptoms. Instruct the examinee to do each of the following volitionally, taking care to avoid inadvertently including an automatic response:
    - Cough.
    - Click the tongue.
    - Blow.
    - Bite the lower lip.
    - Puff the cheeks.
- Elicit numbers *1 through 5* aloud under both volitional and automatic conditions. Compare. If automatic counting is more fluid than purposeful number naming, the finding is remarkable. The two steps that appear below offer suggestions as to how to accomplish this:

- Elicit volitional number naming by holding up two fingers, then asking the person to identify the number of fingers you are holding up. Repeat for the numbers 5, 1, 4, and 3, in that order, or in any order that is not sequential counting.
    - Then, elicit automatic counting by asking the person to count sequentially from 1 to 5.
- Elicit automatic and volitional backward counting. Compare. If automatic backward counting is more fluid than volitional backward counting, this finding is remarkable. The activity offered below is one way to elicit the data:
    - Ask the person to count backward from 20 to 1, beginning with 20 and ending with 1.
    - Since backward counting from 20 to 11 is not usually overlearned or automatic, it requires volitional planning. However, counting from 10 to 1 is the countdown sequence and therefore is overlearned and automatic for most people. So, evaluate fluidity of these two halves separately. If counting from 10 to 1 is markedly more fluid than counting from 20 to 11, the finding is remarkable.
- Compare saying a word in automatic sequence with saying the same word as an answer to a question outside the sequence:
    - Ask the examinee to tell the name of the month of a particular holiday that is known to the person, giving consideration to cultural orientation. Avoid January since it begins a sequence. For example, Thanksgiving is a holiday that most North Americans observe regardless of religion or culture. A person's birthday month is another suggestion.
    - Then ask the person to say the months of the year, beginning with January.
    - Compare the fluidity of the person's pronunciation of *November* (or relevant month of Thanksgiving holiday) or the month of birth under both volitional and automatic circumstances. If saying

the name of the month in sequence is more fluid compared with answering a question, then this finding is remarkable.

- Compare fluidity for pronouncing words of increasing length and complexity:
  - Ask the person to say the word triads shown on the recording form. Each triad includes words of increasing length and complexity. If shorter, simpler words are pronounced with more fluidity than the longer, more complex words, then the finding is remarkable.

Discretionary Clinical Observation 15: Screening for Submucous Cleft

Resources that were consulted and integrated with clinical experience when designing a plan for submucous cleft screening include Bzoch (2004), Kummer (2008), Kummer and Lee (1996), Reiter, Brosch, Wefel, Schlömer, and Haase (2011), Riski (n.d.), and Shprintzen, Schwartz, Daniller, and Hoch (1985).

When to Screen for Submucous Cleft

Consider screening for submucous cleft if noting any symptom flagged in the corresponding decision box on the recording form. Because screening for submucous cleft can be mildly invasive, safety precautions appear in Box 3–9.

Clinical Question Associated With Submucous Cleft Screening

Clinical Question 32 (see Table 0–3) asks, "When examining individuals for whom integrity of the hard palate is questionable, who also exhibit signs of hypernasal speech or difficulty with obstruent consonants, does evidence strengthen a medical referral?" An affirmative response is remarkable. The procedures are helpful for responding to the clinical question.

Equipment Needed for Submucous Cleft Screening

- Examination gloves
- Penlight

Procedures for Submucous Cleft Screening

- Identify the finger that you plan to use to palpate the palate. We recommend the third finger (i.e., ring finger) of the nondominant hand because it is the weakest finger that

---

Box 3–9. Special Notice About Screening for Submucous Cleft

Screening for submucous cleft is mildly invasive and requires considerable care to prevent injury to the examinee. If suspecting submucous cleft, and concerns linger as to whether the screening can be performed safely, then refer the individual to a physician for medical evaluation without performing the screening, but provide the physician with the clinically relevant evidence gathered during speech and during palatal inspection (Routine Clinical Observation 5).

Because the screening can provide additional information that may strengthen the referral or recommendations, whenever submucous cleft screening can be performed safely for a person with questionable palatal integrity, completing it and reporting the results is preferred.

Because most examinees who are subject to this screening are young children, procedures refer to the examinee as a child. However, because of the occult nature of submucous cleft, the condition may not yet be verified in some older children and even young adults. Therefore, the basic procedures appear in this section, with minor adaptations for the very young appearing in Chapter 4.

can extend far enough into the oral cavity to perform the examination. The weakest finger is selected to minimize the risk of injury. First finger and fourth finger options may also be considered:

○ For very young children, the fourth finger (i.e., pinky) may be long enough, and some recommend using it instead.

○ Some recommend using the first finger (i.e., index finger) because controlling its movement and sensing tactile differences can be easier. If using the index finger, extra caution is recommended to prevent injury, especially for less experienced clinicians.

• Use the penlight to verify the location of suspicious palatal coloring.

• For the tactile inspection, use finger-tip action instead of wrist or arm action. In fact, rely on this method throughout the procedure to avoid the possibility of accidental injury should you encounter an area of the palate that is not supported by bone.

• Begin tactile inspection by rubbing the child's anterior-maxillary gums gently. Massaging the gums in this way is done to familiarize the child with the sensation of an examiner's finger inside the mouth. Also since the gums are typically supported by bone, this action can give the examiner a baseline sensation that is somewhat consistent with the normal amount of tactile resistance for an intact hard palate.

• When the child seems reasonably tolerant of having an adult's finger inside the mouth, proceed by gliding the finger in a posterior direction across the maxillary incisors and palpate the alveolar ridge, continuing to use finger-tip action only. Again, rubbing the alveolar ridge is a way to further acclimate the child to the sensation.

• Then continue by gliding the finger in a posterior direction along the medial dental arch all the way back to the last molar.

• Proceed by gliding the finger across the posterior border of the hard palate. At

midline, use sense of touch to check for the nasal spine. If a notch is noted instead, this is remarkable.

• Then, proceed by gliding the finger in a forward direction along the median palatal raphe. It is possible that you will feel a bony protuberance at midline (i.e., palatal torus). If found, this may be remarkable but typically not clinically relevant with regard to submucous cleft.

• Finally, glide the finger along the palate from back to front on either side of the median palatal raphe.

• If any palpated area is found to have decreased tactile resistance, this is remarkable.

Discretionary Clinical Observation 16: Screening for Surplus Nasal Airflow During Speech

A variety of techniques exist for gathering superficial evidence relative to surplus nasal airflow during speech. All involve equipment of some type, from mirrors or shiny plates to listening tubes or straws. When formalizing the procedures for this section, various resources were consulted (Brescovici & Roithmann, 2008; Duffy, 2013; Lowit & Kent, 2011; Kummer, 2008; Kummer & Lee, 1996; Riski, n.d.; Yorkston et al., 2010).

Then a decision was made to endorse the one method deemed easiest to perform based on clinical experience, while still yielding reasonably reliable results. Other methods are available, and if an experienced clinician prefers them, that person is encouraged to substitute the preferred method in place of the procedures offered herein.

When to Screen for Surplus Nasal Airflow

The procedure is designed to call attention to atypical nasal airflow emission, if it occurs, for speech sounds that require intraoral pressure. Consider this screening if noting any symptom flagged in the corresponding decision box on the recording form.

Clinical Question Associated With Screening for Surplus Nasal Airflow

Clinical Question 33 (see Table 0–3) asks, "For individuals who will be referred for evaluation of velar structure or function, does evidence strengthen a referral for more in-depth testing?" An answer of *yes* to the question implies a remarkable finding. The procedures that follow are useful for answering the question *and* for estimating the extent to which any anomaly influences resonance or articulation.

Equipment Needed for Surplus Nasal Airflow Screening

- Examination gloves
- Examination mirror

Procedures for Surplus Nasal Airflow Screening

The procedure for this particular screening has a long-standing clinical history, is simple to execute, and allows for considerable flexibility. Simply hold the mirror under the examinee's nares during speech and simultaneously examine the mirror for evidence of untimely nasal airflow emission that manifests in the form of mirror condensation. Any of the following techniques or combination thereof may be used to obtain the speech sample. Choose the one that seems most appropriate for the examinee. A second or third may be needed to confirm findings, but only one is required. Any mirror condensation for oral phonemes is remarkable.

- Instruct the person to say the plosive consonants /p/, /t/, or /k/ in simple CV or VC syllables. Mirror condensation is remarkable.
- Instruct the examinee to name objects or pictures of words that combine voiced early developing obstruent consonants and vowels only (e.g., bib, baby, bubble, bow, bee). Care should be taken to avoid words with nasal consonants. Any mirror condensation is remarkable.

- If a person's repertoire does not yet include obstruent consonants, guide the examinee to say vowels imitatively. Mirror condensation is remarkable.
- Place the mirror under the person's nares during connected speech. Watch for bursts of condensation, which should occur during nasal consonant production only (/m/, /n/, and /ŋ/) and evaporate for all other sounds. This option may be the most desirable for children who do not reliably follow simple directions. Continuous, excessive, or untimely mirror condensation is remarkable.

Discretionary Clinical Observation 17: Observations for Dysarthria

Some existing oral-facial examinations focus on neurogenic-communication disorders, such as the dysarthrias and apraxia of speech. In developing the procedures for this section, several were consulted (Bunton, Kent, Duffy, Rosenbek, & Kent, 2007; Bunton, Kent, Kent, & Rosenbek, 2000; Duffy, 2011, 2013; Duffy & Kent, 2001; Edmiaston, Connor, Loehr, & Nassief, 2010; Fuller, Pimentel, & Peregoy, 2012; Hegde & Freed, 2013; Yorkston et al., 2010). Clinical experience with motor-speech disorders was also taken into account.

For clinicians who work regularly in the area of motor-speech disorders, procedures from a different resource (e.g., Duffy, 2013), can easily be substituted for those offered in this section. The procedures proposed herein, however, are likely to be useful to clinicians doing a generic oral-facial inspection.

When to Observe for Dysarthria

Dysarthria is described in Box 3–10. The routine observations provide ample opportunity to identify those likely to benefit from observations for dysarthria (i.e., Discretionary Clinical Observation 17). Refer to the corresponding decision box on the recording form to identify candidates for this procedure.

Box 3–10. Dysarthria Described

Dysarthria is a collective name for a family of motor-speech disorders resulting from damage to the central nervous system or peripheral nervous system. As a result, disturbed muscular execution interferes with the person's control of the speech mechanism for speech.

Several basic types of dysarthria are identified, and each can occur in isolation or in combination with one or more of the other types (i.e., mixed dysarthria). Dysarthria can also occur concomitant to apraxia of speech, aphasia, language of confusion, dementia, or any other neurogenic communication disorder.

It is noteworthy that dysarthria can result from a number of etiologies, including cerebrovascular accident; traumatic brain injury; various neurologically based diseases, many of which are progressive in nature; injury to the immature nervous system; or compromised development of any relevant part of the nervous system. However, although etiology is important, etiology does not generally determine the type of dysarthria that the person experiences. Instead, symptoms more closely correlate to site or sites of lesion.

Because the dysarthrias all present differently, differential diagnosis can be complicated and requires specific clinical and academic preparation. However, in general, any or all of the dysarthrias can result in abnormalities relative to strength, speed, range, steadiness, tone, or accuracy of muscle movements required for speech production. Furthermore, these abnormalities can affect all dimensions of speech production, including respiration, phonation, resonance, articulation, and prosody.

Clinical Questions Associated With Dysarthria Observations

Clinical Question 34 (see Table 0–3) asks, "When routine inspection reveals symptoms of dysarthria, does evidence confirm or rule out a diagnosis?"

If the answer supports a diagnosis of dysarthria, the finding is relevant. Because the term *dysarthria* is a collective name for a family of motor-speech disorders, identifying or ruling out dysarthria is only the beginning. Therefore, Clinical Question 35 is added to facilitate a more specific diagnosis relative to type: "If evidence supports diagnosis, does it provide enough data to reliably identify the type of dysarthria?" For experienced clinicians who practice in the area of motor-speech disorders, answering Clinical Question 35 is not difficult; however, less experienced clinicians may find this question more challenging, even when dysarthria occurs in the absence of comorbid symptoms.

Furthermore, for some, the evidence may not clearly support or rule out a diagnosis. When this happens, Clinical Question 36 should be asked: "If neither question yields an affirmative response, does evidence support referral for more in-depth testing?" An affirmative response suggests a need for referral.

The procedures that follow are useful for responding to the proposed questions. They may also facilitate identifying specific symptoms of dysarthria if it is diagnosed.

Clinical Intent of the Dysarthria Observations

The findings can be useful for suggesting or ruling out a diagnosis, and in some cases, they can give insight that may lead to identifying an exact type of dysarthria. They can also corroborate a recommendation or referral for more in-depth testing. For clinicians who have limited experience in this important area of clinical practice, the structured dysarthria observations in this manual are useful for providing structure that can facilitate data collection that may lead to clinical decisions or possibly referral for specialist consultation.

Equipment Needed for Dysarthria Observations

The dysarthria observations require no special equipment.

The Procedures

The dysarthria observation entails two parts. The first requires the examiner to carefully reflect on audible cues given during the conversational speech sample and other speech production activities completed during the routine inspection. The second requires evaluating the same parameters while the examinee reads aloud. The three passages shown in Box 3–11 are provided for convenience.

General Symptoms of Dysarthria. In general, dysarthria affects all aspects of speech production:

articulation, prosody, resonance, phonation, and respiration. Neuromuscular symptoms that characterize dysarthria include reduced range of motion, reduced strength, compromised rate and coordination of movement, poor muscle tone, and compromised ability to vary muscular tension. These symptoms can affect any structural part that participates in accomplishing any aspect of speech. Speech production features that characterize dysarthria appear in Table 3–2 for convenience.

Classifying Dysarthria by Type According to Speech Symptoms. Dysarthria is not a single motor-speech disorder but a family of disorders, all having a neurologic etiology. Again, for the sake of convenience, seven types of dysarthria are described according to speech symptoms in Table 3–3.

When Dysarthria Co-Occurs With Other Neurogenic Disorders of Speech, Language, or Cognition. When symptoms of dysarthria co-occur with other neurogenic symptoms, teasing out all variables that lead to a complete and accurate diagnosis is not necessarily within the scope of this manual and should be left to the discretion of those with expertise in neurogenic communication disorders.

Box 3–11. Selected Reading Passages

Three reading passages are provided to supplement observations for dysarthria (i.e., Discretionary Clinical Observation 17) and are considered useful for literate examinees. They are presented in alphabetical order, by title. Note that "My Grandfather" has a time-honored history of universal acceptance and in fact was the reading passage used when differentially describing each dysarthria according to symptom pattern (Darley, Aronson, & Brown, 1975).

To provide options, however, two additional passages with differing degrees of history and acceptance are also shown. Any of the three pas-

sages, if read aloud, is likely to reveal symptoms of dysarthria if present. When considering which passage to select, consider the examinee's reading level as well as potential for interest in the topics. Note that paragraph divisions have been added to all three passages to facilitate reading efficiency.

The Caterpillar

Do you like amusement parks? Well, I sure do. To amuse myself, I went twice last spring. My most *memorable* moment was riding on the Caterpillar, which is a gigantic rollercoaster high above the ground. When I saw how high the Caterpillar rose into the bright blue sky I knew it was for me.

After waiting in line for thirty minutes, I made it to the front where the man measured my height to see if I was tall enough. I gave the man my coins, asked for change, and jumped on the cart.

Tick, tick, tick, the Caterpillar climbed slowly up the tracks. It went SO high I could see the parking lot. Boy was I *scared*! I thought to myself, "There's no turning back now." People were so scared they screamed as we swiftly zoomed fast, fast, and faster along the tracks.

As quickly as it started, the Caterpillar came to a stop. Unfortunately, it was time to pack the car and drive home.

That night I dreamt of the wild ride on the Caterpillar. Taking a trip to the amusement park and riding on the Caterpillar was my *most* memorable moment ever! (Patel et al., 2013, p. 9)

My Grandfather

You wished to know all about my grandfather. Well, he is nearly 93 years old; yet he still thinks as swiftly as ever.

He dresses himself in an old black frock coat, usually minus several buttons. A long flowing beard clings to his chin, giving those who observe him a pronounced feeling of the utmost respect.

When he speaks, his voice is just a bit cracked and quivers a little. Twice each day he plays skillfully and with zest upon our small organ. Except in the winter when ooze or snow or ice prevents, he slowly takes a short walk in the open air each day.

We have often urged him to walk more and smoke less, but he always answers, "Banana oil!" Grandfather likes to be modern in his language. (Van Riper, 1963, p. 484)

The Rainbow Passage

When the sunlight strikes raindrops in the air, they act as a prism and form a rainbow. The rainbow is a division of white light into many beautiful colors. These take the shape of a long round arch, with its path high above, and its two ends apparently beyond the horizon.

There is, according to legend, a boiling pot of gold at one end. People look, but no one ever finds it. When a man looks for something beyond his reach, his friends say he is looking for the pot of gold at the end of the rainbow.

Throughout the centuries people have explained the rainbow in various ways. Some have accepted it as a miracle without physical explanation. To the Hebrews it was a token that there would be no more universal floods. The Greeks used to imagine that it was a sign from the gods to foretell war or heavy rain. The Norsemen considered the rainbow as a bridge over which the gods passed from earth to their home in the sky.

Others have tried to explain the phenomenon physically. Aristotle thought that the rainbow was caused by reflection of the sun's rays by the rain. Since then physicists have found that it is not reflection, but refraction by the raindrops which causes the rainbows.

Many complicated ideas about the rainbow have been formed. The difference in the rainbow depends considerably upon the size of the drops, and the width of the colored band increases as the size of the drops increases.

The actual primary rainbow observed is said to be the effect of super-imposition of a number of bows. If the red of the second bow falls upon the green of the first, the result is to give a bow with an abnormally wide yellow band, since red and green light when mixed form yellow. This is a very common type of bow, one showing mainly red and yellow, with little or no green or blue. (The Rainbow Passage is a public domain text.)

Table 3–2. General Symptoms of Dysarthria[a]

Symptom Category	Specific Speech Manifestations That May Result From Dysarthria	Neuromuscular Defect That May Explain
Articulatory inaccuracy	<ul><li>Imprecise consonants</li><li>Irregular articulatory breakdown</li><li>Distorted vowels</li></ul>	Breakdown in coordinating activities required for articulation
Prosodic excess	<ul><li>Slow speech rate</li><li>Excess and equal stress</li><li>Prolonged phonemes</li><li>Prolonged intervals</li><li>Inappropriate silences</li></ul>	Slowness in executing repetitive movements
Prosodic insufficiency	<ul><li>Monopitch</li><li>Monoloudness</li><li>Reduced syllable and word stress</li><li>Short phrasing</li></ul>	Restricted range of movement
Articulatory-resonatory incompetence	<ul><li>Imprecise consonants</li><li>Distorted vowels</li><li>Hypernasality</li></ul>	Impaired force of muscle contraction, combined with reduced range of movement
Phonatory stenosis	<ul><li>Low vocal pitch</li><li>Harsh voice</li><li>Strained-strangled voice quality</li><li>Pitch breaks</li><li>Interruptions in voice flow</li><li>Excessive loudness variation</li><li>Slow speech rate</li><li>Short phrasing, possibly compensatory</li></ul>	Physiologic narrowing of the laryngeal passage
Phonatory incompetence	<ul><li>Breathy voice</li><li>Audible inspiration</li><li>Short phrasing</li></ul>	Reduction in force of muscular contraction
Resonatory incompetence	<ul><li>Hypernasal resonance</li><li>Nasal-airflow emissions</li><li>Imprecise consonant production</li><li>Short phrasing</li></ul>	Reduction in force of muscular contractions, combined with failure to close the velopharyngeal valve
Phonatory-prosodic insufficiency	<ul><li>Monopitch</li><li>Monoloudness</li><li>Harsh voice quality</li></ul>	Hypotonia

[a]Table is not intended to substitute for clinical experience with motor-speech disorders.

Table 3–3. Seven Dysarthrias Classified by Speech Symptoms[b]

Type of Dysarthria	Type of Symptom	Audible Speech Symptoms
Spastic dysarthria (associated with pseudobulbar palsy)	Articulation	• Imprecise articulation, especially as complexity increases
	Resonance	• Hypernasal resonance, usually in the absence of audible nasal-airflow emissions
	Voice (i.e., phonation)	• Low and monotonous vocal pitch • Harsh voice quality, can include strained-strangled quality
	Prosody	• Monotone
Flaccid dysarthria (associated with bulbar palsy)	Articulation	• Imprecise articulation, due to failure to achieve intraoral pressure secondary to velopharyngeal incompetence • Imprecise articulation, due to consonant and vowel distortions secondary to tongue and lip immobility
	Resonance[a]	• Hypernasality, with nasal-airflow emissions during speech
	Prosody	• Short phrasing (may be due to air wastage)
	Respiration	• Audible inspiration • Breathy exhalation
Mixed spastic and flaccid dysarthria (associated with amyotrophic lateral sclerosis)	Articulation	• Impaired articulation
	Resonance	• Hypernasal resonance with nasal airflow emissions
	Voice (i.e., phonation)	• Low vocal pitch • Hoarse quality • Strained-strangled quality
	Prosody	• Slow speech rate • Short, highly distorted phrases
	Overall impression	• Tremendous effort to rise above overpowering muscle weakness
Ataxic dysarthria (associated with cerebellar disorders): Pattern 1	Articulation	• Intermittent articulatory breakdown
	Prosody	• Dysrhythmia
	Voice (i.e., phonation)	• Irregularities in pitch and loudness
	Overall	• Symptoms are especially noticeable on verbal diadochokinetic activities

Table 3–3. *continued*

Type of Dysarthria	Type of Symptom	Audible Speech Symptoms

Ataxic dysarthria (associated with cerebellar disorders): Pattern 2	Prosody	• Altered prosody, characterized by
		  ○ Sound prolongations
		  ○ Equal syllable stress
		  ○ Prolongation of intervals between syllables and words
		  ○ Artificially uneven speech with a seemingly measured pace

Hypokinetic dysarthria (associated with Parkinson disease)	Articulation	• Imprecise articulation, due to incomplete muscle excursion • Difficulty initiating articulation
	Voice (i.e., phonation)	• Breathy voice • Reduced loudness, sometimes inaudible voice
	Prosody	• Reduced vocal emphasis • Peaks and valleys of pitch • Variations of loudness that flatten out monotonously • Short rushes of speech, with illogically placed pauses and variable rate, even accelerated rate • Inappropriate silences • Repetition of initial sounds
Hyperkinetic dysarthria (associated with dystonia)	Articulation	• Unpredictable articulatory breakdown, secondary to involuntary movement • Unpredictable vowel distortions, secondary to involuntary movements
	Voice (i.e., phonation)	• Unpredictable interruptions in vocal flow, secondary to involuntary movements • Unpredictable and excessive variations in loudness, secondary to involuntary movements • Reduced variation in pitch and loudness, perhaps in anticipation of involuntary movements
	Prosody	• Slowed speech rate, perhaps in anticipation of involuntary movements • Prolonged interword intervals, perhaps in anticipation of involuntary movements • Inappropriately placed silences, perhaps in anticipation of involuntary movements

continues

Table 3–3. *continued*

Type of Dysarthria	Type of Symptom	Audible Speech Symptoms
Hyperkinetic dysarthria (associated with choreoathetosis)	Articulation	• Sudden articulatory breakdown
	Voice (i.e., phonation)	• Sudden bursts of loudness • Sudden elevations of pitch • Increased overall loudness
	Prosody	• Rate variations, possibly to manage anticipation of breakdowns; these may include prolonged pauses and equal stress on all syllables and words
	Respiration	• Involuntary movements alter the normal breathing cycle, resulting in sudden gusts of exhaled breath and contributing to the above symptoms

[a]The prominent symptom.
[b]Table is not intended to substitute for clinical experience with motor-speech disorders.

Discretionary Clinical Observation 18: Speech Sound Stimulability Screening

Speech sound stimulability screening is frequently completed routinely as a part of a comprehensive communication evaluation and does not need to be repeated if it has already been done. Because the results can interface with oral-facial evaluation findings, instructions for speech sound stimulability screening are included as a discretionary procedure.

Speech sound stimulability screening has been described in a variety of clinical and academic resources (Bankson et al., 2009; Bauman-Waengler, 2011; Goldman & Fristoe, 2000; Gordon-Brannan & Weiss, 2007; Hegde & Pomaville, 2013). These resources were consulted and information was integrated with professional experience when developing this manual's protocol for stimulability screening.

When to Apply Speech Sound Stimulability Screening

Speech sound stimulability screening is often an appropriate objective when the assessment has identified an atypical speaking pattern for which the person does not presently compensate. If formal stimulability testing was not done prior to the oral-facial inspection, the screening provided herein may be useful when ascertaining whether clinical teaching can result in strategies to adequately compensate for a structural or physiologic anomaly or even facilitate when no organic etiology seems apparent. Use the corresponding decision box on the recording form to determine whether the stimulability screening is appropriate for the individual examinee.

Clinical Question Associated With Speech Sound Stimulability Screening

Clinical Question 37 (see Table 0–3) asks, "For individuals with atypical speech sound production, when clinical teaching opportunities are presented, does the examinee respond by improving or changing the speaking pattern?" An answer of *yes* indicates that the person demonstrates stimulability for the speech sounds probed.

Equipment Needed for Speech Sound Stimulability Screening

The only necessary equipment is a full-face-view mirror that should be present in any diagnostic or therapy room. If one is not in the room, make arrangements to supply one.

Procedures for Speech Sound Stimulability Screening

- Identify consonant sounds that the examinee produces in error. If there are many error consonants, select four to six possible therapy targets. Plan to explore stimulability for each selected phoneme, one at a time.
- Refer to Table 3–4, which contains a list of CV syllables that correspond to standard consonant phonemes of American English. Write the phonemes that you plan to probe in the appropriate place on the recording form.
- Seat yourself and examinee in the vicinity of a mirror that is large enough for full-face viewing.
- Facing the examinee, instruct as follows:
  - I will say a syllable aloud.
  - I will look directly at you while I say the syllable.
  - Look directly at me, and listen carefully. You will be asked to say the syllable in exactly the same way as I say it. I may say the syllable in a way that is different from the way that you usually do, so watch and listen carefully. Try to say it exactly the way that I do.
  - After you say the syllable, sometimes I may suggest a way to change what you do in order to say it like I do.
  - When we are through with one syllable, we will do exactly the same with another until we finish.
  - Are you ready?
- Then, facing the examinee, present the first syllable. Make sure your articulatory movements are clear but not overly exaggerated.
- Ask the examinee to turn and face the mirror, then imitate the word or syllable exactly.
- If the examinee reproduces the target exactly, then consider the target phoneme *stimulable with imitation*.
- If the examinee does not approximate the target, you may find that by careful

Table 3–4. Probes for Speech-Sound Stimulability Screening

Consonant Target	Syllable Probe
/p/	/pʌ/
/b/	/bʌ/
/m/	/mʌ/
/w/	/wʌ/
/f/	/fʌ/
/v/	/vʌ/
/θ/	/θʌ/
/ð/	/ðʌ/
/t/	/tʌ/
/d/	/dʌ/
/s/	/sʌ/
/z/	/zʌ/
/l/	/lʌ/
/n/	/nʌ/
/ʃ/	/ʃʌ/
/tʃ/	/tʃʌ/
/dʒ/	/dʒʌ/
/ɾ/	/ɾʌ/
/j/	/jʌ/
/k/	/kʌ/
/g/	/gʌ/

listening and clinical intuition, you are able to identify an articulatory placement adjustment that could improve the way the person says the consonant. Give the examinee that instruction and suggest trying again while facing the mirror (e.g., If a person has an interdental lisp and continues to protrude the tongue between the teeth, it may be helpful to ask the examinee to see what happens if the tongue stays behind the teeth, and say it again.). If the examinee makes the suggested adjustments with this type of verbal prompting, consider the target sound *stimulable with imitation and instruction.*

- If the examinee does not amend the target for either of the stimulability activities, then consider the target *not readily stimulable.*

Experienced clinicians may check stimulability for other parameters of speech production, such as voice and resonance, and this exercise is likely to yield information that is clinically useful overall. However, the procedures may be more organic than those described in this section, extending beyond the scope of the manual.

Discretionary Clinical Observation 19: Screening for Laryngeal and Respiratory Efficiency (i.e., S:Z Ratio)

When defining the procedures and scope of this particular screening, a number of resources were consulted and integrated with clinical experience. These include Eckels and Boone (1981), Gelfer and Pazera (2006), Prater and Swift (1984), Shipley and McAfee (2008), and van der Meer, Ferreira, and Loock (2010).

Clinical Question Associated With Screening for Laryngeal and Respiratory Efficiency

Clinical Question 38 (see Table 0–3) asks, "For examinees who exhibit symptoms of laryngeal or respiratory inefficiency, does the S:Z ratio provide additional information that strengthens a medical referral for more in-depth testing?" An answer of *yes* is clinically significant.

When to Screen for Laryngeal and Respiratory Efficiency

Routine procedures described in Chapter 2 provide sufficient opportunity to detect laryngeal and respiratory inefficiency in speech and nonspeech activi-

ties; therefore, a medical referral for either vocal or respiratory inefficiency can be made without calculating the S:Z ratio.

In the case of medical referral for more in-depth vocal or respiratory evaluation, this particular screening may be considered, although it is not required. You are strongly encouraged to use professional judgment in making the decision about whether S:Z ratio data are likely to add meaningful information to routine findings. Additional notes about using the S:Z ratio as a clinical tool appear in Box 3–12.

Box 3–12. Note on S:Z Ratio

The S:Z ratio has been used to distinguish between individuals with and without laryngeal pathology (Prater & Swift, 1984; Shipley & McAfee, 2008; van der Meer et al., 2010). More specifically, van der Meer et al. (2010) describe the S:Z ratio as a "simple, reliable, time-efficient test" (p. 492) with "excellent potential as a screening tool" (p. 492) because it "requires minimal clinical training" (p. 490) and yields a "reliable and simple measure of laryngeal dysfunction that can be easily used by clinicians."

Yet, we cannot ignore that some experts disagree (Gelfer & Pazera, 2006), reporting sufficient overlap when comparing ratios for those with and those without vocal pathology, and that difference between the groups may become even more confusing when data collection fails to control for such variables as vocal intensity, respiratory effort, vocal effort, and laryngeal or airway resistance.

With this in mind, we issue a strong caveat for extreme caution when collecting and applying S:Z ratio data. And we further acknowledge that the S:Z ratio is never intended to substitute for a medical referral when audible vocal or respiratory symptoms present themselves.

Equipment Needed When Screening for Laryngeal and Respiratory Efficiency

- Stopwatch
- Recording device

Procedures for Gathering Laryngeal and Respiratory Efficiency Data

This screening requires that the examinee sustain the /s/ and /z/ consonants each for as long as possible on a single breath, and for three trials, while the examiner records the sustained speech sounds, timing their duration. Elicit the phonemes as follows.

- Instruct the person to sustain /s/ for as long as possible, maintaining a constant intensity, respiratory effort, vocal effort, and airflow resistance. Modeling is recommended. Repeat for three trials. Record the vocalizations, making it possible to recheck duration later. The longest measurement of the three is the one to use.
- Repeat the same procedure for the consonant /z/.

Making S:Z Ratio Calculations

Use the longest measured /s/ duration as the numerator, and use the longest measured /z/ duration as the denominator. Divide. For example:

- Suppose the durations of /s/ and /z/ are the same number—for instance, 20 seconds; then the ratio is 20:20, also expressed 20/20 or 20 ÷ 20. When you divide 20 by 20, the result is an S:Z ratio of 1.0. Traditionally, a ratio of 1.0 is considered the norm.
- When the /s/ and /z/ durations are different numbers, the calculation procedures are still the same, but arriving at the outcome may be somewhat more complicated, and a calculator may be helpful. For example:
  - An /s/ duration of 20 seconds and /z/ duration of 25 seconds is 20:25, also expressed as 20/25 or 20 ÷ 25. When you divide, the result is an S:Z ratio of 0.8.

  - Similarly, if the /s/ duration is 25 seconds and the /z/ duration is 20, the ratio is 25:20, which may be expressed as 25/20 or 25 ÷ 20. The resulting numerical expression for the S:Z ratio in this case is 1.25.

See Chapter 5 for information on how to interpret S:Z ratio results.

Discretionary Clinical Observation 20: Gag Reflex Stimulation

Methods for stimulating gag reflex vary. In deciding on the exact procedures to recommend, expert opinions were consulted (Bankson et al., 2009; Duffy, 2013; Miller, 2002; Ramsay, Smithard, Donaldson, & Kalra, 2005; Terré & Mearin, 2006), and clinical experience was also taken into consideration.

Clinical Question Associated With Stimulating Gag Reflex

Clinical Question 39 (see Table 0–3) asks, "For individuals who will be referred for neurologic or genetic evaluation, does response to gag reflex stimulation provide additional information to corroborate the referral?" If the answer is *yes*, the finding is potentially remarkable. The procedures that follow are useful for evaluating whether gag reflex is elicited *and* for distinguishing types of atypical gag reflexes if they occur.

When to Perform Gag Reflex Stimulation

It is not necessary or even advisable to stimulate the gag reflex for every examinee. Many individuals exhibit hyperactive, asymmetrical, or absent gag reflexes with no impact on speech production and no indication of physical or neurologic pathology; therefore, stimulating gag reflex on most people has no clinical purpose.

However, whenever the velum or pharynx exhibits signs of paresis or compromised innervation, the procedure may augment the data collected during routine inspection and thereby supplement a neurologic or genetic referral. Consider screening for gag reflex if noting any symptom listed in the corresponding decision box of the recording form.

The gag reflex procedure is considered mildly invasive. Therefore, so as not to disrupt rapport, doing it last is strongly recommended. Notes appear in Box 3–13.

Equipment Need for Stimulating Gag Reflex

- Examination gloves
- Extra-long cotton-tipped swab, individually wrapped

Procedures for Stimulating the Gag Reflex

- Remove the wrapping from the cotton-tipped swab. An extra-long cotton-tipped swab is preferred to a tongue depressor because it is a gentler implement. Furthermore, being narrow, the swab can accomplish the job efficiently, and many examinees are familiar with the cotton-swab probe due to its similarity to procedures used in medical offices when testing for strep.
- Ask the examinee, "Do you gag easily?"
  - If more specificity is needed, you may assist with questions such as, "Do you gag when brushing your teeth?" or "When the dentist examines your teeth?"
  - If the examinee acknowledges not knowing the term *gag*, describe it as an unpleasant feeling in the throat that makes a noise; then demonstrate or approximate the noise.
  - If someone claims to have a hyperactive gag reflex, being prepared is always helpful.
- If you believe that stimulating the gag reflex is important but the examinee refuses or reports a hyperactive gag reflex, do not force the issue. Then document that gag reflex stimulation was offered and refused, along with the person's reason for refusing the procedure (e.g., hyperactive reflex, fear of vomiting).
- Instruct the willing examinee to open the mouth.
- Before entering the mouth with the cotton swab, visually locate the pharyngeal wall and velum.
- Quickly and lightly touch the base of the tongue or posterior pharyngeal wall with the tip of the swab. A normal gag reflex manifests as a strong, symmetrical contraction involving the entire pharyngeal wall and velum, and it occurs simultaneous to the swab's contact with the base of the tongue or posterior pharyngeal wall.
- Stop immediately upon eliciting the reflex. If no reflex occurs upon contact, stop immediately; do not repeatedly attempt to elicit the response.
- Any response other than a timely and typical contraction as described above is remarkable. Some possible atypical responses may include the following:
  - Absent gag reflex: no response
  - Hypoactive gag reflex: weak response
  - Hyperactive gag reflex: forceful response, which also may be premature
  - Premature gag reflex: response prior to contact
  - Delayed or latent gag reflex: delay between contacting the pharyngeal wall and reflex

---

Box 3–13. Note on Gag Reflex Procedure

Stimulating the gag reflex has the potential to be mildly invasive. For that reason, if you deem that gag reflex stimulation is necessary, save it for last to avoid any potential for confounding the clinical rapport needed to obtain meaningful findings in other areas.

Rarely, in extreme cases, a hyperactive gag reflex may be so intense that it induces retching or even vomiting. Individuals with potential for a severe response typically self-identify and refuse the procedure. However, be prepared to handle the unexpected gracefully and calmly before you begin.

Discretionary Clinical Observation 21: Prompt for Dysphagia Screening

Resources consulted for this section include Donovan et al. (2013), Eadie (2007), Edmiaston et al. (2010), Fucile et al. (1998), Leder, Suiter, Murray, and Rademaker (2013), Mann (2002), Martino et al. (2009), McCullough et al. (2005), Terré and Mearin (2006), and Trapl et al. (2007).

Clinical Questions Associated With Prompt for Dysphagia Screening

Clinical Question 40 (see Table 0–3) asks, "Does evidence support the need for dysphagia screening in aging adults?" An answer of *yes* leads to the immediate termination of an oral diet to be followed directly by scheduling a dysphagia screening.

Equipment Needed to Perform the Prompt

No equipment is needed to identify individuals who are at risk for dysphagia.

Purpose and Procedures Associated With the Prompt for Dysphagia Screening

The purpose of the prompt is to identify individuals who, although not mandated for dysphagia screening, present symptoms that indicate a high risk. That is, law requires dysphagia screening for all patients with suspected cerebrovascular accident; furthermore, persons with recent laryngectomy are also at risk for dysphagia. For these two groups, dysphagia screening should be completed regardless of symptoms, as soon as the person is alert and healthy enough to participate and before resuming an oral diet. Because these individuals are screened regardless of symptoms, the prompt for dysphagia screening does not apply to them.

However, all other aging adults should participate in the prompt. In fact, although the observation is called *discretionary*, this is because it does not

routinely apply to all examinees. Yet when evaluating older adults, consider the dysphagia screening prompt to be a routine inspection procedure. For that reason, it appears with routine clinical observations on the recording forms for all three categories that address the examination needs of older adults.

The procedure associated with the prompt is simply to observe for symptoms during conversation for all examinees, regardless of age. The symptoms are listed in the appropriate decision box on the recording form.

Follow-Up to Dysphagia Screening Prompt

If the prompt identifies a person who is as at risk for dysphagia, discontinue an oral diet and immediately make arrangements for the screening to be completed by a person who is either fully trained or under the direct supervision of a person who is. Regulations require that the health care provider administering the screening is fully trained and competent to complete it, although not necessarily a dysphagia expert.

Dysphagia Screening Tools. A number of dysphagia screenings are available. Practitioners are apt to prefer a particular tool. Furthermore, no one screening has been identified as best for all patients. Therefore, we defer selection of the screening tool to the professional who uses it.

When any screening indicates a need for dysphagia testing, instrumentation is required. Diagnosing and treating dysphagia is reserved for those whose academic and clinical education prepared them specifically for that area of practice.

Concluding the Oral-Facial Inspection

Refer to the Chapter 2 conclusion for information on how to end the oral-facial inspection.

4

Suggested Adaptations for Examinees With Special Needs

The vast majority of candidates for oral-facial inspection present with a special need in some area; otherwise, no one would have referred them for communication evaluation. Yet most people with a communication disorder are able to participate in a meaningful oral-facial inspection using the procedures described in the previous chapters. Even so, some physical, cognitive, and age-related challenges are capable of confounding a clinician's ability to derive meaningful results when using the routine and discretionary procedures alone. For that reason, the present chapter suggests adaptations that are intended to facilitate evidence gathering for a select group of special-needs populations.

The Overarching Clinical Questions for Special Populations

Bear in mind that although some procedural changes are suggested herein, the overarching clinical questions that have been applied throughout (see Table 0–2) remain unchanged. Furthermore, the process shown in Figure 2–1 also applies to individuals whose needs are addressed under the topic of special needs.

Three Types of Adaptations

The adaptations offered for special populations generally fit into one of three categories. They are modifications, accommodations, and considerations.

The term *modification* refers to changes in either content or minimal expectation and may include deleting or adding a procedure or allowing for a lesser response due to disability or age. On the other hand, *accommodations* are slight procedural changes that can simply facilitate the inspection and may include minor adjustments, such as preferential seating or use of manual language for communication. The difference between modification and accommodation is that for modifications, content or expectations change, whereas for accommodations, content and expectations remain the same.

The third type of adjustment, *considerations*, for all intents and purposes refers to ways that clinicians may extend appropriate sensitivity to examinees with special needs to facilitate a more effective or courteous experience overall, without changing the protocol in any way. Considerations tend to include minor enhancements, such as use of props and pretend play when working with young children or gestures of respect shown to older adults.

General Comments on Procedural Changes

For the purpose of simplicity, the terms *adaptation*, *adjustment*, or *change* may be used interchangeably when generally referring to adjustments described in this chapter. In the interest of clarity, however, whenever the specific terms *modification*, *accommodation*, and *consideration* appear in the text, the above-noted definitions apply.

Special Recording Forms

Since adaptations for some special groups entail augmenting, truncating, or deleting certain portions of the general protocol, special recording forms are available to assist with data collection. Refer to Appendix A for a full array of available recording forms.

Suggested Protocol Changes for Very Young Examinees: Birth-to-5 Years

The birth-to-5 age group comprises a widely heterogeneous population that requires adjustments to procedure, content, and expectation, even under normal developmental circumstances. Furthermore, many young children who receive services exhibit symptoms of or are at risk for developmental delay or physical anomaly that can influence their developmental progress, increasing the heterogeneity of the group.

Normally, birth-to-5 children progress quickly from neonates who are preverbal and do not follow instructions to toddlers who may be quite verbal and follow simple commands well. Furthermore, with the passage of time, infants and toddlers become preschoolers who engage socially and are in the process of gaining skills that directly prepare them for literacy and academic work.

In most cases, when examining the oral-facial region for very young children, obligatory adjustments correlate to age and responsiveness. For convenience, the manual addresses the needs of three age groups separately: infants, toddlers, and preschoolers, yet the boundaries between the groups are not always readily discernible. In fact, for many young children who require communication evaluation, normal development has been interrupted; consequently, many young examinees persist in displaying all or some of the characteristics of a chronologically younger age group. For this reason, the age-limit boundaries frequently have limited value and are rightfully trumped by behavioral-descriptive boundaries. However, approximate age ranges can be useful, so they are provided along with descriptive information.

Infants: Preverbal Children

For the purpose of the inspection, let us loosely define infants as preverbal children or, more specifically, children who *have not yet begun* to use words for communication. Similarly, as a rule, this group is preambulatory and has limited capacity to understand spoken language. Invariably, the preverbal phase begins at birth, and for normally developing children, it ends within the vicinity of the child's first birthday.

To complicate matters, many young children who receive services are unlike normally developing children in the way they progress through infancy and early development. That is, for some, the preverbal phase extends well beyond the first birthday, and often there is a temporal gap between the emergence of first words, reliable language comprehension, and achieving gross and fine-motor milestones.

The standard oral-facial inspection relies heavily on the examinee's ability to understand and respond to verbal instructions, execute oral movements, and engage in nonspeech and speech activities. This renders the routine and discretionary clinical observations somewhat limited in usefulness for an infant population when considered in an unmodified form.

The infant-focused adjustments offered in this chapter are appropriate for nearly all children before their first birthday. The exact upper age limit boundary for which these changes should be applied for special-needs children is a matter of professional judgment, depending on developmental progress. When it is time to execute the inspection, a competent clinician ordinarily has adequate information on which to base a decision concerning whether a child older than 12 months would benefit from infant-like adjustments.

Toddlers: Children With Limited Language

Let us define toddlers as children who have limited expressive language skills that include first words, holophrastic sentences, words supplemented by gestural communication, and simple sentences. As a general rule, this group of children has begun to walk using a characteristic gait, aptly described as *toddling*. And most toddlers comprehend simple, concrete language and can follow one- to two-step commands.

The phase generally begins with the emergence for first true words and ends when complex sentence structures begin. For normally developing children, toddlers are 1- and 2-year-olds, with the phase ending in the neighborhood of the third birthday.

As with infants, children with communication disorders are at risk for both late onset of toddlerhood and persisting toddler-like behaviors beyond the 36th month of life. Consequently, toddler-like adjustments may be needed for children older than 36 months, and the decision is based on the child's performance mingled with professional judgment.

Preschoolers

As a rule, normally developing preschoolers are engaging conversationalists, and many can follow multistep directions. They are able to climb, jump, run, draw, count, name shapes and colors, recite the alphabet and poems, sing songs, manipulate objects, and perform many other social and preacademic activities.

Preschoolers are generally playful and respond best if the oral-facial inspection is carried out as if it were a game. Furthermore, they have preferences with regard to the types of play they enjoy, and it is often expedient to consult with parents about toys or activities they are inclined to choose before the day of the evaluation arrives.

By law, children with special needs transition to preschool when they graduate from early intervention (i.e., between the ages of 33 and 36 months), and the classification stands until the child enters kindergarten and becomes a school-age child (i.e., sometime between the fourth and sixth birthday, depending on district rules and month of birth). However, children with special needs who are within the age boundaries for preschool may function at a much lower level. Flexibility in determining which types of adjustments to make is important to a successful clinical experience.

Whether the examinee requires the adjustments noted for preschool-age children is again a judgment call based on child-centered evidence and clinical experience. The evaluating clinician should have adequate information to make the decision before beginning the oral-facial inspection. Furthermore, some special-needs children even older than 5 years may benefit from the suggestions in this section as well.

General Suggestions for Birth-to-5

When working with the very young, creatively use whatever method works to accomplish the goal for each procedure. This may include using washable puppets, toys, stickers, games, reward systems, flavored tongue depressors, or opportunities for competition whenever it may facilitate understanding or maintain participation. Creativity can also include using a spontaneous crying episode as an opportunity to check for unprompted velar movement during nonspeech activity, inspect the size and condition of the oral chamber, or even gain cursory information on palatal integrity.

Also, appropriate parental involvement is encouraged whenever possible. But parents should receive clear instructions as to their role since some activities they do instinctively in a well-meaning attempt to help could in reality interfere with obtaining accurate results. For example, a parent may draw out a response through imitation, repetition, or prompting before the clinician is ready to forsake the idea of eliciting a spontaneous act.

In addition, many small children usually work best when casually seated on the floor, in a child-sized chair, Rifton chair, or seat designed to accommodate infants but generally not when seated at an adult-sized table in a traditional chair. Furthermore, examiners working with small children should consider abandoning the orderly sequence presented in this manual, instead seizing opportunities as they present themselves. This flexible approach requires a keen understanding of both the oral-facial inspection purposes and processes so that procedures may be applied spontaneously, even while adapting them to suit the client's needs.

Also, we recommend a playful approach to oral-facial inspection for this group. Use props, friendly competition, and informal games. Some examples are found in this chapter and also on the demonstration video.

Specific Adjustments for Routine Clinical Observations When Evaluating Young Children

For the birth-to-5 group, the adaptations lend themselves to being addressed in a step-by-step format. For some procedures, a set of common ideas seems to suffice across all three stages. For others, the suggestions distinctly differ according to the needs of children at the various stages of development. Resources consulted in adapting the procedures for infants and young children include Frankenburg (2002); Frankenburg, Dodds, and Archer (1990); Frankenburg, Dodds, Archer, Shapiro, and Bresnik (1992); and Guddemi and Case (2004).

Preparing the Work Area for Birth-to-5 Children

Due to the natural curiosity that nearly all young children bring to the process, the entire set of equipment and supplies should be handy for examiner access but completely outside the child's reach and preferably outside the child's visual field. Instead of laying supplies on the table as shown in Figure 1–1, consider sanitizing a plastic box (i.e., about the size of a small shoebox or large pencil box) along with the equipment; then retrieve supplies from it as needed. Otherwise, with regard to equipment, supplies, and preparations, follow the instructions shown in Chapter 1 and Appendix B.

Instructing the Examinee or Guardian for Birth-to-5 Children

As soon as a child is alert enough to engage socially, address the child directly for all social and instructional interaction. Use simple language and an engaging tone, without ignoring guardians who are present, and recognize that they benefit from direct communication as well.

On the whole, when working with younger infants, some of the explanations are given for the benefit of the adult guardian, not the baby. Yet an infant's response to direct social engagement may provide insight relative to the child's needs and may even elicit oral-motor behaviors that are of interest.

Furthermore, young children understand varying degrees of what adults do and say, so use very simple, concrete, and reassuring language, and focus comments in the direction of the child whenever possible. Also, routinely address older toddlers and preschoolers directly, using developmentally appropriate language.

Never ignore guardians and significant others who may be present. Moreover, provide a reasonable amount of additional information for any family member who requests it, even if that family member is a child (e.g., the examinee or a sibling).

Routine Clinical Observation 1: Conversational Speech Sample

By way of review, the overall purpose of any conversational speech sample is to perceptually judge whether intelligibility, resonance, voice, speech sounds, syntax, fluency, and pragmatics are appropriate for the examinee's age and gender. With regard to oral-facial inspection, only intelligibility, resonance, voice, and speech sounds are of concern (see Box 2–1).

Furthermore, when working with preverbal children and children with limited language, one may question the use of the term *conversation*, replacing it with terminology that recognizes the child's verbal output as more accurately resembling *vocal play*, and the term *comprehensibility* may rightfully replace the term *intelligibility* since intelligible speech is not a fixed expectation for this group. Nonetheless, the goal of the social interchange described in Routine Clinical Observation 1 is to elicit either conversation or spontaneous interactive vocal play and to make judgments with regard to the age appropriateness of the child's comprehensibility or intelligibility, volubility, voice, resonance, and speech sound production.

Since judgments that result are based on perception, not instrumentation, general familiarity with children in the birth-to-5 population is essential for competently eliciting the sample while at the same time making meaningful judgments about the child's speech development.

Although syntax, fluency, and pragmatics should be carefully observed during a conversational speech sample from an overall diagnostic perspective, their relevance to the oral-facial findings are minimal. Thus, they are not addressed specifically in this section, and examiners are encouraged to consult other published standards to evaluate.

Collecting Vocal Play Sample for Preverbal Children. Most preverbal children vocalize during social engagement and play, spontaneous nonsocial play, or even during crying and fussing. If at all possible, use these opportunities to make relevant judgments about volubility, resonance, voice, speech sound repertoire (i.e., phonemic, phonetic, and phonological inventories), and flow.

Collect the Conversational Speech Sample for Toddlers and Preschoolers. Frequently, children with limited language and verbal preschoolers receive a formal language sample as part of the diagnostic process. If a formal sample was collected, it replaces the conversational speech sample, provided it was preserved in such a way that the judgments mentioned in Chapter 2 can be drawn from it. If a formal language sample was not collected or was not adequately preserved, the obligatory judgments can be made in the context of simple and brief age-appropriate social engagement during informal play.

Evidence the Conversational Speech Sample Yields. The conversational speech sample provides a venue for systematically judging comprehensibility or intelligibility, resonance, voice, phonology, and prosody, all of which should be considered when interpreting oral-facial inspection results. In addition, other areas such as language and fluency can be judged using a connected speech sample, but since these judgments do not typically affect oral-facial region inspection, they are not discussed in this section.

Intelligibility has no direct relevance to preverbal children. However, many preverbal children communicate comprehensively without words, and others do not. Therefore, although making a *comprehensibility* judgment may not directly affect the oral-facial inspection, the rating is exceedingly relevant when judging the child's performance as a communicator. Principles for rating intelligibility (see Table 2–1) can be applied when rating comprehensibility, even for preverbal children.

Regarding verbal children and children with limited language, the intelligibility rating is more obviously significant to the oral-facial evaluation objectives. Refer to Table 4–1 for normative data on intelligibility for children in these groups.

Any evidence of atypical *resonance* is noteworthy for young children (Box 4–1). Experience with normally developing children of similar age is the best way to acquire an internal-auditory comparison model in preparing to judge whether a young child's resonance is within the normal range.

Voice, as with older children and adults, should be clear. Note any evidence of harshness, hoarseness, breathiness, weakness, tension, tremor, deterioration with use, inappropriate pitch, or other vocal difference. Similarly, it is experience with normal and atypical birth-to-5 voices that prepares one to make the kinds of judgments that are needed.

Table 4–1. Intelligibility Estimates for Young Children by Age

Age in Months	Estimated Intelligibility Perceptions for Familiar Communication Partners (e.g., Family), %	Estimated Intelligibility Perceptions for Communication Partners Who Are New to the Child, %
24–30	85–90	25–50
30–36	Nearly 100	50–70
36–42	100	75–90
42–48	100	100

Box 4–1. Resonance Development

Due to the high position of the newborn's larynx, as well as the disproportionately large size of the tongue in relation to the oral cavity, resonance during infancy is uniquely recognizable by its distinctly nasal focus. As the child's vocal mechanism matures, the larynx drops, lengthening the pharyngeal chamber. This and other anatomic changes allow for the size of the oral cavity to more adequately accommodate the tongue as well as oral resonance, while also permitting room for velopharyngeal closure.

The larynx begins to descend about halfway through the first year of life and arrives at its childhood elevation, usually by the third birthday (Thom, Holt, Hixon, & Smith, 2006). As a result of these anatomic developments, the child's resonance gradually changes over time with a decrease in nasal resonance and corresponding increase in oral and pharyngeal resonance.

Evaluating speech sounds for preverbal children requires knowledge of *preverbal phonological development*. Table 4–2 provides general information in this area. Note that by the end of the first year, although speech is far from complex or even comprehensible, in the context of jargon, normally developing children demonstrate the ability to produce the full repertoire of speech sounds for their native language, using prosodic patterns and syllable structures that also reflect knowledge of the language they have been hearing since birth. At this point, however, few sounds are available for meaningful linguistic contexts.

Once children begin using true words and short utterances, consonants for early words should be consistent with the age-of-mastery information provided in Table 4–3. Furthermore, phonological development should be consistent with Table 4–4.

Prosody essentially develops in the first year of life, such that by the time first words emerge, the child's jargon-like utterances strongly resemble the adult model with regard to inflection and flow. Stages of babbling suggest an organized development of speech prosody; thus, the basic stages of babbling are displayed and described in Table 4–2.

Atypical prosodic patterns may manifest as frequent starts and stops, audible or silent groping, or unusual stress patterns. Any prosodic pattern that calls attention to itself as different from normally developing children learning to use the same native language is remarkable. Furthermore, a paucity or absence of babbling during the appropriate developmental period is clinically significant and should be noted.

Routine Clinical Observations 1: Facial Region Inspection and Respiratory Observations

Routine Clinical Observation 1 also directs the examiner to inspect the facial region and observe respiratory patterns. Since neither requires a response from the examinee, the inspection can be done without modification or adaptation when the child is at rest.

Routine Clinical Observation 2: Lip and Tongue Mobility and Strength

Infants. For preverbal children, delete Routine Clinical Observation 2 if the child is judged as not yet capable of following the instructions or not able to tolerate. As an alternative, provide opportunities and encourage vocal play. Then carefully observe the movements of the tongue, lip, and jaw during these activities.

Toddlers and Preschoolers. Many toddlers and preschoolers may be able to perform activities required for Routine Clinical Observation 2. To encourage participation, it is often expedient to recruit a washable friendly-looking puppet with moveable mouth, some semblance of teeth, and a tongue that moves. Playfully allowing the child to pretend to perform a parallel evaluation on the puppet can be very effective. This may require that the clinician provide a child-friendly representation of the certain items (e.g., penlight, stopwatch, pediatric tongue depressor, or cotton-tipped swab).

Table 4–2. Brief Summary of Preverbal Phonological Development in Infancy

Approximate Age in Months	Sound Repertoire	Babbling Stage
0–1	• Predominantly reflexive vocalizations (e.g., crying, fussing, coughing, sneezing, and burping) • Occasionally, some quasi-resonant nuclei (vowel-like vocalizations) and syllabic nasals	
1–2	• Simple, irregularly timed syllables that contain sounds resembling back vowels and back consonants	
3–5	• Add vocal play that includes squeals, growls, yells, raspberries, or vowel-like sounds that are more adult-like (fully resonant nuclei) and friction noises • Resonance has become more oral	Marginal babbling emerges and is characterized by CV and VC sequences that are somewhat irregularly timed and comprise vowel-like and consonant-like sounds that more closely resemble the adult model
6–8	• Add stops, nasals, glides, and the lax vowels /ɛ/, /ɪ/, and /ʌ/ • Alveolar and bilabial consonants have replaced velars	Canonical babbling is characterized by regularly timed CV syllable sequences comprising consonants and vowels that closely approximate the adult model
9–12	• Full speech-sound repertoire available for jargon but not for meaningful speech • Prosody reflects primary language	Variegated babbling comprises a wide variety of syllable sequences that resemble adult speech in intonation. Strings of syllables mimic real statements, questions, and exclamations prosodically, but they do not contain real words.

Table 4–3. Approximate Age of Mastery for American English Consonants

Age of Child in Years	Consonants in Speech-Sound Repertoire for Most Children
2	/p/, /m/, /w/, /n/, /d/, /h/
3	/b/, /t/, /k/, /g/ (in addition to all of the above)
4	/f/, /j/, /ŋ/ (in addition to all of the above)
5	/v/, /s/, /z/, /ʃ/, /tʃ/, /dʒ/, /l/ (in addition to all of the above)
6	/ʒ/, /r/ (in addition to all of the above)
7	/ð/ (in addition to all of the above)
8	/θ/ (in addition to all of the above)

Table 4–4. Selected Natural Phonological Processes and Approximate Ages of Suppression

Age of Child in Years	Naturally Occurring Phonological Processes Suppressed by Most Children		Example
2	Denasalization		Moo → /bu/
2½	Reduplication		Water → /ˈwɔ wɔ/
	Diminutization		Apple → /ˈæ pi/
3	Assimilation	Labial	Boat → /boʊp/
		Alveolar	Soup → /sut/
		Velar	Dog → /gɔg/
		Nasal	Mouse → /maʊn/
	Stopping of	/f/	Fish → /pɪʃ/
		/v/	Very → /ˈbɛ ri/
		/s/	Sick → /tɪk/
		/z/	Zoo → /du/
		/ʃ/	Show → /toʊ/
		/tʃ/	Chicken → /ˈtɪk ən/
		Postvocalic devoicing	Nose → /noʊs/
		Prevocalic voicing	Cup → /gʌp/
	Affrication		Shoe → /tʃu/
	Final consonant deletion		Cup → /kʌ/
	Unstressed syllable deletion		Banana → /ˈnæ nə/
	Initial consonant deletion		Cup → /ʌp/
4	Fronting of initial velar singles		Key → /ti/ Go → /doʊ/
	Deaffrication		Chicken → /ˈʃɪk ən/
	Cluster reduction (without /s/)		Frog → /fɔg/ (cluster reduction) Frog → /ɔg/ (cluster deletion)
	Stopping of	/dʒ/	Jump → /dʌmp/
4½	Depalatalization of final singles		Wish → /wɪs/
	Vowelization		Staple → /ˈste po/

Table 4–4. *continued*

Age of Child in Years	Naturally Occurring Phonological Processes Suppressed by Most Children		Example
5	Depalatalization of initial singles		Sheep → /sip/
	Alveolarization		Pie → /ta͟ɪ/
	Velar fronting		Cow → /ta͟ʊ/
	Cluster reduction (with /s/)		Stair → /tɛɚ/
6	Labialization		Thing → /fɪŋ/
	Stopping of	/θ/	Thing → /tɪŋ/
		/ð/	That → / dæt/
7	Gliding with initial liquids		Lamb → /jæm/ Rabbit → /'wæ bɪt/
	Vowelization of prevocalic liquids		Red → /u 'ɛd/
8	Epenthesis		Blue → /bə 'lu/
9	Consonant cluster substitution		Thread → /twɛd/

Some examiners subject themselves to an imaginary inspection that the child performs in an effort to secure engagement and decrease stress. However, allowing the child to playfully perform a child's interpretation of the procedures on a puppet is preferred as the remote opportunity for accidental harm to the clinician is removed.

When evaluating the data, bear in mind that young children normally have difficulty elevating and otherwise manipulating the tongue on command (Ozanne, 1992; Williams & Stackhouse, 2000). Therefore, perfectly smooth and accurate control of lingual movements is not expected, although symptoms of compromised motor control are noteworthy if evident.

Routine Clinical Observations 3 and 4: Dental Alignment, Bite, and Occlusion

Routine Clinical Observations 3 and 4 are irrelevant for newborns. That is, humans typically arrive edentulous at birth, or nearly so. For that reason, evaluating incisor alignment, bite, and occlusion is not performed on infants.

The lower central incisors normally erupt between the ages of 6 and 10 months. Once the teeth begin to emerge, alignment and bite may be evaluated as tolerated by the young examinee. Occlusion, however, cannot be evaluated until an ipsilateral set of first molars is fully erupted, which is anywhere between the ages of approximately 15 and 20 months. A full set of deciduous teeth can typically be viewed by the third birthday.

Refer to Figures 2–8 through 2–26 as needed. Also, the birth-to-5 recording forms include a dental diagram with approximate ages for primary teeth eruption and shedding.

Routine Clinical Observations 5 and 6: Oral Interior and Velar Movement

Infants. Examining the oral interior of infants can be challenging since the infant does not reliably follow verbal instructions. Furthermore, clinicians must be resourceful and efficient to gather needed information during the brief window of time while the child's mouth is open for viewing.

We have a few suggestions for provoking the desired open-mouth posture for small children. They are described in Box 4–2, beginning with least invasive.

None of the suggestions in Box 4–2 is guaranteed to elicit mouth-open posture sufficient to completely inspect an infant's oral interior. The clinician who is completely familiar with the oral interior is prepared to make the most of the opportunity if a quick one presents itself. Moreover, it is possible that some parts of the inspection may need to be tabled.

When viewing the inside of the infant's mouth, anticipate that the general landmarks and condition are the same as those described in Chapter 2, with a few exceptions. That is, expect to see a tongue that is disproportionately large for the oral cavity, the absence of teeth, and for newborns whose larynx

---

Box 4–2. Suggestions for Achieving Mouth-Open Posture for Young Children

Many young children resist efforts to view the inside of the oral cavity. Although there is no guarantee that the following suggestions will produce the desired result, they may be very helpful in many instances.

- Because infants naturally imitate the facial expressions of adults during social interaction, engaging in social play that involves open-mouth posture may yield the desired result. Recruiting a parent to elicit an imitated open-mouth position in this manner may also work.
- Many young children can be encouraged to open the mouth and allow the examiner to take a look by imitation, mirror play, or taking turns with the puppet.
- Lay the child down in a parent's lap in a supine position, with feet or buttocks resting on the parent's stomach and head resting over the parent's knees, lower than the rest of the body. In this position, the child's mouth tends to open naturally due to gravity, until the child begins to object, allowing a short window for viewing the oral interior. The best viewing angle results if you position yourself above the child and across from the parent. Your view of the oral interior under this circumstance is upside down. If the tongue falls back when the child is in this position, use a tongue depressor

to move it out of the way so that you may take a look at the pharynx, if this can be done without traumatizing the child.
- Place a tongue depressor between the child's maxillary and mandibular incisors and gently apply firm and steady downward pressure. Eventually, the muscles used to elevate the mandible tire. At that point, if you lightly stimulate the gag reflex, the child's mouth will open completely, again giving a short window of opportunity for viewing.
- Gently occlude both nares, forcing the mouth to open for breathing.
- If all else fails, it is probable that the young child will spontaneously cry heartily at some point during the session, naturally assuming a mouth-open posture. If no other attempt has yielded a reasonable opportunity for oral viewing, taking advantage of a spontaneous cry for cursory inspection is a legitimate way to gather only the most superficial of evidence. Spontaneous nonspeech velar action may be seen during a cry if the child's protest occurs with a mouth-open posture. Of course, spontaneous velar action shows that the velum is capable of movement, but this information cannot be tendered as evidence of adequate velar movement for speech.

has not yet descended, the epiglottis may be viewable. Findings are remarkable if they deviate from those described in this paragraph as combined with Chapter 2 comments.

Toddlers and Preschoolers. Some preschoolers and toddlers cooperate heroically while a clinician views the oral interior; however, many are not inclined to do so. Conveniently, the suggestions in Box 4–2 apply to these groups as well.

While the child's mouth is open, check to verify that all parts are present and intact, and check for function if the child tolerates. Refer to information provided in Chapter 2 for details.

Then, if the occasion presents itself while the child's mouth is still open, check velar movement. Surprisingly, many young children are able to complete this screening if it is done in a friendly, noninvasive way. This may be because older toddlers have been asked to say /ɑ/ at the doctor's office and are familiar with the routine.

Routine Clinical Observation 7: Verbal Diadochokinesis

Infants, Toddlers, and Younger Preschoolers. Performing verbal diadochokinesis with children in the birth-to-3 population (i.e., infants and toddlers) is not clinically practical; the task is quite abstract and requires oral agility that is not in place for most children at that age. Even for normally developing 3-year-olds, reliability is questionable, accuracy errors are common, and performance variability is high (Green, Moore, Higashikawa, & Steeve, 2000; Green, Moore, & Riley, 2002; Howlin & Cross, 1994; Williams & Stackhouse, 2000). Therefore, we suggest customarily foregoing the procedure for any child younger than 4 years.

Older Preschoolers. Many 4-year-olds are able to follow the instructions and perform verbal diadochokinesis activity, and in general, normally developing 5-year-olds complete the procedure with little or no difficulty (Williams & Stackhouse, 2000). A way to encourage participation is to control a small vehicle that only moves when the child says the target syllable or syllables and to change the vehicle for the various syllables and sequences that

are a part of this portion of the test. For example, in the manual's companion video, the child examinee moved one car forward toward a goal by saying /pə/ repetitively, moved a different car forward by saying /tə/ repetitively, and moved a third car when saying /pə tə/ repetitively. He was not asked to say any syllables with the /k/ sound because he had not yet produced the phoneme /k/ spontaneously in syllables or words.

Moreover, consider that both 4- and 5-year-olds produce rapid-alternating or rapid-sequential syllables more effectively when the syllable combinations form real words (e.g., buttercup or pat-a-cake), not nonsense syllable sequences (e.g., /pə tə kə/). However, two problems with real words are noted in Chapter 2 and reiterated here. That is, when meaning is ascribed to the rapid-alternating or rapid-sequential syllables forming a word, the activity is modified considerably, and it becomes a linguistically influenced speech event. Furthermore, since English is a stress-timed language (see Box 2–19), producing multisyllabic words with even rate and stress is unnatural for native English speakers, further modifying the activity. Therefore, although multisyllabic words can be used when checking rate and precision for rapid-alternating articulatory movements, the act of introducing real words tactically modifies the activity, making it quite different from the standard verbal diadochokinesis task.

Furthermore, there are problems associated with rate data norms for the very young that may result from differences in data collection techniques or high degree of performance variability among children (Cohen, Waters, & Hewlett, 1998; Williams & Stackhouse, 2000). For these reasons, rate evaluation criteria may not necessarily apply to data collected using modifications described herein. Instead, the results of data collected for 5-year-olds may be most useful when exploring whether the child has difficulty with verbal programming and sequencing, articulatory precision, or other symptoms of neuromuscular involvement (Canning & Rose, 1974; Fletcher, 1972; Henry, 1990; Williams & Stackhouse, 2000).

Therefore, if a clinician chooses to collect verbal diadochokinetic data for a 4- or 5-year-old, it may be best to forego calculating the rate and look more closely at the programming and accuracy of the syllable productions. The decision with regard to attempting verbal diadochokinesis should be based on experience with the individual child. Refer to Chapter 2 for basic instructions.

Routine Clinical Observation 8: Vowel Prolongation

Newborns, infants, and toddlers (i.e., birth-to-3) and many young preschoolers (i.e., 3-year-olds) are not likely to participate meaningfully in the vowel prolongation activity; therefore, omit it for them. Normally developing 4- and 5-year-olds, however, should be able to follow the instructions and playfully complete the activity as it is presented, with the need for few age-motivated considerations if any.

Discretionary Clinical Observations

Discretionary Observations to Automatically Exclude for the Birth-to-5 Age Group

Several discretionary clinical observations do not appear on the birth-to-5 recording forms. They should be deleted for reasons stated beside each one named below.

- Omit screening for temporomandibular joint disorder (i.e., Discretionary Clinical Observation 11) since young children do not typically have mandibular constriction.
- Omit tongue-thrust swallow procedure (i.e., Discretionary Clinical Observation 12). Tongue-thrust swallow is the typical swallow pattern for infants; thus, testing for it is generally accepted as inapt for children younger than 5 years.
- Omit observation for acquired apraxia of speech (i.e., Discretionary Clinical Observation 14). When young children exhibit symptoms of apraxia, the observation for developmental apraxia of speech (i.e., Discretionary Clinical Observation 13) is the appropriate tool.
- Omit prompt for dysphagia screening (i.e., Discretionary Clinical Observation 21). The prompt for dysphagia screening that appears

in this manual is designed for adults. Any infant who exhibits symptoms of feeding or swallowing difficulties should receive a specialist evaluation that explores all areas of concern relative to age-appropriate feeding and swallowing matters.

Discretionary Clinical Observations That May Be Appropriate, With Procedural Adjustment

Screening for Nasal Cavity Clearance: Discretionary Clinical Observation 9. Nasal cavity clearance screening is appropriate for any person who exhibits associated symptoms listed on the recording form, even if that person is a young child. The instructions in Chapter 3 are essentially unchanged for children who tolerate the screening. For most young children, however, omit the part that involves occluding each naris alternately while the examinee expels air through the nose, unless guardians report that the child is already capable of blowing the nose.

Facial Dimension Estimates: Discretionary Clinical Observation 10. Facial dimension estimates should be considered if noting symptoms of facial dysmorphia shown on the recording form or in Table 2–2. Although submitting to facial dimension estimates is largely a passive activity for the examinee, it requires holding still and closing the mouth. Some young children may not tolerate; in that case, ballpark estimations may substitute for the procedures described in Chapter 3. Any suspected deviation is noteworthy and may lead to recommendation or referral.

Observation for Developmental Apraxia of Speech: Discretionary Clinical Observation 13. The observation for developmental apraxia of speech should be considered for any child who displays associated symptoms listed on the recording form. The procedure as described in Chapter 3 can be applied to both preverbal and verbal children as tolerated.

Screening for Submucous Cleft: Discretionary Clinical Observation 15. The screening for submucous cleft is described in Chapter 3. The procedure can and should be performed if associated symptoms displayed on the recording form are noted and if the child tolerates. Always refer a child for medical evaluation whenever suspecting that palatal or velar integrity may be compromised.

Screening for Nasal Airflow Emissions: Discretionary Clinical Observation 16. By and large, this discretionary screening can only be performed on young children who are capable of volitionally producing some speech sounds. Many older toddlers and preschoolers comply with procedures as they appear in Chapter 3. The symptom list that appears on the recording form may serve as a guide when identifying children for whom the screening is needed.

Dysarthria Observation: Discretionary Clinical Observation 17. Omit the reading passage from Discretionary Clinical Observation 17 when considering symptoms of dysarthria in young children. Otherwise, dysarthria observations as described should be possible for any child who can participate in a conversation.

Speech Sound Stimulability Screening: Discretionary Clinical Observation 18. Apply the speech sound stimulability screening procedures described in Chapter 3 if age-inappropriate speech sound errors are noted and if the child tolerates. The list of indicators shown on the recording form can be used to determine whether screening is appropriate.

Laryngeal and Respiratory Efficiency: Discretionary Clinical Observation 19. Most infants, toddlers, and younger preschoolers are not inclined to submit to laryngeal and respiratory efficiency screening. If the procedure is needed, however, many older preschoolers (i.e., 4- and 5-year-olds) perform the activity without significant need for procedural changes.

One way to facilitate laryngeal and respiratory screening in an older preschooler is to use props and friendly competition to playfully elicit and prolong the /s/ and /z/ consonants. That is, using representations of two small friendly-looking snakes, where you take the role of speaking through one snake and the child takes the role of speaking through the other, use the props to compete in a friendly way to determine which snake can make the longest hissing sound (i.e., /s/). Then put away the snakes and introduce two small friendly-looking bumblebees who are in competition to produce the longest buzzing sound (i.e., /z/). Measure duration for the child's consonant productions, select the longest /s/ and /z/ durations, and after the session, calculate ratio as described in Chapter 3.

Bear in mind, even if the child completes the activity, if vocal pathology is even a slight possibility, more scientific measures are needed. This requires referral to otorhinolaryngology.

Gag Reflex Stimulation: Discretionary Clinical Observation 20. Gag reflex stimulation is a passive activity, only requiring that the subject open the mouth and allow a person to touch the base of the tongue or posterior pharyngeal wall with an extra-long cotton swab. If a neurologic referral is anticipated, the gag reflex findings may be helpful; however, it may not be worth the cost in lost rapport with young examinees. Clinical judgment should guide this decision on a case-by-case basis.

Discretionary Clinical Observations Not Introduced Previously

Discretionary Clinical Observation 22: Screening for Amblyopia. The clinical question associated with amblyopia screening, Clinical Question 41 (see Table 0–3), asks, "Does the young child exhibit signs that suggest referral for amblyopia testing?" An answer of *yes* is clinically significant and results in a referral to ophthalmology.

Equipment needed for amblyopia screening is minimal. It includes examination gloves and an eye test paddle.

Amblyopia symptoms may be observed during social interaction. In fact, social interaction (i.e., Routine Clinical Observation 1) has much potential to reveal the most obvious symptom of amblyopia: the wandering eye. However, many children with amblyopia do not display such an obvious symptom. Therefore, the procedure is suggested for all children younger than 6 years, regardless of symptoms. See Box 4–3 for more information on amblyopia.

The *amblyopia screening procedure* is not complicated. Acquire an eye test paddle or simply attach half a small index card to a tongue depressor, and

---

Box 4–3. Why Screen for Amblyopia

Amblyopia, the leading cause of monocular vision, is usually correctable up to the end of the critical period for visual development (i.e., approximately 5–6 years of age) and affects 3% of the population. A quick screening for amblyopia is easy to perform, does not require special certification or training, and may identify children who should be referred for ophthalmology evaluation and for whom there is still hope for binocular vision. More information on amblyopia appears in Box 4–5.

use it to cover each eye one at a time, as discreetly as possible. The normal response to the screening is for the child to show no sign of distress when either eye is covered, although many children display evidence of noticing the paddle in front of the eye.

If the child shows any signs of distress while either eye is covered (e.g., crying, change in demeanor, determined attempt to see around the visual obstruction), it is possible that the procedure has blocked the only eye that communicates well with the brain. This response is remarkable and should lead to a specialist referral for vision testing.

Furthermore, some children may exhibit signs of distress when either eye is covered, without evidence of a preference for a particular eye. Children who exhibit this symptom should also be referred to ophthalmology.

Discretionary Clinical Observation 23: Screening for Select Primitive Reflexes. For infants, as well as some toddlers and preschoolers, add a screening for select primitive reflexes (i.e., also called neonatal reflexes, infantile reflexes, and newborn reflexes). In building the screening procedure, the following resources were consulted: Duffy (2013), Gupta (1999), Jones, Morgan, Shelton, and Thorogood (2007), Shipley and McAfee (2008), and Zafeiriou (2004).

The clinical question associated with primitive reflex screening, Clinical Question 42 (see Table 0–3), asks, "For infants, toddlers, and some preschoolers

suspected of possible neurologic involvement, does evidence show that primitive reflexes are present and suppressed at developmentally appropriate ages?" An answer of *no* suggests that follow-up is needed.

Procedures for screening selected primitive reflexes are described in Table 4–5, along with a description of each reflex. Check all five reflexes for infants. When examining a toddler, consider checking the primitive reflexes if the child exhibits signs of late talker, feeding disorder, swallowing problems, difficulty learning to walk, discoordination, or cognitive delay (Capute, 1979; Gupta, 1999; Jones et al., 2007; Shipley & McAfee, 2008; Zafeiriou, 2004).

Adaptations for People With Social and Cognitive Challenges

People with cognitive and social limitations comprise a sizable portion of the population receiving speech-language services. Many times, they are younger than 21 years of age and receive special services through an individualized education plan (IEP) or individualized family service plan (IFSP) in the public education or public health system.

As a heterogeneous group, individuals may present with concomitant disabilities, such as visual impairment, physical immobility or limited mobility, autism, deafness, hard of hearing, and the like. Comments in this section only apply to protocol adjustments relative to cognitive and social-language difficulties; use the recording form for general use unless concomitant concerns indicate otherwise.

Consult Accommodation Plan if One Is in Place

By and large, the routine and discretionary procedures provided should serve as an adequate guide, with some highly individualized modifications and accommodations being necessary in some cases. If an accommodation plan exists for the individual, this trumps any recommendation offered herein, so it should be consulted and followed when planning an oral-facial exam.

Table 4–5. Selected Primitive Reflexes

Reflex	Age Boundaries	How to Stimulate	Normal Response	Comments
Rooting	Present at birth and inhibited between ages 6 and 12 months	Place infant in supine position. Then, lightly stroke cheek with an outward motion. If evaluating an older child, an upright position is acceptable.	Infant turns head toward stimulus and displays sucking motion	• Rooting reflex is important to feeding • If persists, may interfere with movements needed for speech • Can recur in adults with certain neurolesions
Sucking	Present at birth and up to the age 2 to 3 months	Place infant in supine position. Then, place gloved finger, pacifier, or nipple on the roof of the infant's mouth. If evaluating an older child, an upright position is acceptable.	The baby sucks on finger, pacifier, or nipple. Tongue moves forward and backward while jaw moves up and down.	• Sucking reflex is necessary for feeding • If absent in a newborn who exhibits feeding problems, contact health care provider immediately • If persists, may interfere with movements needed for speech • Can recur in adults with certain neurolesions
Palmar grasp	Birth to 6 months	With infant's head at midline, place a finger or object into the infant's palm on the ulnar side (i.e., little finger)	Infant grasps the object	Reflex that persists past 6 months of age has been associated with delayed speech as well as swallowing problems
Tongue-thrust reflex (not to be confused with tongue-thrust swallow)	Birth to about 6 months	Place infant in prone position; then touch the tip of the infant's tongue	Infant protrudes tongue	• Provides protection against choking in early months • Must fade before successful introduction of solid foods
Babinski	Always abnormal	Place infant or child in supine position. Then stroke lateral surface of the sole, extending from the heel to the head of the fifth toe.	(1) Upward flexion of great toe (2) Fanning outward of other four toes	• The reflex is observed if two extensor responses occur simultaneously

General Adaptations for People With Cognitive Limitations

If giving an oral-facial evaluation to a person with cognitive or social limitations, when setting up equipment, most of the time it is necessary to keep the materials out of reach or even out of sight as was explained for the birth-to-5 population. Furthermore, when instructing the examinee, it is very important to use language that the person understands while speaking directly to the person. Box 4–4 provides a list of suggestions that may be helpful throughout

> ### Box 4–4. Suggestions for Giving Instructions to Any Person With Compromised Comprehension
>
> - Maintain appropriate eye contact throughout.
> - Be aware of nonverbal cues that may indicate confusion or need for more information (e.g., facial expression, distraction).
> - Use simple, concrete language.
> - Use short but not truncated sentences.
> - Insert meaningful pauses to allow for more processing time (i.e., chunk).
> - Consider inserting a brief pause prior to content words; then emphasize the content word slightly, without interrupting the flow of speech.
> - If the examinee follows directions incorrectly or incompletely, when reinstructing be cautious to redirect with a positive tone. For example, say something like, "Great! Now, let's try it a different way." Then provide more information as needed.
> - Use demonstration if necessary, and document it.
> - It is absolutely not appropriate to proceed with any part of the evaluation without reasonable meaningful explanation and an attempt to achieve understanding.

the evaluation for anyone who exhibits signs of compromised comprehension.

The remainder of the inspection can be performed for this group as described in Chapters 2 and 3, taking care to ensure that the examinee is treated respectfully throughout. Also, the oral-facial evaluation can be administered in parts or over a period of days if participation wanes.

General Adaptations for People With Social Language Disorder or Tactile Aversion

Although individuals with autism spectrum disorder are frequently described according to the condition's social motivational and social emotional traits, emerging evidence supports the idea that the condition may in fact be associated with motor difficulties that can be noticed through oral-facial inspection activities such as those described in this manual (Belmonte et al., 2013). This finding highlights the importance of oral-facial inspection for individuals suspected of having social language disorder but does not suggest that oral-facial evaluation results can be used to diagnose the condition.

Furthermore, individuals with autism spectrum disorder may be hypersensitive to oral stimulation, and in fact, the inspection may trigger symptoms of tactile aversion in individuals with increased tactile sensitivity (Belmonte et al., 2013). This is true not only for those with autism spectrum disorder but also for other groups, such as individuals with genetic anomalies such as Kabuki syndrome, fear of dentists, or embarrassment about poor dental hygiene or craniofacial abnormality.

In cases where tactile aversion is evident, accommodations may include giving the person more time, augmenting the instructions with additional explanation, allowing the examinee to perform the procedure on a doll or puppet before expecting compliance, or encouraging the examinee with a playful attitude (for child) or verbal praise. However, when compliance is not achieved, the examiner must be willing to modify the protocol and perhaps even omit the activities that cause discomfort.

Note that on the instructional video that accompanies the manual, the child with Kabuki syndrome demonstrated tactile resistance during screening for primitive reflexes and during the screening for submucous cleft. In both cases, the clinician appropriately made a reasonable attempt to complete the procedure but did not sacrifice rapport to do it.

When Oral-Facial Evaluation Is Not a Relevant Test

The oral-facial evaluation is not relevant for clients who are nonverbal and are judged to have no potential for spoken language due to previously identified physical or cognitive limitations. The inspection should only be administered to people for whom the four overarching clinical questions are answerable and relevant (see Table 0–2).

Adaptations for People With Sensory and Physical Limitations

Sensory and physical limitations can obligate adjustments when inspecting the oral-facial mechanism. For the purpose of this manual, we offer suggestions for addressing the needs of people who present limitations in three categories: auditory, visual, and physical-mobility. Any accommodation plan that is in place takes precedence over the following recommendations and suggestions.

Auditory Limitations

Individuals with auditory limitations include the deaf and hard of hearing, whether aided or unaided, regardless of preferred mode of communication or cultural orientation (i.e., Deaf or hearing culture). Whenever a hard-of-hearing or deaf person, or a parent of a hard-of-hearing or deaf child, seeks speech-language services, due to the speech-language pathology scope of practice, one may safely presume that potential for spoken communication is under consideration.

As a rule, deaf and hard-of-hearing individuals find spoken-language learning challenging, primarily because hearing is the modality through which

spoken language is learned naturally. Although many deaf and hard-of-hearing people enhance their hearing through technology (e.g., hearing aid, cochlear implant, assistive listening device), the auditory signal that the person receives through the device is different from the signal received through natural hearing and is therefore difficult to interpret in the absence of strategic listening practice (Cole & Flexer, 2011).

Regardless, if spoken language is a potential goal, the oral mechanism must be inspected to determine that all parts are present, intact, and functioning adequately for speech, as is true for any other speech-therapy candidate. For these purposes, routine and discretionary procedures provided in this manual should suffice as a general guide.

However, some considerations can facilitate a more meaningful outcome. For example, if both clinician and examinee use American Sign Language (ASL) or any other manual communication system at a level that is at least functional, the manual system should be the preferred mode of communication *for giving instructions and for general communication*. In many cases, however, gesture, visual prompting, *and* interpreting services may be necessary if the clinician and examinee do not comfortably share a common communication mode.

Bear in mind that written instructions and speech reading may not yield a successful outcome due to the potential for ambiguity unless the examinee is known to have high proficiency in these areas. If an interpreter is needed to ensure that instructions are clearly understood, one should be hired.

Typically, other than finding a common communication modality and taking measures to ensure comprehension, no modifications are needed to perform the procedures. However, the examiner should be alert to potential findings that may indicate a particular therapy plan, and these are discussed in Chapter 5.

Visual Limitations

Vision problems that may affect a person's ability to participate in an oral-facial evaluation include blindness of any kind, tunnel vision, macular degeneration, cataracts, monocular vision, hemispatial neglect, hemianopia, and amblyopia. Individuals with serious visual problems may need accommodations when administering an oral-facial evaluation. Mostly, this involves preferential seating, respectfully informing the examinee of the procedures and your location throughout, and sensitivity to the possibility that the person with visual limitations may be unnecessarily surprised if the procedure is not explained sufficiently and if satisfactory warning is not given before initiating physical contact or proximity.

In addition, a few inspection procedures require the examinee's visual attention, and individuals with low vision may require deleting that portion of the evaluation or finding an alternative method for prompting. For example, observation for acquired apraxia of speech (i.e., Discretionary Clinical Observation 14) suggests finger counting using a visual prompt. If low vision prevents this, a tactile prompt may be substituted. Likewise, for watch-and-do activities, substituting a verbal explanation may suffice but should be documented as having been done in the absence of visual prompting.

These general suggestions are useful for most people with limited vision. For your convenience, the manual distinguishes between certain types of vision problems, as shown in Box 4–5.

Physical Mobility Limitations

Physical and mobility limitations can manifest in a wide variety of ways; therefore, modifications and accommodations are similarly varied. For example, stroke patients may experience hemiplegia or hemiparesis, and individuals with cerebral palsy or other neurologically based problem may experience anything from mild weakness or discoordination to a lifetime of being wheelchair bound or even bedridden.

If the mobility limitations affect the oral-facial mechanism, the focus is on the extent to which the concerns are likely to affect speech or potential for compensatory movements. For physical limitations that do not affect speech, the inspection procedures that appear in Chapters 2 and 3 should be useful as written. However, if physical challenges seem predisposed to interference with data collection in any way, consultation with special services may be help-

ful. In general, it is important to remember that the examinee should be in a seated and upright position if at all possible.

Suggested Adaptations for Older Adults

Often, when older adults receive a communication evaluation, there has been a cerebrovascular or traumatic incident resulting in brain injury, neurologic infection or degenerative disease, or surgery to remove all or part of the larynx. Lesser vocal pathologies not leading to laryngeal excision can also cause an adult to seek voice evaluation, and a smaller number of older adults are seen for a plethora of other reasons.

Regardless of grounds for evaluation, by virtue of age alone, older adults present unique needs that warrant consideration as well as a few protocol modifications. Therefore, before moving on to specific populations, the manual presents some general guidelines for inspecting the oral-facial region in older adults.

General Protocol Modifications for Older Adults

When working with older adults, plan to omit four discretionary clinical observations. They are deemed unnecessary for this age group:

- Facial dimension estimates (i.e., Discretionary Clinical Observation 10)
- Tongue-thrust swallow procedure (i.e., Discretionary Clinical Observation 12)
- Observations for developmental apraxia of speech (i.e., Discretionary Clinical Observation 13)
- Screening for submucous cleft (i.e., Discretionary Clinical Observation 15)

Recording forms for older adults omit all references that correspond to these discretionary clinical observations. Furthermore, cup of water should be eliminated from the materials list since it is only needed for a procedure that is planned for exclusion.

Box 4–5. Vision Problems

Blindness

The term *blindness* applies to any person whose vision is either absent or compromised and cannot be corrected to a functional level as diagnosed by a vision specialist. Examinees in this category experience seriously blurred vision even with correction, possibly no perceptible vision at all, or any level of low-vision function between these two anchors. The general instructions for low-vision examinees apply to this group.

Visual Field Deficits

Tunnel Vision

Tunnel vision results in a decreased visual field that eliminates all or nearly all peripheral vision. The etiology can be genetic (e.g., Usher syndrome), neurologic reaction to assault, disease, or chronic long-term stress. More recently, people who spend their lives in front of a computer screen are at risk for developing a type of tunnel vision called *computer vision syndrome* (Godnig, 2003).

Macular Degeneration

Macular degeneration, also a visual field problem, is considered a leading cause of legal blindness. The macula is at the center of the retina, and its integrity is crucial to focused vision. When the macula deteriorates or is compromised due to age or disease, the central visual field is not available; consequently, focused vision is not possible (Takeda et al., 2009).

Hemispatial Neglect

Hemispatial neglect is a condition that occurs most often in brain-injured patients whose cerebral infarct involves right cerebral hemisphere areas that interpret visual information, although it can result from left cerebral infarct in rare cases. Essentially, patients with hemispatial neglect experience reduced recognition or response to stimuli presented to the left visual field and may even behave as if the left half of their visual space does not exist. For instance, if asked to draw or copy a picture, the patient may draw only the right side; if asked to bisect a line, the patient may place the line of bisection on the far right instead of in the middle; when eating, the person may only attend to and eat the food that is on the right side of the plate; when reading, the patient may read only the right half of the page; or when shaving, the person may shave only the right side of the face (Buxbaum, 2006; Lundervold, Bergmann, & Wooton, 2005).

Approximately 10% of right hemisphere strokes result in hemispatial neglect syndrome. In the early stages, the condition is easy to detect, with much spontaneous recovery within the first few weeks after the stroke and some adaptation due to learning. However, when the effects persist, they can have a long-term impact on activities of daily living.

Visual Field Cuts

People with neurologic impairment can experience a variety of types of visual field cuts, including hemianopia or hemianopsia. When both eyes are affected, the condition results in complete loss of the visual field on one side. Similarly, visual field loss may also include quadrantanopia or scotoma, to name a few examples.

Accommodations for Visual Field Deficits

Accommodations for visual field deficits depend entirely on the portion of the visual field that is lost and the extent to which it is lost. Visual field deficits described above are discussed separately with regard to accommodations.

CHAPTER 4

Individuals with tunnel vision may or may not have clear vision, but their visual field is so limited that it is as if they were viewing the world through a narrow tunnel. When examining a person with tunnel vision, position yourself so that the person can find you in the central visual field; also place visual prompts within the boundaries of that same area.

Macular degeneration, on the other hand, takes away the central portion of the visual field, which is the portion that enables focused vision. Therefore, general adaptations suggested for low vision are useful for this group.

When working with persons who have hemispatial neglect or hemianopia, preferential seating becomes the key issue. Sit on the person's preferred side and present all stimuli from that side, as the person may not even detect your presence if you position yourself on the deficit side.

Monocular Vision

Monocular vision occurs when an individual has functional use of only one eye. Physically, this can result from amblyopia, neuropathology, injury, cataracts, disease, infection, or other impairment. Although persons with monocular vision have nearly the same visual field as persons with binocular vision, the quality of the signal is reduced, and three-dimensional vision is not possible. Accommodations for monocular vision apply to any person who has the functional use of only one eye.

Amblyopia

Amblyopia affects approximately 3% of the population and is the leading cause of monocular vision. It results from a significant disparity between the perceptual signals sent to the brain from the two eyes. Although most often associated with poorer vision in one eye, amblyopia can result from having two eyes with dissimilar refractive errors. As a result, to avoid double vision, the child's brain trains itself to ignore the signal sent to it from one of the two eyes.

Frequently, treatment involves placing a patch over the dominant eye, which forces the brain to receive and interpret the signal from the nondominant eye. If amblyopia is not corrected by the end of the critical period for visual development (i.e., approximately 5–6 years of age), in most people, the brain trains itself to permanently ignore visual information that the nondominant eye sends to it, regardless of whether the nondominant eye is structurally capable of functioning. The person becomes functionally blind in one eye or functionally monocular. Normally, this condition is not correctable after the critical period for visual development, although there are exceptions (Astle, Webb, & McGraw, 2011; Engel-Yeger, 2008).

Screening for amblyopia is included in the birth-to-5 section of this chapter because the condition can be fairly obvious during oral-facial inspection, the screening is simple, and early identification can remarkably improve quality of life for young examinees. As a rule, there is no need to screen for amblyopia in school-age children and adults because in most cases amblyopia is only treatable if caught before the school-age years; furthermore, school-age children are screened for vision problems annually in the public and private education systems.

Accommodations for Monocular Vision

Preferential seating is a universally applied adaptation for persons with monocular vision regardless of the etiology. Because visual field boundaries are essentially unchanged regardless of whether the person benefits from the vision in one eye or two, most people with monocular vision function reasonably well if approached from either side but most likely are more comfortable if accommodated by preferential seating. Because quality of vision is compromised for monocular individuals and three-dimensional vision is not possible, depending on the visual acuity of the one eye that remains, the monocular person may need additional processing time when working with visual prompts.

Cataracts

Cataracts are generally a temporary condition because they can be corrected surgically in most cases. When present, cataracts cloud a person's vision in the affected eye. General accommodations suggested for low vision are useful for this group. If cataracts affect only one eye, then the accommodations for monocular patients are appropriate.

Common Considerations When Serving an Adult Population

As a rule, the three groups to be discussed require immediate medical care, which takes precedence over the rehabilitation services that inevitably ensue once the acute stage of the illness has passed. Many times, the first visit takes place in the intensive care unit when the person may or may not tolerate even minimal interaction. Ordinarily, the complete assessment occurs after the person's medical condition is stable.

Health and Physical State

Even when not acutely ill, health or other physical complications can have a profound impact on findings, the person's ability to participate, or even clinical dynamics. For example, examinees in this age group may exhibit signs of aging voice, propensity for fatigue, dementia, cognitive and memory disorders, ischemia, physical pain or immobility, concomitant health problems, psychiatric conditions, effects of medication or even polypharmacy, degenerative processes, sensory deterioration, functional decline, fear, depression, weight change, grieving, adjustment to loss, facing end-of-life issues, effect of facing fewer options, family dynamics (e.g., spouses, significant others, adult children, even grandchildren), and compromised dignity.

Communication Needs Common to Older Adults

Many adult patients, having led full and dignified lives, now face the discomfort of a communication disorder confounded by the reality of much younger health care providers who often casually assume first-name familiarity and speak with a perceived condescending tone and unnecessarily loud voice. To counter potential for perceived disrespect, take every measure possible to demonstrate respect, stopping short of patronizing the older person.

One act that can go a long way toward communicating respect is to use the person's preferred title (e.g., Mr., Mrs., Ms., Miss, or even Dr.) followed by surname. In fact, as a general rule, it is considerate to never assume a first-name relationship with any older client. Instead, consider calling the person by title and surname, unless the older person initiates a request for a more familiar form.

Also, speak directly to the person, using appropriate eye contact. Avoid conversations that ignore the person's presence and discourage family members and other staff from doing the same. Instead, address the examinee directly whenever this can be done without being rude to the family member. Always offer the examinee the opportunity to ask questions before checking with other individuals who may be present.

General Considerations When Preparing the Work Area for an Older Adult

As for preparing the work area, most adults refrain from touching the materials so the equipment and supplies can be placed in an easily accessed location on the work table. There are exceptions, and always take precautions if in doubt.

General Considerations When Instructing an Older Adult

When instructing the examinee or family member, take special care to address the client directly, not the family members. Use appropriate language for the person's education and communication abilities, as you would for any client. Refer to Box 4–4 if suspecting comprehension difficulties.

General Considerations When Inspecting an Older Adult's Dentition and Oral Interior: Routine Clinical Observations 3 to 5

When inspecting an older adult's oral interior, there is always the possibility of dentures, partial plate, crowns, other dental work or prostheses, or missing teeth. Usually, if a prosthetic device is worn, any alignment, bite, and occlusion concerns do not require your attention. However, if dentures are present and do not seem to fit well, if consonants are imprecise or slushy, or if the examinee reports pain or discomfort related to a dental appliance, refer for prosthodontic follow-up.

Many dental appliances cover the palate, preventing inspection. There is no need to remove the appliance when inspecting the oral interior, as palatal integrity is generally not a concern with older adults who have an acquired communication disorder.

Some adult examinees are edentulous or display multiple edentulous spaces. Consider this condition significant only if it interferes with speech. In many cases, it does not.

Prompt for Dysphagia Screening: Discretionary Clinical Observation 21

Although the prompt for dysphagia screening is a discretionary procedure for all other populations, it becomes a routine procedure whenever working with older adults. Therefore, special recording forms associated with these populations place the dysphagia prompt with routine inspection procedures, even though it has discretionary status for other groups.

Modifications and Accommodations for Special Adult Populations

Many adult patients can participate in the oral-facial inspection as described in Chapters 2 and 3, with consideration given to general suggestions offered in the preceding paragraphs. Yet, for older adults with neurogenic etiology or laryngectomy, specific additional modifications and accommodations should be taken into account. For that reason, the next several paragraphs are devoted to meeting the oral-facial inspection needs of individuals in these categories.

Adaptations for Adults With Neurogenic Etiology or Suspected Neurogenic Etiology

The comments that follow specifically relate to adults who have experienced a neurologic episode, such as cerebrovascular accident, traumatic brain injury, neurosurgery, or disease. Although there are notable differences between these groups relative to clinical needs, adaptations for oral-facial evaluation can be addressed collectively. For the most part, oral-facial evaluation procedures described in Chapters 2 and 3 can be performed without modification, provided the examinee understands the instructions and tolerates the evaluation. Some suggestions for facilitating the inspection are offered.

Instructing the Examinee or Family Member. When evaluating a person who has experienced a neurologic episode, be aware that aphasia may interfere with an examinee's ability to understand the directions and perform activities. Whenever suspecting compromised comprehension, the suggestions in Box 4–4 may facilitate communication, not only during the initial instructions but also throughout the inspection.

Routine Clinical Observation 1: Conversational Speech Sample. Consider that a conversational speech sample may be difficult to elicit for people with aphasia or motor-speech disorder. Some examinees may not be capable of engaging in meaningful conversation at all.

Situational picture cards or reading sample (see Box 3–11) can be useful for eliciting speech for this group. Omit the conversational speech activity for anyone who does not engage socially.

Adaptations for Laryngectomees

A number of sources were consulted when considering the oral-facial examination needs of laryngectomized people. They include Berlin (1963); Chone, Gripp, Spina, and Crespo (2005); Eadie (2007); Lewin et al. (2008); Maclean, Cotton, and Perry (2009); Pawar, Sayed, Kazi, and Jagade (2008); and Shipley and McAfee (2008).

Comments on adaptations for laryngectomized adults are divided into two categories: preoperative laryngectomy and postoperative laryngectomy. Typically, the preoperative group has been diagnosed with laryngeal disease that necessitates surgical removal of the larynx or a portion of it. If the opportunity to evaluate the oral-facial mechanism for structure and function presents prior to surgery, preoperative inspection can provide information that is useful for planning postoperative care. However, since the surgery to remove the diseased tissue may be urgent, and depending on the philosophy of the referring surgeon, a preoperative visit may or may not occur.

The postoperative laryngectomee is quite different from the preoperative laryngectomee in that postoperatively, the examination takes place without a larynx and without the benefit of oral and nasal airflow. So the oral-facial inspection needs of these two groups are discussed separately. Relevant physical changes resulting from laryngectomy can be found in Box 4–6. Furthermore, vocal restoration options are discussed in Box 4–7.

Preoperative Laryngectomy. For the preoperative layngectomee, although the person still has a larynx, it is not functioning well and is scheduled for removal. The oral-facial inspection comprises only one small part of the preoperative assessment session that also includes interview and testing, as well as education.

Our interest in the preoperative laryngectomee's oral-facial region excludes any effort to evaluate the function of the laryngeal mechanism. And the inspection's focus is on judging whether all parts assumed to remain after surgery are present, intact, and functioning and to anticipate any anatomic or physiologic conditions that may potentially impede vocal rehabilitation using the method chosen by the person, as well as its alternatives.

By and large, the procedures described in Chapters 2 and 3 can be performed as written. Some exceptions and deletions are described.

The preoperative laryngectomee conversational speech sample (Routine Clinical Observation 1) requires some additional considerations. That is, unless there are other interfering factors, such as severe respiratory distress, conversation should be achievable. Furthermore, you should be able to judge relevant aspects of speech production, including intelligibility, resonance, speech sounds, syntax, prosody, and pragmatics.

Box 4–6. Relevant Physical Changes Resulting From Laryngectomy

Laryngectomy, by definition, is the removal of the larynx, which rules out any possibility of laryngeal speech. Postoperative airflow for speech, however, depends on the method selected for voice restoration and is addressed in Box 4–7.

Breathing for the laryngectomee is no longer accomplished via the nasal and oral egresses but through a surgically constructed tracheostoma. To be exact, when the surgeon detaches the larynx from the trachea's uppermost boundary, the incised superior end of the trachea is brought forward, a corresponding stoma is created at the base of the neck, and the trachea is sutured to it. The resulting tracheostoma becomes the ingress and egress for life-sustaining air, eliminating the role that the respiratory tract above the trachea normally plays in both respiration and speech production.

For individuals whose laryngeal disease triggered respiratory distress, the surgery may bring about welcome relief relative to that symptom. On the contrary, an adverse effect of the surgery may be a compromised ability to laugh, cry, or swallow.

Box 4–7. Vocal Restoration Options for Laryngectomized Individuals

The most common vocal restoration options are tracheoesophageal speech with artificial valve, esophageal speech, and electronic larynx.

Tracheoesophageal Speech With Artificial Valve

Tracheoesophageal speech is most frequently the first choice for laryngectomized individuals, but it cannot be implemented immediately after laryngectomy surgery as it requires a second surgical procedure. Furthermore, it is not always successful for the long term.

To qualify for the tracheoesophageal procedure:

- Patient must be fully healed from the laryngectomy surgery and pronounced cancer free.
- The tracheoesophageal wall must be healthy.
- Stoma should be at least 1.5 cm in diameter, located at the manubrium just above the jugular notch of the sternum.
- Manual dexterity, coordination, adequate respiratory reserve, ability to learn a new skill, visual acuity, alertness, hygiene habits, and motivation are judged adequate to manage and maintain the device over time.

The tracheoesophageal surgery, called a tracheoesophageal puncture, creates a tracheoesophageal fistulus. That is, at the location of the stoma, the surgeon creates a fistulus that penetrates the wall that the trachea and esophagus share. The small hole is then fitted with a prosthetic device. When the stoma is fully occluded, the prosthesis redirects air from the lungs into the esophagus, where it vibrates the pharyngeal-esophageal segment, thereby creating a sound source that is capable of being modified in the vocal tract, resulting in speech. The stoma can be occluded either manually using a thumb or finger or by inserting a prosthetic valve.

Although most patients initially express a preference for tracheoesophageal speech, complications can interrupt or even prohibit the long-term use. Pharyngeal-esophageal segment spasm is one potential obstacle that may thwart success and can be tested using the Blom-Singer insufflication test kit that is not part of the standard oral-facial inspection but is readily available to those who treat laryngectomy patients. A second possible barrier to success is the potential for *candida* or other microbial colonization, infecting the small prosthesis that occupies the tracheoesophageal fistulus. And third, a valve that is too long for the person's anatomy may leak, necessitating temporary removal so that it can be replaced with a properly fitted prosthesis.

When tracheoesophageal puncture fails or is temporarily interrupted, the patient needs an alternative communication mode. Therefore, learning how to use an electronic larynx or esophageal speech is important, even if the patient elects the tracheoesophageal puncture option.

Esophageal Speech

Esophageal speech requires no additional surgery or appliance, making it less invasive and the most readily accessible alternative. To accomplish esophageal speech, the person uses the tongue to inject air into the mouth of the esophagus and uses that air to set the pharyngeal-esophageal segment into vibration, creating a buzz-like sound that can travel the vocal tract and be modified using the same resonating and articulatory systems that are used for laryngeal speech.

To successfully learn esophageal speech:

- The esophagus must be structurally sound.

- Tongue must have sufficient strength and coordination to inject air into the mouth of the esophagus.
- Client should have the following:
  o Hearing that is adequate for spoken-language comprehension as well as self-monitoring
  o Ability to learn the new skill, as well as motivation to follow through on it
  o Ability to phonate reliably on demand using an alaryngeal voice
  o Short latency between the inflation of the esophagus and vocalization (i.e., able to phonate within 0.6 seconds after inflating the esophagus for 10 trials)
  o Ability to use esophageal voice to sustain /ɑ/ for a minimum of 2.2 seconds for 10 repeated trials
  o Ability to sustain phonation during articulation (i.e., articulate the syllable /dɑ/ 8–10 times on one injection for five repeated trials)

Esophageal speech candidates who have not yet achieved the above-listed performance goals should not be discouraged from making an effort to achieve them and may proceed with esophageal speech training that includes efforts to achieve these goals. Laryngectomized individuals should not eliminate esophageal speech from their voice restoration options without taking time to attempt these performance objectives.

Electronic Larynx

The electronic larynx is a handheld vibrator that creates an external sound source. When held properly against the neck, the device directly vibrates the skin that it contacts and thus indirectly disturbs the air that is in the nearby resonating chambers, creating a sound that can be modified for speech using the supralaryngeal valves along the vocal tract.

Most laryngectomees are able to use the electronic larynx option. Prerequisite skills are as follows:

- Very precise articulation for intelligible speech when using an electronic larynx
- Manual dexterity
- Motivation and ability to learn the new skill

A number of types of electronic larynges with a wide price range are available from a variety of manufacturers. Candidates should evaluate the options on a trial basis before purchasing one.

Expect to note audible symptoms of vocal pathology, but since the larynx is scheduled for removal, there is no need to describe or address the exact vocal symptoms. Pay careful attention to all other aspects of speech production though, since postoperative speech quality may be similar to but will not exceed the preoperative quality.

In fact, it is rare to find an alaryngeal speaker whose speech is 100% intelligible. Therefore, judging speech intelligibility preoperatively is particularly important if you have the opportunity, since it may be considered a baseline when establishing speech intelligibility goals postoperatively. Also, identifying any barriers to precise articulation preoperatively is very useful when establishing goals for the long term.

Although *breath-support judgments* that result from Routine Clinical Observation 8 and from connected speech (Routine Clinical Observation 1) can provide helpful information for preoperative laryngectomees, these measures are not sensitive enough to discern capacity needed for some types of alaryngeal speech. That is, if a candidate for laryngectomy plans to use tracheoesophageal speech, the device requires adequate pulmonary reserve. Furthermore, since some pathogens that placed the person at risk for laryngeal disease are also capable of negatively affecting pulmonary function, laryngectomees are normally at risk for pulmonary function that does not adequately support tracheoesophageal alaryngeal speech. Therefore, routine referral for scientifically

CHAPTER 4

based pulmonary testing is in the client's best interest (Pawar et al., 2008).

Postoperative Laryngectomy. The recently laryngectomized patient requires medical clearance to begin speech pathology services. The amount of time required after surgery varies, depending on the patient's health and physical recovery.

Once cleared, the ensuing assessment includes far more than oral-facial inspection. Yet the oral-facial region should be examined for structure and function as a part of the overall postoperative evaluation process.

Modifications to Chapter 2 and 3 procedures are significant. For example, since the patient no longer has a larynx, does not use the respiratory tract above the larynx, and has not yet participated in vocal restoration therapy, there is no need to complete any procedure that requires vocalization. Therefore, exclude the following:

- Conversational speech sample (i.e., part of Routine Clinical Observation 1)
- Velar movement (i.e., Routine Clinical Observation 6)
- Verbal diadochokinesis (i.e., Routine Clinical Observation 7)
- Vowel prolongation (i.e., Routine Clinical Observation 8)

Also, any other oral-facial inspection procedure that was performed preoperatively does not need to be repeated unless the surgery somehow changed the structure or function needed to perform the act. An obvious example of a situation requiring reinspection is the occasional individual who experienced a cerebrovascular accident since preoperative inspection.

With regard to protocol additions, if the patient was not seen preoperatively and has not yet been evaluated for pulmonary reserve, this issue should be tended as soon as the person receives medical clearance, particularly if tracheoesophageal speech is under consideration. This step is accomplished through medical referral.

Additional procedures for patients planning to use esophageal speech (i.e., Discretionary Clinical Observation 24) are inserted to give consideration to the person's candidacy for esophageal speech training. Clinical Question 43 (see Table 0–3) asks, "For the laryngectomized patient who plans to learn esophageal speech, does the evidence suggest candidacy for this method of alaryngeal speech?" An answer of *yes* is a positive prognostic indicator for examinees. Some guidelines that may be useful for evaluating candidacy for esophageal speech are provided.

Many laryngectomized patients select esophageal speech as their long-term vocal restoration goal. Furthermore, patients who choose tracheoesophageal puncture generally need an alternate mode of communication. Many choose esophageal speech for that purpose, and some find that they prefer esophageal speech over tracheoesophageal speech once they have learned both methods.

A few skills are potentially useful in predicting whether a person is a good candidate for esophageal speech (Berlin, 1963). These should be interpreted as guidelines only and are not intended to eliminate potential candidates without giving them the opportunity to make progress with the benefit of direct clinical teaching.

The first skill relates to tongue strength and agility. To use esophageal speech, the speaker should demonstrate the ability to use the tongue to inject air into the esophagus while at the same time use it to articulate with precision. Clinical teaching and practice are required.

The next four skills assume that the speaker has already successfully injected air into the esophagus. If the person has not yet done so at the time of the oral-facial inspection, these activities can be tabled until that goal has been accomplished. Since esophageal speech is difficult to learn and requires much practice, the person's success with the following four activities may be helpful in gauging proficiency expectations or anticipated rate of treatment progress.

- The ability to use the esophagus to phonate reliably on demand. Ask the examinee to inject air and use it to phonate the vowel /ɑ/ for as long as possible, preferably for at least 0.4 seconds. Then repeat for 20 trials.
- A short latency between inflating the esophagus and esophageal vocalization. Instruct the person to inject air and use it to phonate /ɑ/ as soon as possible after

injecting the air. Then repeat for 10 trials. The expectation is for the latency time between injection and phonation to not exceed 0.6 seconds.

- Adequate duration of esophageal phonation. Instruct the patient to inject air, use it to say /ɑ/, and hold the vowel for as long as possible. Repeat for 10 trials. The expectation is for the examinee to repeatedly sustain the vowel for 2.2 seconds or more.
- Ability to sustain esophageal phonation during articulation. Instruct the examinee to

inject air, then use it to say the syllable /dɑ/ repeatedly for eight trials. The expectation is for the patient to produce the eight syllables on only one injection.

Conclusion

This concludes the instructions for completing an oral-facial inspection. Proceed to Chapter 5 for information on how to interpret the data once they are collected.

CHAPTER 4

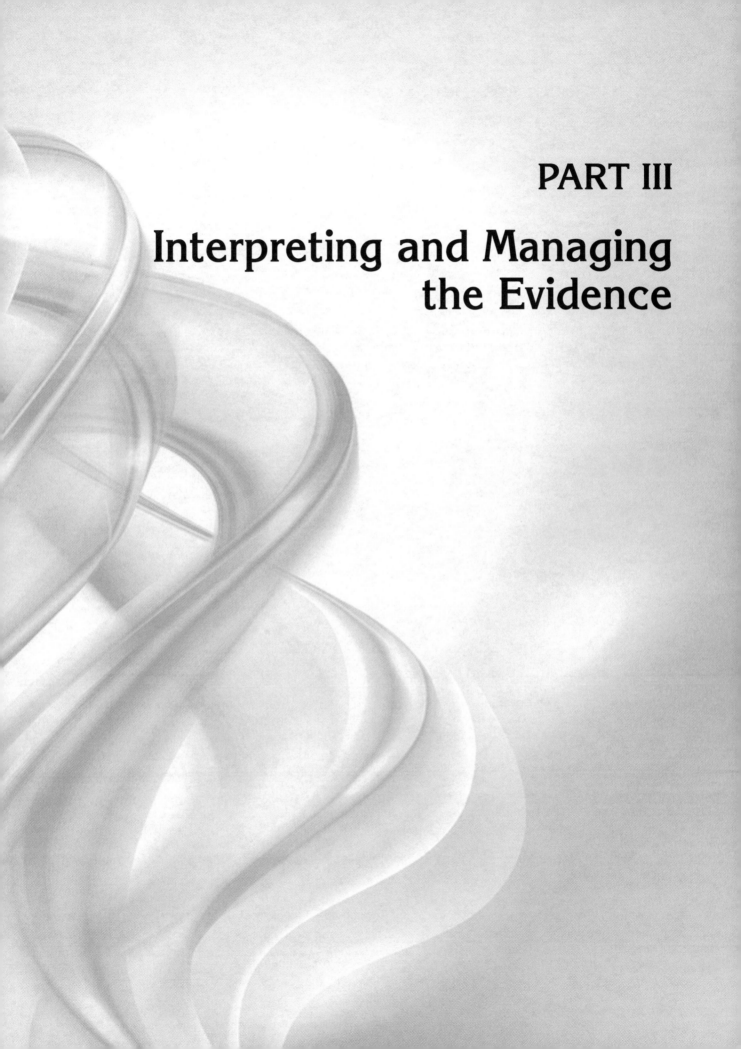

PART III
Interpreting and Managing the Evidence

5

Interpreting the Findings

Chapters 1 through 4 propose a structure that is useful for gathering evidence associated with basic oral-facial inspection according to a series of relevant clinical questions. The crux of Chapter 5, then, is to support clinicians for assessing and interpreting findings, so as to facilitate individualized evidence-based clinical decisions.

By way of review, oral-facial inspection may or may not result in remarkable findings. When it does, consider that more information is often needed for the sake of drawing accurate conclusions that lead to meaningful and relevant clinical decisions. One important feature of this chapter is that, while guiding interpretation of noteworthy findings, it distinguishes between findings that are diagnostic, findings that prompt additional within-discipline testing, and findings that alert the examiner to a need for external referral.

Overview of the Interpreting Process

The flowchart in Figure 5–1 illustrates one perspective of the interpretation process. It assumes routine procedures are performed along with any discretionary procedures deemed necessary, the proper recording form is completed, and the full array of evidence is available for consideration. The first act of interpreting the evidence is to judge whether recording form data support the statement that *all anatomic parts presumed necessary for speech are present, intact, and functioning* (Figure 5–1 and Table 0–2). Visually scan the completed recording form for minus signs (–) to make this determination.

Since the oral-facial inspection is only a small part of the comprehensive communication evaluation (see Table 0–1), results of *all* testing must be considered in concert to arrive at meaningful insight relative to the presenting communication disorder. That is, consider all evidence before making clinical decisions. Furthermore, recognize that the oral-facial inspection has potential to identify or rule out physical symptoms that explain disordered speech or call for special attention, highlight a need for referral, or even call attention to idiosyncrasies that have no relevance to speech.

When All Parts Are Present, Intact, and Functioning

Whenever the recording form highlights no feature as noteworthy, the simple lack of physically atypical evidence supports categorizing the person's idiosyncratic speaking pattern as *functional*, not organic. Be aware that the functional category best suits the evidence for most examinees.

For individuals whose oral-facial inspection reveals no physical explanation, evidence that results from other evaluation procedures may become the point of reference when building the foundation of an effective plan of care. Although failure to identify an organic etiology perhaps seems anticlimactic at first glance, the lack of physical evidence eliminates a host of possible next steps, while at the same time it clearly defines certain parameters that affect diagnosis, prognosis, and plan of care.

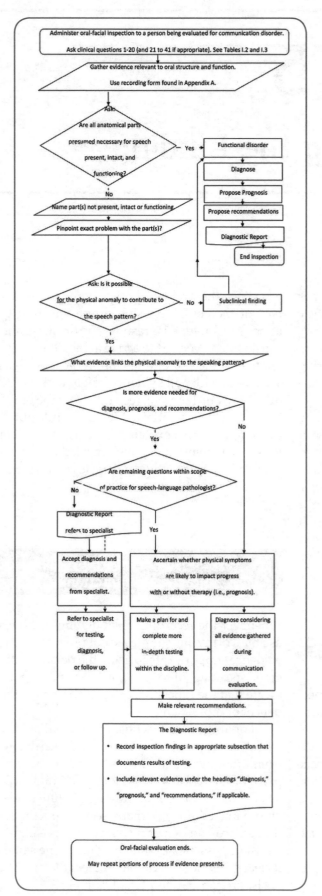

Figure 5–1. Flowchart showing overview of the clinical decision-making process.

When at Least One Anatomic Part Is Not Present, Intact, or Functioning

The recording form is set up to flag remarkable anatomic and physiologic features. Interpreting the findings, then, requires that one judge whether the evidence suggests a relationship between a physical anomaly and a communication disorder.

To do this, identify exactly which anatomic parts are marked as noteworthy and then pinpoint the exact nature of the concern with that part. Once that is done, compare the evidence to identified speech symptoms and judge whether the evidence gathered potentially explains the speaking pattern.

When Atypical Physical Symptoms Are Present But Deemed Not Clinically Relevant

For many people with physical symptoms, evidence does not directly link identified physical traits with speech production irregularities, classifying the exhibited communication disorder as *functional*. For instance, a velum that appears short upon inspection, although atypical, may be judged as a subclinical finding if the examinee displays neither symptoms of hypernasal resonance nor difficulty creating intraoral pressure for obstruent consonants. When physical idiosyncrasies seem to have no clinical relevance, since diagnosis, prognosis, and recommendations address speech symptoms directly, little if any reference may be made to physical structure or function, even though structural anomalies are identified.

When Atypical Physical Symptoms Are Judged as Clinically Relevant

For some individuals, the oral-facial evidence exposes that something is physically awry, *and* the anomaly is judged useful for explaining a particular speaking pattern. The communication disorder in this case is classified as *organic*. Although across the board, this type of diagnosis applies to a minority of examinees, the organic versus functional distinction is consequential to both follow-up and plan of care.

For organic communication disorders, identify exactly which parts show evidence of irregularity, specify the exact nature of the concerns, and describe the presumed relationship between the speaking pattern and physical idiosyncrasy. Sometimes the connection between speech pattern and physical anomaly is obvious. For instance, the observation that an examinee's velar tissue is nearly absent or minimal leaves little or no doubt that the physical feature likely explains hypernasal resonance concomitant to difficulty creating intraoral pressure for obstruent consonants.

Nevertheless, judging the evidence for clinical relevancy can be challenging when symptoms are less obvious, when they occur concomitantly to a host of other symptoms, or when the oral-facial inspection reveals that additional evidence is needed. That is, in the above example, a short or nearly absent velum was observed for an examinee with hypernasal resonance and compromised intraoral pressure for obstruent consonants. For that person, the standard of care is to follow up by referring to otorhinolaryngology or a craniofacial team, which can then evaluate the condition from an interdisciplinary perspective, using instrumentation to definitively describe velar function, thereby adding evidence that sheds substantial light on the person's speech production pattern. In this situation, medical follow-up takes precedence in preparing the immediate within-discipline plan of care, as is often the case whenever oral-facial inspection exposes an organic explanation for speech production idiosyncrasies.

When Additional Testing Is Needed

Referrals That Involve Professionals Outside of the Speech-Language Pathology Discipline. When testing outside of the discipline is needed, the next step is to refer the examinee to the appropriate team or professional, with a recommendation to address a particular clinical question or area of concern, but does not include recommending a specific procedure that is outside the examining clinician's scope. For example, when referring the above-mentioned person to a craniofacial team, the appropriate recommendation requests an assessment of velar structure and function and respectfully omits references to a particular test or follow-up procedure, leaving specific decisions to the discretion of the team. This is done despite the strong possibility that the referring clinician may be well aware of available options.

Furthermore, when referring outside the discipline, it is possible that the formal diagnosis, prognosis, and recommendations need to be tabled until all conclusive evidence is in. Tentative diagnosis, prognosis, and recommendations may be in place pending additional information, and recommendations should clearly include entries that direct the purposeful completion of all data collection. This affects the exact flavor of the diagnostic report that immediately follows the evaluation session, a topic to be addressed in more detail in Chapter 6.

Table 5–1 displays suggestions that link symptom patterns to possible referral recipients. Consult it as needed when considering a referral.

Recommendations for Further Testing Within Speech-Language Pathology. The potential always exists for an oral-facial inspection to end with additional within-discipline questions that should receive a response in the immediate future. Sometimes this happens due to short supply of time or client attention span, which can hamper the goal of completing a full array of tests during the communication evaluation, but it can also result from a need for a procedure that is not part of the oral-facial inspection (Table 5–2).

Regardless, additional within-discipline testing can usually be recommended and completed within the context of diagnostic therapy or even through scheduling an additional session. Again, this situation may affect the amount of detail that can be included in the immediately ensuing diagnostic report, especially with regard to diagnosis, prognosis, and recommendations.

Evaluating Routine and Discretionary Clinical Observations

Chapters 2 through 4 link routine and discretionary clinical procedures to specific clinical questions (see Table 0–3), and the corresponding recording form guides documentation for noteworthy symptoms. The focus of this section is on potential clinical applicability for particular symptoms marked as noteworthy on the individual recording form and using that evidence to address relevant clinical questions.

Consider Evidence Resulting From Routine Clinical Observation 1: Conversational Speech Sample

Unlike all other clinical observations that comprise the oral-facial inspection protocol that we provide, the conversational speech sample does not seek to expose or rule out structural or functional irregularities. Instead, it sheds light on audible manifestations that characterize the communication disorder in connected speech, consequently highlighting concerns with specified anatomic and physiologic features that may become the focal point during the physical inspection.

Implications of an Atypical Speaking Pattern

Clinical Question 1 (see Table 0–3) asks, "Does the conversational speech sample reveal a specific atypical speaking pattern that should be further explored during a later portion of the inspection so as to discover whether the speaking pattern has an organic etiology potentially affecting the plan of care?" An answer of *yes* is remarkable.

Since the oral-facial inspection is done to explore whether there is a physical explanation for an already identified atypical speaking pattern, generally the conversation highlights at least one idiosyncratic pattern in connected speech. The speech pattern may then partially define parameters for the remainder of the inspection.

The nature of the speech concern influences how the evidence is handled. For example, some examinees enter the evaluation process with communication concerns for which there is no known associated pathology. This includes some people who have difficulty expressing themselves through their first language, as well as people requesting assistance with regard to second-language learning or dialectal difference. Conversely, other examinees enter the process with an already identified or suspect pathology that may or may not contribute to the communication concerns. These two groups have markedly different needs, so they are discussed separately.

Table 5–1. When to Refer for External Testing Based on Findings

Specialist to Receive Referral	Symptoms	Comments
Primary care physician (PCP)	Evidence of illness, infection, allergy, or abnormal behavior: these may include inflammation, swelling, rash, excessive mucous or drainage, coughing, sneezing, lethargy, complaints of generalized aches and pains, symptoms of fever, headache, preoccupation with an ear, scratching, redness in the eyes, wheezing or any breathing difficulty, and behavioral concerns such as pica or vocal tic	Since it is outside scope of practice to distinguish between infection and allergy, the referral can be made to the PCP with the understanding that the diagnosis will be made and the patient will be referred if needed as part of the treatment plan
Otorhinolaryngology	Evidence of craniofacial anomaly: this may include compromised integrity of any structural part (e.g., lips, palate, velum) or perceived resonance disorder	If uncertain as to which specialist should evaluate the examinee, refer to the PCP with a report of known evidence and request evaluation and follow-up.
	Perceptible evidence of vocal misuse or vocal pathology	More often than not, a doctor-patient relationship is already in place. Refer for evaluation if it is not; request permission to communicate with the doctor if the relationship is established.
Genetics specialist	Evidence of symptoms appearing in a cluster	
	Evidence of atypical physical traits or facial dimensions	
	Dental symptoms: missing teeth, malformed teeth, transversions (if accompanied by other symptoms)	
Craniofacial team	If considering referrals to both otorhinolaryngology and genetics, the examinee may be well served by a referral to a craniofacial team for multidisciplinary evaluation and follow-up	
Pulmonologist	Any person with shortness of breath	
	Laryngectomee: prior to tracheoesophageal puncture surgery	
Allergist	Any person who reports rhinitis symptoms to be seasonal	
	Any symptoms of contact dermatitis (e.g., recurring rash)	
Oral surgeon	Ankyloglossia	

continues

CHAPTER 5

133

Table 5–1. *continued*

Specialist to Receive Referral	Symptoms	Comments
Neurologist	Evidence of neuromotor involvement: this includes symptoms of apraxia or dysarthria, difficulty swallowing, asymmetry of any kind either at rest or in motion, fasciculation, tremor, spasm, or muscle fatigue	If uncertain as to which specialist should evaluate the examinee, refer to the PCP with a report of known evidence and request evaluation and follow-up. More often than not, a doctor-patient relationship is already in place. Refer for evaluation if it is not; request permission to communicate with the doctor if the relationship is established.
	History of neurologic incident: cerebrovascular accident, traumatic injury, or neurologic disease. Typically, a relationship with a neurologist is already in place for this group; refer if this is not the case.	
Ophthalmologist	Failed amblyopia screening (birth-to-5 population only)	
	Holding visual materials close to the face or away from the face	
	Squinting when working with visual stimuli	
	Complaints about not being able to focus or see clearly	
Orthodontist	Evidence of concerns with dental alignment, bite, or occlusion	Some dental problems can occur in a cluster, thus indicating a need for genetic evaluation. These individuals may best be served by a referral to a craniofacial team, since an orthodontist typically participates as a team member.
Dentist	Evidence of poor dental hygiene	
	Deformed or developmentally absent dentition	
	Supernumary teeth	
	Suspected temporomandibular joint disorder	
	Evidence of bruxism	
Prosthedontist	Evidence of poorly fitted dentures: this may include report of painful dentures, imprecise articulation associated with dentures, or dentures that appear to move during speech or at rest	
Speech-language pathologist with specialized training	Any complex disorder for which the examining clinician does not have specialized training or experience. These may include • Motor-speech disorder • Resonance disorder • Palatal cleft or other anomaly • Deafness • Voice disorders	

Table 5–2. When to Recommend Additional Speech-Language Testing Based on Findings

Referral	Sample Indicators
Speech-language pathologist with specialist training	Suspecting a disorder or condition that the examiner does not have adequate experience or education to diagnose with confidence
Diagnostic therapy	Examinee exhibits evidence of needing desensitization or additional training to participate fully (e.g., child examinee who resists compliance with inspection procedures)
	Not enough time to complete the full evaluation due to attention limitations or complex symptoms

Atypical Speaking Pattern for Which There Is No Known or Suspected Physical Explanation. When an examinee presents with communication idiosyncrasies in a first language and there is no known physical explanation, determining whether there is a physical anomaly that can explain or partially explain the speaking pattern is of particular interest and foundational to interpreting all findings beyond this point. For instance, if hyponasal resonance is noted during connected speech, portions of the inspection that are likely to yield information on nasal cavity clearance take on a high priority once the speaking pattern has been identified. Similarly, imprecise lingua-palatal fricatives and affricates (i.e., /ʃ/, /ʒ/, /tʃ/, /dʒ/) may highlight the need to closely examine tongue size, palatal arch configuration, and tongue mobility.

On the other hand, for people who request assistance with second-language learning or dialect, interpreting the evidence involves no attempt at finding an explanation for a disorder but instead focuses on ruling out physical concerns that may hinder acquiring and applying a new set of speech production rules. Therefore, identifying speech patterns in conversation can lead to exploring whether the differences reflect characteristics of the person's first language or dialect, while also alerting the clinician to use oral-facial inspection to explore whether any physical barriers likely prevent adding features to the person's existing repertoire.

For instance, in an example above, a native-English speaker exhibited symptoms of hyponasal speech. Extend that example to include a person with language or dialectal difference. Even if a lesser degree of nasal resonance were to be a trait of the person's original language or dialect, it behooves the examiner to look into nasal cavity clearance to judge whether American English resonance is physiologically attainable. Furthermore, using a different example, if a native Spanish speaker were to devoice certain voiced consonants of English, one would want to identify exactly which voiced consonants are devoiced and compare them to the phonological system associated with the Spanish language before proceeding with any procedures that look more closely at the laryngeal system.

Atypical Speaking Pattern for Which There Is an Identified or Suspect Physical Explanation. In some cases, the examinee enters the oral-facial inspection having already received a medical diagnosis that places the person at risk for communication disorder, such as craniofacial anomaly, a particular syndrome, or history of a neurologic episode. Since a biologically based irregularity is already identified, the goal is to ascertain the degree to which known physical symptoms contribute to the speaking pattern. This is not to the neglect of the possibility that in some cases, the inspection can serve to unveil previously unidentified structural and functional irregularities that should also be considered.

Implications Relative to Intelligibility Rating

Clinical Question 2 (see Table 0–3) asks, "Is the intelligibility rating in connected speech judged as fair, poor, or unintelligible?" An *affirmative* response is remarkable.

The intelligibility rating is fundamental to any communication evaluation. It can be useful when determining the overall impact that the disorder imposes on communication success, regardless of whether the inspection reveals, confirms, or rules out anatomic or physiologic irregularity. Including intelligibility rating in oral-facial inspection ensures that impact on communication success is considered for all examinees.

Implications Relative to Audible Symptoms Immediately Following a Swallow

Clinical Question 3 (see Table 0–3) asks, "Is a spontaneous swallow while at rest or during speech, followed immediately by cough or noticeable change in vocal quality?" A response of *yes* is remarkable.

For examinees with a history of recent neurologic episode or laryngectomy, dysphagia screening is a routine part of the communication evaluation. So for clients with that history, the prompt for dysphagia screening is not needed. Yet, some adults without laryngectomy or known neurologic history may also present the need for dysphagia screening, and symptoms can be detected during conversational speech. If the prompt for dysphagia screening is flagged, oral feeding should be discontinued, and screening should be performed before making a decision to resume normal eating activities.

Consider Evidence From Routine Clinical Observation 1: Facial Region Inspection

Clinical Question 4 (see Table 0–3) asks, "Does the facial-region inspection reveal any externally observable anomalies of the face or head that may either interfere with speech or guide a specialist referral?" A response of *yes* is remarkable.

When Observable Facial Anomalies Potentially Interfere With Speech

Some facial observations may suggest neurologic involvement, nasal cavity obstruction, a history of oral-facial surgery, evidence of mouth breathing, posture that is disadvantageous to speech production, or the presence of an undiagnosed syndrome. A general set of symptoms, accompanied by relevant commentary, is displayed in Table 5–3.

When Observable Facial Anomalies Lead to Specialist Consultation. Table 2–2 lists selected features of the face and head that may suggest consulting with medical professionals who specialize in genetics or otorhinolaryngology. The list is not comprehensive, and any craniofacial irregularity, even if not listed, normally mandates a genetic referral.

If *facial proportions* are of concern, and if the examinee has no established relationship with otorhinolaryngology or genetics, more detailed information about the exact nature of the facial irregularities can corroborate a referral. Although estimating facial dimensions should not be used to rule out the need for a referral when facial proportions seem atypical, the evidence that results from performing it can strengthen the referral if one is needed.

In some cases of facial dysmorphia, a *syndrome may be suspected*. However, precisely identifying or ruling out a syndrome is outside the scope of practice for speech-language pathologists. Although not all syndromes are genetically based, genetic specialists are best prepared to interpret the evidence when any type of syndrome is under consideration. Genetic consultation may be accomplished through a craniofacial team or through the child's primary care physician, depending on the circumstance.

When Craniofacial Evidence Suggests Compromised Palatal Integrity

Sometimes the external craniofacial evidence suggests a breach in integrity of bony, muscular, and mucosal framework that normally separates the oral and nasal cavities or even another structural anomaly of the head or face, implying the need for reconstructive surgery. Clearly, evidence of this magnitude is normally noticed from a medical perspective prior to speech-language evaluation, and in fact, the speech-language pathologist is more likely to be the recipient of the referral when patently obvious physical symptoms are present.

Table 5–3. Facial-Region Symptoms Sorted by Potential Implications

Possible Clinical Implication	Indicators Noted During Facial Inspection	Suggestions for Follow-up and Other Comments
Neurologic involvement	Facial asymmetry at rest or in motion	• Refer to neurology if patient-doctor relationship is not already established
	Asymmetrical angles of the mouth	• Refer for motor-speech disorders testing
	Ptosis of any feature	• Additional opportunities to observe evidence of motor-speech disorders occur throughout routine inspection
	Jaw that seems to hang open at rest	
	Fasciculations in perioral region	
	Unequal elevation of mouth angles during spontaneous smile	
	Poor saliva management	
Nasal airflow obstruction	Small nares	• Refer for medical evaluation (primary care physician or otorhinolaryngology)
	Flat nasal bridge	• Discretionary-Clinical Observation 9 (i.e., Nasal-Cavity Clearance Screening) may have merit
	Nasal asymmetry	
History of oral-facial surgery secondary to craniofacial anomaly	Flat nasal tip	• Seek clarification relative to medical history
	Scarring of any kind (e.g., scarring of cupid's bow, facial scarring)	• Promote existing relationship with medical service providers
	Flat zygomas	• Ascertain prognosis for additional progress in therapy
Mouth breathing	Open-mouth posture at rest	• Refer to physician if suspecting congestion, allergies
	Poor saliva management	• Refer to otorhinolaryngology if suspecting upper respiratory inflammation associated with adenoid facies
	Visible features associated with adenoid facies (i.e., mouth breathing, shortening of the upper lip, and elongated face)	• Consider Discretionary Clinical Observation 9 (i.e., nasal cavity clearance screening)
	Poor facial muscle tone	• Increase awareness when observing for malocclusion
		• Consider that mouth-open posture may be due to habit secondary to a previous nasal cavity obstruction
		• Consider medical referral since air that does not pass through the nasal passages is essentially unfiltered; mouth breathing can lead to illness, asthma, sleep apnea, and other airway conditions
		• When accompanied by forward-tongue posturing, open-mouth posture can turn out to be one of the many indicators to consider when deciding whether to screen for tongue-thrust swallow

continues

Table 5–3. *continued*

Possible Clinical Implication	Indicators Noted During Facial Inspection	Suggestions for Follow-up and Other Comments
Posture that is disadvantageous to speech production, especially if audible symptoms imply vocal tension, limited mandibular excursion, or concerns with respiration	Stiffness or tightness in the neck, jaw, shoulders, or scapula Habitual shoulder elevation	• Any postural evidence that points to the possibility of jaw or neck tension, or limited mandibular movement should be considered sufficient evidence to perform temporomandibular joint disorder screening (Discretionary Clinical Observation 11) • If postural concerns accompany audible symptoms of vocal tension, evidence is sufficient to mandate screening for laryngeal and respiratory efficiency (Discretionary Clinical Observation 19) • If addressing a voice disorder, postural work may become a treatment target
Syndrome	Craniofacial anomaly co-occurs with other anatomic or physiologic irregularities (e.g., comorbid features, symptom cluster)	• Refer to genetic specialist for evaluation • Consider referral to craniofacial anomaly team

Consider the Evidence From Routine Clinical Observation 1: Respiration at Rest and During Speech

Clinical Question 5 (see Table 0–3) asks, "Do observations of breathing reveal any pattern that may impede normal, fluid, and properly resonant speech?" Evidence that yields an affirmative response is noteworthy.

Normal Versus Atypical Breathing

Normally, resting respiration is accomplished efficiently via the nasal orifices, requiring no conscious effort. The only discernible manifestation, if any, should be a slight inaudible and rhythmic expansion and contraction of the abdomen or possibly the lower thorax.

As a rule, from a speech-language pathology perspective, breathing is only a cause for concern if it calls attention to itself, interferes with normal speech fluidity or resonance, in some way prevents the person from achieving personal or professional communication goals, or if it causes physical strain leading to vocal pathology. If noting breathing patterns that seem to affect speech, consider the types of clinically relevant breathing that are described below.

Clinically Relevant Breathing Patterns. One clinically relevant breathing pattern is *short exhalation cycle*. Normally, the exhalation cycle is at least twice as long as the inhalation cycle, even at rest. During speech, the exhalation cycle can be considerably more than twice the duration of the inhalation phase, depending on the speaking activity (Bauman-Waengler, 2011; Boone, McFarlane, Von Berg, & Zraick, 2010; Seikel, King, & Drumright, 2010).

A short exhalation cycle can be recognized by audible symptoms such as short phrasing, running out of air quickly during speech, or gasping for air at the end of phrases. Short exhalation cycle is often an indicator of shallow breath support (e.g., upper-thoracic or clavicular breathing discussed below). The pattern can be habitual or can have its origin in problems with the person's pulmonary, neurologic, or immune system.

Shallow breath support and short exhalation cycle clearly overlap. Audible manifestations of shallow breath support, however, include not only short phrasing and frequent interruptions for air intake but also features such as low volume and poor voice projection. Generally, breathing is considered shallow if it does not adequately support fluid speech. As with short exhalations for speech, shallow breath support can have its origin in the person's pulmonary, neurologic, or immune systems.

Two types of shallow breathing are relevant to the discussion. They are thoracic and clavicular breathing. Furthermore, some distinguish between upper thoracic and lower thoracic breathing since many individuals function quite well using lower thoracic breathing for speech, whereas upper thoracic breathing is generally too shallow to support free-flowing speech of adequate volume.

Since using *thoracic breathing* habitually to project the voice is not efficient and may lead to vocal pathology, if thoracic breathing is noted for individuals who exhibit symptoms of vocal pathology or misuse, this is clinically relevant, especially for people whose lifestyle or career requires frequent vocal projection (e.g., teachers, public speakers, vocalists, actors). Furthermore, thoracic breathing in children has been associated with symptoms of poorly controlled asthma (Boone et al., 2010; Courtney, 2013). Therefore, if a child presents with aberrant voice quality or possible symptoms of breathing disorder concomitant to thoracic breathing at any level, this should be considered remarkable.

Clavicular breathing is even shallower than thoracic. Clavicular breathers use airflow inefficiently, while also placing unnecessary strain on the accessory neck muscles, particularly the sternocleidomastoid, potentially increasing laryngeal tension. Thus, clavicular breathing not only provides inadequate breath support for speech but also can be associated with phonatory disorders (Boone et al., 2010; Iwarsson, 2001). Clavicular breathing is always remarkable.

Mouth breathing was addressed under a similar heading when considering the topic that spoke to facial observations, since open-mouth posture is a cardinal symptom of using the oral orifice for breathing. Refer to that section and corresponding table (see Table 5–3) if respiratory observations expose a pattern of mouth breathing.

Problems coordinating breathing for speech are also noteworthy. Specifically, we will discuss the impact of using residual air or the inspiratory phase of the breathing cycle when speaking.

The prominent audible features of *speaking-on-residual air* are glottal fry, stridor, short phrasing, weak volume, and inability to project the voice. Laryngeal tension that manifests as strained voice quality is also associated with the pattern. Since many deaf and hard-of-hearing individuals have not had consistent access to strategic listening practice for spoken-language learning, it is common for some deaf and hard-of-hearing people to miss the audible cues that facilitate the coordination of breathing for speech. Essentially, under the circumstance of compromised hearing, speaking on residual air can be considered a habit that the person is capable of unlearning and replacing with a new breathing-for-speech pattern. Prognosis for making this change depends the person's age, motivation, and the extent to which the pattern is habitualized.

Speaking on residual air, specifically at the end of phrases, can also be linked to cultural orientation or even generation. Again, under this circumstance, the pattern is typically habitual and should be addressed therapeutically if associated with vocal abuse or vocal pathology. The pattern can also be associated with some neurologic findings and with shortness of breath.

Few individuals *attempt to speak on the inspiratory phase of the breathing cycle*, and the vocal symptoms are clearly recognizable, distinctly characterized by glottal fry, stridor, and laryngeal tension. Most often this pattern is habitual and one possible vocal attribute associated with deafness due to insufficient access to audible cues for coordinating breathing with speech as described above. Habitual use of this ineffective breath support pattern is vocally abusive and can result in vocal pathology. Immediate attention is warranted.

Breath Support for Alaryngeal Speech. A small subgroup of examinees are about to undergo or recently underwent laryngectomy, and many select tracheoesophageal puncture and hands-free valve as their first choice for alaryngeal speech. One physical requirement for the tracheoesophageal puncture surgery is breath support that is sufficient to force the ascending airflow through the artificial valve for alaryngeal voice production.

Since the need for laryngectomy is often associated with cancer secondary to a long-term history of exposure to toxins, in many cases lung tissue has been compromised by the same chemical-environmental events that led to laryngeal demise, making laryngectomees a high-risk group for pulmonary insufficiency. Any evidence of shortness of breath or shallow breathing is a negative prognostic indicator if tracheoesophageal puncture is being considered.

More evidence related to breath support is gathered throughout the course of oral-facial inspection. However, the most reliable way to evaluate breath support in this population is to refer to a specialist for pulmonary function evaluation.

Referral and Follow-Up for Breathing Concerns

Generally, when a person does not appear to have adequate airflow to support fluid speech, medical referral should be made to assess lung function (e.g., pulmonologist). This is especially true if wheezing or other noises accompany either the examinee's inhalation or exhalation cycle.

Although in many cases, concerns with breath support may be addressed through *pulmonary evaluation*, the full explanation may not be entirely exposed through that measure. That is, if an examinee recently experienced a neurologic episode or exhibits other symptoms of neurologic decline (e.g., myasthenia gravis), and the breathing concerns appeared at approximately the same time, then a *neurologic referral* is advised. This is particularly true if the examinee shows symptoms of neurologic involvement as evidenced by performance on a full range of routine and selected discretionary clinical observations as well as other clinical observations, some unrelated to the procedures described in this manual.

On the other hand, some examinees report or display symptoms of hypersensitive immune system (i.e., allergies). For them, breath support issues may best be addressed by a referral to an *allergist*.

Finally, breathing concerns can occur due to *habit*. If breathing patterns are habitual and if they interfere with speech, then addressing them becomes

part of the examinee's treatment plan. Yet, stating that the concerns stem from no identifiable organic origin may be risky. Thus, perhaps a better practice in many cases may be to refer the person for medical evaluation and medical clearance before proceeding with a therapeutic program, even if suspecting no organic etiology.

Consider Evidence Resulting From Routine Clinical Observation 2: Assess Lips and Tongue for Mobility and Strength

Clinical Question 6 (see Table 0–3) asks, "When inspecting lips and tongue for strength and mobility, does the examinee exhibit irregularities that potentially explain atypical articulation errors noted during speech?" Evidence that results in an affirmative answer to this question is noteworthy.

Lip Symptoms

Two procedures in this section afford opportunity to observe *lip strength*. They are *lip seal* and *lip resistance*. Five procedures provide opportunity to observe the lips in motion. *Lip mobility* procedures include *pucker the lips, spread the lips, sustain an exaggerated /u/ sound, quick repetitions of bilabial consonants,* and *smack the lips.* If any lip strength or mobility exercise yields noteworthy findings, this is clinically relevant under conditions of imprecise bilabial consonants, history of neurologic incident, injury to the immature nervous system, other evidence of neurologic findings, labial asymmetry, relevant scar tissue, or other evidence of lip surgery or labial cleft.

Tongue Strength and Mobility

One procedure focuses on *tongue strength*: *tongue resistance*. The five *tongue mobility* exercises include *tongue protrusion, tongue elevation, tongue lateralization, wiggle tongue* to left and right, and *tongue rotation*.

If any tongue strength or mobility exercise results in a noteworthy outcome, this is clinically relevant if concomitant to imprecise lingual consonants, history of neurologic incident, injury to the immature nervous system, other evidence of neurologic findings, tongue asymmetry, or evidence of surgery to remove the tongue or a portion of it. Clinically relevant tongue symptoms might also include extraneous movements that interfere with discrete and purposeful actions required for efficient connected speech (e.g., jerking, writhing, dystonia, involuntary movements associated with chorea and athetosis), poorly differentiated movements, weakness, flaccidity, or deviation.

Structural Features of the Tongue

When observing the tongue for strength and mobility, be aware of the structural features that may become evident either at rest or in motion. Specifically, *asymmetry* and *atrophy* are both noteworthy if observed.

Clinical Implications of Lip and Tongue Structure, Strength and Mobility

If the examinee displays any of the lip or tongue symptoms described above and is not already under medical care for the condition, a medical referral is in order. Referring to neurology or otorhinolaryngology depends on whether symptoms affect performance or structure. Also, observations for apraxia should be considered when motor programming seems to be the main concern, whereas observations for dysarthria are appropriate when concerns relate to strength and mobility.

Ankyloglossia

Tongue mobility activities give opportunity to examine the length of the frenum, shape of the tongue tip, and freedom of tongue movement. These observations are useful for identifying individuals who display symptoms of ankyloglossia.

Symptoms of ankyloglossia are only of clinical concern when occurring concomitant to poorly articulated tongue-tip sounds since the condition does not always interfere with speech. As stated previously, humans have an excellent capacity to compensate for anatomic idiosyncrasy. Thus, it is entirely possible for a person to produce the standard lingua-alveolar, lingua-palatal, and lingua-dental consonants without elevating the tongue to the alveolar

ridge; furthermore lingua-dental consonants require minimal tongue-tip elevation.

Speech-language pathologists are quite capable of reliably recognizing ankyloglossia by viewing the tongue tip, lingual frenum length, and freedom of movement, yet ankyloglossia is a medical condition that should be evaluated by a physician who should also be involved in plan of care. Therefore, when observing the features of ankyloglossia, a medical referral is the next appropriate step (e.g., oral surgeon).

In some cases, as a result of the referral, the specialist arranges for surgery to clip the lingual frenum and thereby improve freedom of tongue movement. In other cases, the child is referred back to speech-language pathology with a suggestion to use exercises to stretch the lingual frenum, freeing up the tongue for movement without surgery. Generally, regardless of whether surgery is used, most children with clinically significant ankyloglossia return for speech therapy to address the articulatory problems that resulted from years of tongue immobility.

Consider the Evidence Resulting From Routine Clinical Observation 3: Dental Bite and Alignment

Clinical Question 7 (see Table 0–3) asks, "Does a systematic inspection of dentition reveal bite or alignment irregularities that potentially influence an identified atypical speaking pattern or imply a need for specialist referral?" If evidence supports an affirmative response to the question, the findings are noteworthy.

For the vast majority of examinees, atypical dental alignment and bite are subclinical findings. That is, most people naturally compensate when dentition is not optimal for speech. In some cases, however, follow-up is needed to resolve dental issues, facilitate compensatory strategies, or both.

Alignment and Bite Irregularities Not Affecting Speech

Even when dental alignment or bite is judged as clinically insignificant from a speech-language perspective, more often than not, from dental hygiene and cosmetic perspectives, misaligned dentition calls for orthodontic evaluation. Furthermore, if dental decay or poor dental hygiene is apparent, this is frequently revealed through inspecting the dentition and should result in referral for dental evaluation accompanied by a sensitively worded recommendation for oral hygiene education.

Evidence of bruxism can be recognized if biting surfaces appear worn down. Although not usually directly affecting speech, a dental referral is appropriate.

Alignment and Bite Irregularities That Influence Speech Sound Production

Depending on the way that alignment and bite irregularities influence airflow efficiency for sibilants, if they correspond to a speaking pattern that may be linked to the identified dental arrangement, speech sound stimulability screening can facilitate exploring whether effective compensatory strategies are within the examinee's immediate grasp. And if dental alignment or bite seems to contribute to the atypical communication pattern, an orthodontist should be consulted. Some possible ways that dental anomalies may partially explain atypical speaking patterns are shown in Table 5–4.

Since many people compensate well for dental irregularities, speech sound stimulability screening can provide an opportunity to observe the person's response to clinical teaching. If compensation is readily achieved, then this is a positive prognostic indicator, suggesting that the person is likely to benefit from therapy, regardless of orthodontic referral, and the referral for orthodontic evaluation can become optional. However, if stimulability is not achieved through clinical teaching, then an orthodontic referral could take a higher priority and perhaps become a recommendation as opposed to a simple suggestion.

Furthermore, some bite and alignment concerns can correspond to tongue-thrust swallow. Refer to that section for more information.

Table 5–4. Dental Alignment and Bite Irregularities That May Be Associated With Atypical Speaking Patterns

Speaking Pattern	Dental Alignment and Bite Irregularities That May Be Associated
Frontal lisp or imprecise or inefficient sibilants	• Open bite • Flared bite • Overjet • Frontal-edentulous space(s) • Generous frontal diastema • Large interdental space(s) between maxillary incisors or cuspids
Lateral lisp	• Infraversion of the lateral-central incisors or cuspids • Lateral open bite • Large interdental spaces on either side of the lateral incisors or cuspids
Imprecise articulation	• Supernumary teeth medial to the dental arch • Distoclusion or mesioclusion that results in improper lingua-palatal alignment

Dental Concerns That Lead to Genetic or Otorhinolaryngology Referral

Bear in mind that some dental concerns can be part of a symptom cluster that indicates a need for genetic or otorhinolaryngology referral. Some of these include edentulous spaces resulting from unerupted teeth past the expected time of eruption, malformed teeth, supernumary teeth, and dental transversions.

Dental Hygiene or Decay

While examining dentition, evidence of poor dental hygiene or even decay may become apparent. If either poor hygiene or decay is noticed, the observation is not only remarkable but, for reasons of health, mandates referral. Although the condition of the teeth rarely if ever interferes with speech, refer the examinee to the proper specialist for evaluation and follow-up.

Dental Appliances

The presence of a dental appliance may be noticed when inspecting the dentition as well. For most people who wear an appliance, such as dentures, the typical alignment, bite, and occlusion observations are not needed. However, if a person wearing an appliance reports pain, if imprecise articulation seems to be associated with the appliance, or if the prosthetic device is observed to move during speech or at rest, the person should be referred back to the prosthodontist to address the concerns.

Consider Evidence for Routine Clinical Observation 4: Dental Occlusion

An improper maxillary-mandibular relationship is relatively common. Although the condition can be associated with craniofacial anomaly or syndrome, malocclusion has no relationship to adverse clinical implications in and of itself. In fact, many people speak very well and demonstrate no need for specialist referral while exhibiting features of Class II or Class III malocclusion.

Four clinical questions are asked relative to occlusion. They are designed to help identify individuals for whom malocclusion is potentially clinically relevant.

Dental Occlusion and Craniofacial Anomaly

Clinical Question 8 (see Table 0–3) asks, "Does inspecting dental occlusion reveal a maxillary-mandibular relationship that implies craniofacial anomaly?" An affirmative response is remarkable.

For individuals whose maxillary-mandibular relationship is conspicuously out of the ordinary, specialist evaluation is in order. Facial dimension estimates may provide additional evidence to supplement the referral. Generally, otorhinolaryngology, orthodontics, or genetics should be considered as referral recipients when dental occlusion is misaligned.

When Maxillary-Mandibular Relationship Implies Symptom Cluster

Clinical Question 9 (see Table 0–3) asks, "Does inspecting dental occlusion reveal an atypical maxillary-mandibular relationship that may be considered one symptomatic element of a syndromic cluster to be diagnosed by a specialist?" An affirmative response is remarkable.

Class II and Class III malocclusions can contribute to diagnosis or referral relative to more complex issues when co-occurring with other atypical features of the face and head. Clusters of symptoms, as a general rule, suggest a need for referral to genetics or otorhinolaryngology for more in-depth testing and diagnosis.

When Maxillary-Mandibular Relationship Restricts Lingual Movement

Clinical Question 10 (see Table 0–3) asks, "Does inspecting dental occlusion reveal a maxillary-mandibular relationship that seems to reduce intraoral space available for tongue excursion?" An affirmative response is noteworthy.

In cases of extreme maxillary-mandibular misalignment, malocclusion decreases the amount of intraoral space, preventing the tongue from moving about freely for articulation and resonance. Refer to an otorhinolaryngologist or an orthodontist for evaluation if this is noted.

When the Maxillary-Mandibular Relationship Changes the Relationship Between Tongue and Palate

Clinical Question 11 (see Table 0–3) asks, "Does inspecting dental occlusion reveal a maxillary-mandibular relationship that seems to result in an improper alignment between the tongue and palatal surface, potentially affecting articulatory precision?" An affirmative response is noteworthy.

In extreme cases, malocclusion may result in tongue location that is out of alignment with the palatal and velar points of articulatory contact. For example, normally the tongue tip resides directly below the alveolar ridge, the bulk of the tongue blade resides directly below the palatal arch, and the posterior tongue blade resides directly below the velum. If severe Class II or Class III malocclusion is noted concomitant to articulatory imprecision for sound requiring lingua-alveolar, lingua-palatal, or lingua-velar contact, then the possibility of occlusion contributing to the articulatory imprecision should be considered, and otorhinolaryngology or orthodontic referral may be appropriate.

Consider Evidence for Routine Clinical Observation 5: Oral Interior

Mandibular Excursion

Clinical Question 12 (see Table 0–3) asks, "When asked to lower the jaw, does the examinee's mandible move with adequate excursion to allow for viewing the oral cavity?" A negative response is remarkable.

To examine the oral interior, the examinee must first lower the jaw and thereby open the mouth. If noting limited mandibular excursion or pain associated with movement, that symptom should lead to screening for temporomandibular joint disorder.

Mandibular Strength

Clinical Question 13 (see Table 0–3) asks, "When lowering and raising the jaw while the examiner manually applies resistance, does the examinee exert adequate strength to overcome the resistance and do to it symmetrically?" A negative response is noteworthy.

Also, before beginning to formally inspect the oral interior, observe mandibular strength. Note the examinee's response to examiner-imposed resistance, while attempting to open and close the jaw. Failure to overcome resistance in this way suggests muscular weakness, either bilaterally or unilaterally, and this flags the person as a possible candidate for neurology referral and dysarthria observations.

Structure and Function of the Oral Interior

Clinical Question 14 (see Table 0–3) asks, "Does inspecting the oral interior expose any structural irregularities, such as absent, damaged, or malfunctioning parts that may potentially explain or partially explain the examinee's idiosyncratic speaking pattern?" An affirmative response is noteworthy.

Coloring of Oral Interior. As a rule, abnormal coloring does not typically affect speech. Chapter 2 flags it as noteworthy because of the relationship between health of the mucosa and its physical appearance. Since the cause and treatment of mucosa color changes are not within the purview of speech-language pathologists for diagnosis or treatment, whenever color deviates from a healthy shade of pink, a medical referral is in order. The primary care physician is normally the most logical referral recipient.

The Tongue. Chapter 2 describes normal *tongue-surface texture* and then provides a short list of potentially remarkable surface textures. Deep grooves, deep crevices, or shriveled texture are all noteworthy because they may imply atrophy. If concomitant to symptoms of motor-speech disorder or history of neurologic episode and occurring with imprecise articulation, these findings may contribute to the diagnosis or result in referral for additional testing.

Other textural observations, although unlikely to affect speech, are potentially noteworthy for health reasons. Medical referral is appropriate.

As stated in Chapter 2, variations in tongue size are only considered remarkable if they co-occur with imprecise articulation, are associated with differences in resonance balance, or appear to be responsible for forced changes in the dental arch. Since humans have a remarkable capacity to compensate for variations in tongue size, clinical relevance is rare (Flipsen, Bankson, & Bernthal, 2009).

Small tongue size, also called *microglossia*, may result from heredity, atrophy, syndrome feature, or surgical excision, or in some cases, it may be a physical trait that has no tangible explanation. More often than not, the characteristic is clinically insignificant. In fact, many people who have little or no tongue can produce clear speech (Flipsen et al., 2009).

For some individuals, however, small tongue size is associated with atrophy secondary to neurologic incident or injury to the immature nervous system. In this case, a shriveled or grooved texture is likely to be apparent as well. When this occurs concomitantly to imprecise articulation, this may be considered a potential etiologic factor relative to the person's speaking pattern. Furthermore, this finding may lead to observations relative to dysarthria.

On the other hand, an excessively large tongue, also called *macroglossia*, can result in dental arch changes. Therefore, if large tongue size co-occurs with open bite, flared bite, overjet, or other dental arch or misalignment concerns, this may in some cases be consistent with the oral cavity's attempt to accommodate the exceptionally large tongue. Referral to otorhinolaryngology is advised so that changes in dental arch or alignment can be investigated. Furthermore, exploring whether the candidate compensates in response to clinical teaching can also provide clinically useful information.

Chapter 2 lists and illustrates some *tongue shapes* that may be considered remarkable if associated with articulatory imprecision (see Figures 2–4 through 2–6). A tongue tip that *is heart shaped* is typically associated with a short frenum, which may be first noticed when evaluating tongue elevation and should result in a medical referral; a *pointed tongue tip*, if concomitant to difficulty with tongue-tip sounds, may imply the need to explore speech sound stimulability. Furthermore, a tongue that is noted to be *asymmetrical* either at rest or in motion may be associated with neurologic findings, leading to dysarthria observations and possibly neurology referral.

Other idiosyncrasies of the tongue may also be observed. For example, *fasciculations*, intention or resting *tremor*, and *extraneous movements* are potential neurologic indicators, implying the possible need for neurologic consultation. If noted while at rest or in motion and if co-occurring with changes in articulation or resonance, they give reason to observe for symptoms of dysarthria.

Scar tissue is also a possible tongue observation and if observed should lead to a line of questioning to discover the origin of the scar. Although scar tissue has no clinical relevance when there is no corresponding impact on speech, if the location of the scar or its effect on tongue movement suggests a connection between it and the person's speaking pattern or a need for specialist referral, there is reason to explore whether clinical teaching results in compensatory strategies that improve articulation.

The Hard Palate. Observable features of the hard palate comprise the alveolar ridge, palatal arch, median palatal raphe, and mucous membrane (see Figure 2–27). These visible parts are described according to typical findings in Chapter 2, along with some information on findings that are remarkable.

Any *palatal feature marked as grossly irregular*, if associated with hypernasal speech or difficulty with pressure consonants, may suggest cleft (see Figure 2–28A), fistulus (see Figure 2–28B), or even submucous cleft of the hard palate. In this case, medical referral (e.g., otorhinolaryngology or genetics) is needed unless already established or in process, and screening for submucous cleft can provide useful information to augment the referral.

Ideally, the *spatial relationship between the alveolar ridge and tongue tip* was ascertained when inspecting dental occlusion, with an additional opportunity to take a look at it when inspecting the hard palate. The clinical relevance of atypical alignment is clearly related to whether distortions are noted when listening to consonants that require lingual contact or approximation with the alveolar ridge, hard palate, or velum. Speech sound stimulability screening and otorhinolaryngology referral should be considered if it appears that the tongue is not adequately aligned with the palate for precise articulation, in addition to referral for medical evaluation.

As stated in Chapter 2, normally the *shape of the palatal arch* is neither shallow nor severely vaulted. If either shallow or vaulted arch is noted, the configuration may possibly explain imprecise articulation; therefore, this is a remarkable finding.

Shallow palatal arch is unlikely to affect articulation noticeably, but it is possible for a low arch to allow inadequate space to accommodate tongue mobility (Kummer, 2008). Similarly, in most cases of *high-palatal arch*, the person uses compensatory strategies, resulting in little or no impact on articulation (Bankson, Bernthal, & Flipsen, 2009). However, if vaulted or shallow palatal arch occurs concomitant to imprecise production of sibilants and affricates, the shape of the palate may be considered a possible contributor to the speech concerns.

Speech sound stimulability screening can provide helpful information on the examinee's response to clinical teaching. In addition, for those with a highly vaulted palatal arch co-occurring with speech symptoms, a referral to otorhinolaryngology or genetics may be appropriate.

The *median palatal raphe* is an excellent landmark indicator for visually estimating palatal symmetry. Any deviation from a slightly indented, straight, centrally located line can suggest problems with palatal integrity if associated with hypernasal resonance or difficulty with pressure consonants.

Likewise, whenever bluish coloration is in close proximity to the median palatal raphe, this can indicate possible submucous cleft if associated with hypernasal resonance or difficulty with pressure consonants. Bluish color in that area suggests the possibility of blood supply that is abnormally close to the surface and is likely associated with incomplete bony structure (Bankson et al., 2009). Otorhinolaryngology and genetic referrals should be considered, as should screening for submucous cleft.

Some *mucosal traits* that are potentially remarkable include *discoloration*, *translucency*, and *shading* not consistent with normal palatal contour. Remarkable features of the palatal mucous membrane, if

associated with hypernasal resonance or difficulty with pressure consonants, should result in a consideration for otorhinolaryngology or genetic referral as well as screening for submucous cleft.

When observing the hard palate, be alert to evidence of *scarring* or *discoloration*. If noting that either co-occurs with hypernasal resonance or difficulty with pressure consonants, this may call for consultation with genetics or otorhinolaryngology, or in the case of discoloration, a referral to the examinee's primary care physician may be an appropriate measure, especially in the case of inflammation or other disease indicators.

Note, though, that bluish coloration on the palatal plates that is not proximal to the median palatal raphe may simply indicate extra bony growth and is not generally associated with speech disorder (Bankson et al., 2009). Even so, unexplained discoloration at any palatal location, to be safe, can potentially result in medical referral.

If the *posterior nasal spine* is not visually detected during the inspection, there is no need for alarm, since the landmark is not always superficially visible. If, however, hypernasal resonance or difficulty with obstruent consonants and other noteworthy palatal traits co-occur with this, proceed with a screening for submucous cleft.

Likewise, whether *foveae palati* are evident is irrelevant to the clinical findings. The landmark is mentioned to alert examiners to their occasional visible presence so that they will not be mistaken for miniscule palatal fistuli.

Clinical Significance of Submucous Cleft. In the preceding paragraphs, the possibility of submucous cleft was mentioned repeatedly. Yet, bear in mind that submucous cleft is more often than not clinically insignificant. That is, any time the location of a submucous cleft is above the level of the velum, it is unlikely to negatively affect resonance or pressure consonants, and this is the case for the majority of people with submucous palatal cleft.

The Velum at Rest. For individuals with hypernasal resonance or difficulty with obstruent consonants, any remarkable feature of the resting velum as mentioned in Chapter 2 potentially indicates a need for otorhinolaryngology, neurology, genetic, or primary care referral. That is, since involuntary movements and asymmetry are possible indicators of neurologic involvement, these often lead to consultation with neurology as well as observations for dysarthria. On the other hand, irregularity in size or shape is more likely to be the concern of otorhinolaryngology or genetics. Discoloration, however, may have its origin in infection or disease and should be referred to the examinee's primary care physician.

The Uvula and Faucial Pillars at Rest. The uvula and faucial pillars, in and of themselves, do not contribute remarkably to speech production. However, the shape and condition are capable of providing tangible relevant clues relative to diagnosis and planning.

That is, if *uvular or pillar asymmetry* is noted at rest and is concomitant to hypernasal resonance or difficulty with pressure sounds, this can be an indicator of either neurologic involvement or structural malformation. Both should be considered.

Also, *uvular dysmorphia* (see Figure 2–30) or *absent uvula*, as described in Chapter 2, is potentially clinically relevant if associated with hypernasal resonance or difficulty with obstruent consonants. This is because these features are frequently associated with submucous palatal cleft and can be associated with genetic abnormality.

Palatine Tonsils. From a speech-language pathology perspective, *enlarged palatine tonsils* are only of clinical relevance if they are so large that they hinder one's ability to either (1) transmit speech sounds or (2) move the velum satisfactorily for the purpose of balancing nasal and oral resonance (Kummer, 2008). Yet when individuals present with tonsils that are enlarged or *enflamed*, from a health perspective, a medical referral is appropriate. Furthermore, when noting any tonsillar *discoloration*, the person should be referred for medical evaluation.

For examinees with tonsil symptoms, the referral to otorhinolaryngology can lead to tonsillectomy and adenoidectomy, which involves the surgical removal of both the palatine tonsils and the pharyngeal tonsil. Since making a medical decision about surgery of any kind is outside of the scope of practice for speech-language pathologists, the referral to otorhinolaryngology neither mentions nor sug-

gests the potential for surgical removal. However, speech-language pathologists can address possible precautions with regard to tissue removal if suspecting that either or both types of tonsillar tissue should be spared for the sake of preserving capacity for velopharyngeal closure. For example, excessively large palatine tonsils that obstruct velar movement may leave a gap if removed, possibly compromising velopharyngeal sufficiency that is needed for oral-nasal decoupling. Another example may be the person who displays symptoms of minor problems with achieving intraoral pressure; removing that person's tonsils has potential to exacerbate resonance and obstruent difficulties if tonsillar tissue participates in achieving closure.

Since the pharyngeal tonsil is not normally visible via the oral orifice, oral-facial inspection does not provide concrete evidence to support or refute whether the examinee needs it for velopharyngeal closure. Yet if noting any externally visible indicator of possible velar weakness or structural inadequacy, it is best to put the concerns in writing in the recommendations section of the clinical report, so that the examining physician can take the concerns into account when developing a plan of care.

When the two *palatine tonsils are grossly different in size*, this may be an indicator of disease or even malignancy. Referral to the primary care physician is the next appropriate step, regardless of the condition's impact on speech or resonance.

Furthermore, if the difference in size is extreme, the larger tonsil can impede symmetrical velar movement, possibly interfering with resonance (Kummer, 2008). Thus, if tonsillar asymmetry is associated with hypernasal resonance or difficulty with obstruent consonants, the examinee may be best served by specifying the medical referral to otorhinolaryngology so that proper evaluation of velopharyngeal competence can be examined using instrumentation.

When the *palatine tonsils are absent bilaterally*, this typically suggests a history of chronic tonsillitis resulting in tonsillectomy. Generally, no follow-up is needed, unless the examinee displays symptoms of hypernasal resonance or difficulty with pressure consonants. In that case, an otorhinolaryngology consult should be requested so that potential for velopharyngeal competency in the absence of tonsillar tissue can be explored.

If only *one tonsil is missing*, this may imply remarkable medical history that should be explored by asking relevant questions (e.g., surgical removal of one tonsil secondary to cancer or other disease). Although the absence of one tonsil is rarely significant from a speech-language pathology perspective, if associated with hypernasal resonance or difficulty with obstruent consonants, an otorhinolaryngology referral should be made to determine whether the tonsillar asymmetry interferes with symmetrical closure.

Posterior Pharyngeal Wall. When inspecting the posterior pharyngeal wall, remarkable features that may lead to referral include *discoloration, close proximity to the posterior tongue, excessive size of the pharyngeal opening,* or *observable catarrh*. The referral may be sent to the client's primary care physician if symptoms imply inflammation, infection, diseased tissue, or allergy, while otorhinolaryngology should have an opportunity to evaluate any noteworthy structural anomalies.

Consider Evidence From Routine Clinical Observation 6: Velar Movement

Asymmetrical Velar Movement

Clinical Question 15 (see Table 0–3) asks: "When prompting velar movement through /ɑ/ phonation, does the examinee's velum appear to move symmetrically and with adequate excursion?" An answer of *no* is noteworthy.

Asymmetrical velar movement is noteworthy because it may bring about incomplete velopharyngeal closure unilaterally. If associated with hypernasal resonance or difficulty with obstruent consonants, there are two possible referrals to consider. That is, asymmetrical velar movement, when associated with other neurologic, symptoms can indicate a neurologic referral, and observations for dysarthria should be completed. However, if no neurologic symptoms are noted, and if the examinee displays enlarged tonsils or indicators of palatal structure difference, the proper referral is otorhinolaryngology.

When *inadequate velar excursion* is observed concomitant to perceived hyponasal resonance, the pos-sibility of a prominent pharyngeal tonsil, secondary symptoms of repaired cleft, and shallow nasopharynx should be considered (Kummer, 2008; Riski, n.d.). The possibility of compromised function of the levator palatini muscle and other neuromotor dysfunction should also be taken into account. A referral to otorhinolaryngology or neurology is in order, depending on the symptoms.

Misplaced Velar Dimple

Clinical Question 16 (see Table 0–3) asks, "Is the velar dimple observed to be properly located during /ɑ/ phonation?" A negative response is noteworthy.

Chapter 2 describes a range of standard locations for the velar dimple. If noting that the velar dimple seems farther forward than what is typical, it is possible that the bend in the velum may not be posterior enough to accommodate an adequate seal with the posterior pharyngeal wall, potentially resulting in velopharyngeal insufficiency. On the other hand, if the dimple is judged to be abnormally proximal to the uvula, this can thwart a satisfactory velopharyngeal contact, potentially resulting in velopharyngeal insufficiency (Kummer, 2008; Riski, n.d.). Misplaced velar dimple, if associated with hypernasal resonance or obstruent problems, should lead to an otorhinolaryngology referral.

Consider the Evidence From Routine Clinical Observation 7: Verbal Diadochokinesis

Generally, the associated clinical questions potentially expose two types of remarkable responses to verbal diadochokinetic testing. They are problems with planning and sequencing, as well as difficulty with muscular movements. Four clinical questions are asked.

Clinical Question 17 (see Table 0–3) asks, "For speech-alternating motion, are the syllables produced with steady rate and articulatory precision?" A negative response is noteworthy and may be indicative of motor-speech disorder.

Clinical Question 18 (see Table 0–3) asks, "For speech-sequential motion, are the three distinctly different syllables produced accurately, rapidly, and in sequence?" A negative response is noteworthy and may indicate motor-speech disorder.

Clinical Question 19 (see Table 0–3) asks, "For speech-alternating motion and speech-sequential motion, are the syllables produced with a rate and volume that do not deteriorate?" A negative response is remarkable and may indicate motor-speech disorder.

Clinical Question 20 (see Table 0–3) asks, "For speech-alternating motion and speech-sequential motion, are at least five syllables produced per second?" Slow rate is remarkable and may indicate motor-speech disorder.

Interpreting Verbal Diadochokinesis Findings

Whenever noticing difficulty with volitional planning and sequencing of movements for speech, plan to complete observations of apraxia. If the client is not already in the care of a neurologist, initiate the referral so that the relationship can be established.

Furthermore, whenever the procedure exposes difficulty with muscular strength, coordination, excursion, endurance, or precision, observe for features of dysarthria. Then follow up with a neurology referral, unless that patient-doctor relationship is already established.

Consider the Evidence From Routine Clinical Observation 8: Vowel Prolongation

Laryngeal Implications

Clinical Question 21 (see Table 0–3) asks, "When sustaining a vowel, does the examinee exhibit vocal pitch, quality, loudness, and evenness that are perceived to be within normal limits?" A negative response is remarkable.

Aberrations in pitch, loudness, or quality may indicate vocal pathology or symptoms of motor-speech disorder, prompting referral to otorhinolaryngology or neurology. Furthermore, deterioration of any kind may indicate fatigue, suggesting the possible need to observe for dysarthria.

Breath Support Implications

Clinical Question 22 (see Table 0–3) asks, "When sustaining a vowel, do duration and loudness suggest breath support that is adequate to sustain connected speech?" A negative response is remarkable.

For adults, sustaining a vowel for fewer than 20 seconds may imply inadequate breath support for connected speech, and fewer than 10 seconds may imply inadequate breath support in children. This is especially noteworthy for examinees who exhibit other symptoms associated with respiratory concerns.

Referral for respiratory symptoms depends on the exact nature of the symptoms. As with vocal quality judgments, any indication of deterioration or fatigue with successive trials potentially calls attention to possible neurologic involvement and warrants consultation with a neurologist. In the absence of neurologic symptoms, an otorhinolaryngologist, a pulmonologist, a primary care physician, or an allergist may be the most appropriate referral recipient.

Consider Evidence From Discretionary Clinical Observation 9: Screening for Nasal Cavity Clearance

Clinical Question 23 (see Table 0–3) asks, "For examinees with perceived hyponasal resonance, does viewing the nasal cavity provide evidence of clinically relevant obstruction?" An affirmative response is noteworthy.

If nasal cavity clearance screening exposes any of the remarkable features pointed out in Chapter 3, it is reasonable to conclude that nasal cavity obstruction is a possible factor contributing to a resonance problem. However, because the nasal passageway is mostly hidden from view without instrumentation, when hyponasal resonance is perceived and no obstructions are observed, there is always the possibility of an occult explanation. For instance, enlarged pharyngeal tonsil or hypertrophied nasal conchae can interfere with nasal airflow, but neither is fully observable without instrumentation.

Therefore, although on occasion the procedure successfully identifies an obstruction that should be considered medically, the screening is not regarded as failsafe for ruling out more in-depth testing to identify the source of the resonance problem. Hence, the screening is helpful in that it adds information to the routine inspection findings, but the conclusive evidence confirming or ruling out obstruction or determining the extent of an obstruction lies beyond the scope of simple oral-facial inspection.

Generally, then, a medical referral is in order for most examinees with perceived hyponasal resonance. Evidence resulting from nasal airflow clearance screening is useful for more clearly defining the problem and even pinpointing whether the examinee should be evaluated by an otorhinolaryngologist or a primary care physician.

As a general rule, if a structurally based obstruction is found, then otorhinolaryngology evaluation is the logical next step. Also, individuals with hyponasal resonance for whom no explanation is observed should also be evaluated by otorhinolaryngology since the obstruction may be occult in nature. Bear in mind that some examinees exhibit symptoms of temporary obstruction due to congestion, and these individuals should see their primary care physician or allergist for medical treatment if symptoms persist.

Consider Evidence From Discretionary Clinical Observation 10: Facial Dimension Estimates

Clinical Question 24 (see Table 0–3) asks, "When facial dysmorphia is noted upon superficial inspection, does evidence augment or support a specialist referral?" An affirmative answer is remarkable.

Since facial dimension estimates are performed due to suspected facial dysmorphia based on visual impression, we urge caution in ruling out a referral even if measurements seem to be within the normal range or borderline. This conservative view allows the proper professional the opportunity to decide whether the cursory observations are clinically relevant from a genetic or otorhinolaryngology perspective.

Furthermore, if facial dimension measurements suggest a need for more in-depth testing, these data cannot be tendered as a diagnostic finding. That is, an otorhinolaryngology, genetic, or craniofacial team referral should follow.

Yet as a result of having performed the screening, the rationale for referral can include comments on forehead, midface, and jaw proportions; maxilla and mandible proportions; eye size and position; facial profile angle; and height relationship between the ears and the eyes. In most cases, the physician who receives the referral repeats the measurements if necessary and makes additional observations that extend beyond the scope of speech-language pathology testing. However, augmenting a referral with data only serves to strengthen the recommendation for more in-depth testing.

Consider Evidence From Discretionary Clinical Observation 11: Screening for Temporomandibular Joint Disorder

Clinical Question 25 (see Table 0–3) asks, "For individuals for whom a medical referral is planned due to reduced mandibular excursion or associated pain, does the evidence augment the referral?" An affirmative response is remarkable.

The screening does not diagnose temporomandibular joint disorder, which is a medical diagnosis requiring instrumentation. Magnetic resonance imaging is considered the standard for diagnosing the condition, and this type of testing is outside of the conventional scope of clinical practice for speech-language pathologists. Furthermore, speech-language pathologists do not typically treat temporomandibular joint disorder since as a medical condition, it falls under the purview of medical providers such as dentists and oral surgeons. The screening, however, can result in information that strengthens the referral by adding detail to it.

Consider Evidence From Discretionary Clinical Observation 12: Tongue-Thrust Swallow Procedure

Identifying Tongue-Thrust Swallow Pattern

Clinical Question 26 (see Table 0–3) asks, "For examinees identified as at risk for tongue-thrust swallow, does the evidence support a diagnosis of clinically significant tongue-thrust swallow?" An affirmative response is remarkable.

Findings that indicate tongue-thrust swallow are clearly described in Chapter 3. Essentially, indicators include forced break in labial seal and forward tongue movement during the swallow procedure. For very few examinees, it is possible that the evaluation procedure may interfere with the person's natural swallow pattern, potentially masking a tongue-thrust swallow; therefore, if the procedure does not expose symptoms and if doubts linger as to whether tongue-thrust swallow can be ruled out, refer the examinee for a formal swallow study. Generally, though, the tongue-thrust swallow procedures described in Chapter 3 are effective for identifying the condition.

Obligatory Versus Habitual Tongue-Thrust Swallow

Clinical Question 27 (see Table 0–3) asks, "If tongue-thrust swallow is identified, does the evidence suggest a habitual or obligatory pattern?" Either pattern is noteworthy; however, plan of care may be distinctly different, depending on which pattern is observed.

If tongue-thrust swallow is identified, the next step is to determine whether the pattern is obligatory or habitual. If physical obstruction, alleged temporomandibular joint disorder, or palatal malformation is suspected concomitant to an observed tongue-thrust swallow pattern, the tongue-thrust swallow may be of the obligatory type, and the physical difference should be assessed and addressed medically before initiating therapy. In-depth testing likely includes instrumentation. Tending to the physical cause first is fundamental to proper treatment when obligatory tongue-thrust swallow is suspected.

Implications Resulting From Tongue-Thrust Swallow Procedure

For individuals whose residual tongue-thrust pattern appears to have no physical cause, a habitual tongue-thrust swallow pattern can be diagnosed. With habitual tongue-thrust swallow, appropriate therapy can be very effective in the absence of further medical assessment or intervention. If tongue-thrust swallow pattern is clearly identified without evidence of physical cause, the resulting speech ther-

apy may include a recommendation for treatment to address tongue-thrust swallow, which resides under the larger heading of myofunctional therapy.

If results are inconclusive or if a physical cause cannot be ruled out, then a medical referral for further testing should be included in the plan.

Consider Evidence From Discretionary Clinical Observation 13: Observations for Developmental Apraxia of Speech

Oral-Facial Inspection Can Identify Developmental Apraxia of Speech for Some Children

Clinical Question 28 (see Table 0–3) asks, "For child examinees who exhibit superficial symptoms of developmental apraxia of speech, does evidence support or rule out a diagnosis?" An affirmative response is remarkable.

Diagnosing developmental apraxia of speech is within the scope of practice for speech-language pathologists. Yet, there is no cardinal symptom that distinguishes between young unintelligible speakers with developmental apraxia of speech and those who do not have the condition, and not all speech-language pathologists have the experience to reliably diagnose or rule out developmental apraxia of speech (Duffy, Waumbaugh, Fredrickson, & Haley, 2013).

For clinicians who are experienced with developmental apraxia of speech, Discretionary Clinical Observation 13 provides adequate opportunity to ascertain whether the child's symptoms are consistent with a diagnosis. Therefore, findings in this section can lead to a diagnosis, or they may support ruling out developmental apraxia of speech. We also recognize that experienced clinicians who specialize in motor-speech disorders usually have their own diagnostic protocol that can be used either in lieu of or in tandem with Discretionary Clinical Observation 13.

At Times, More Information Is Needed for Diagnosis

Clinical Question 29 (see Table 0–3) asks, "If not, does the evidence support a referral for more in-depth testing?" An affirmative response is remarkable.

For less experienced clinicians the procedure offers a structure for eliciting symptoms that are capable of leading to a diagnosis but *often* require expert consultation to confirm or rule out the condition. Even if all findings in this section are unremarkable, if doubts about dismissing developmental apraxia of speech from consideration linger, the safest route for the less experienced clinician is to refer for expert opinion, requesting a complete battery to test for developmental apraxia of speech.

Consider Evidence From Discretionary Clinical Observation 14: Acquired Apraxia of Speech

Oral-Facial Evaluation Can Identify Acquired Apraxia of Speech for Some Adults

Clinical Question 30 (see Table 0–3) asks, "When routine inspection reveals symptoms that imply acquired apraxia of speech, does the evidence support or rule out a diagnosis?" An affirmative response is noteworthy.

Motor planning and programming difficulties that may be noted are highlighted on the recording form. The procedure can clearly identify acquired apraxia of speech in an examinee when it is administered by a clinician who has experience with making the distinction, yet experienced clinicians often recognize symptoms readily and proceed directly to diagnostic measures that provide more detail.

More Information May Be Needed for Diagnosis

Clinical Question 31 (see Table 0–3) asks, "If not, does the evidence support a referral for more in-depth testing?" An affirmative response is remarkable.

The procedure provides a framework for less experienced clinicians. When clinicians lack extensive practice with diagnosing and treating acquired apraxia of speech, a definitive diagnosis may not be entirely possible without further training and experience and may even require expert consultation (Duffy et al., 2013). Even experienced clinicians may be inclined to recommend more in-depth testing to discover the exact idiosyncratic manifestations of acquired apraxia of speech in a particular examinee. Therefore, remarkable findings may yield or rule out a definitive diagnosis of acquired apraxia of speech, and the procedure can lead to additional testing.

Consider Evidence From Discretionary Clinical Observation 15: Screening for Submucous Cleft of the Palate

Clinical Question 32 (see Table 0–3) asks, "When examining individuals for whom integrity of the hard palate is questionable, who also exhibit symptoms of hypernasal speech or difficulty with obstruent consonants, does the evidence strengthen a medical referral?" An affirmative response is remarkable.

By and large, persons who receive the submucous cleft screening do not display obvious physical symptoms of oral-facial anomaly (e.g., cleft lip, open palatal cleft, or palatal fissure); otherwise, their palatal difference would have been identified a priori. Nevertheless, audible symptoms co-occurring with suspicious palatal appearance may imply compromised palatal integrity in some cases; thus, individuals with poor resonance and palatal irregularity should be referred for more in-depth testing and medical evaluation. The screening is meant to provide information to augment referral that is likely to prompt appropriate in-depth testing.

Therefore, if submucous cleft screening fails to uncover palpable compromise in palatal integrity, that does not rule out the possible need for medical evaluation. Likewise, if inspection identifies an area with perceived compromised tactile resistance, this does not confirm the presence of a cleft in the palate. Medical evaluation is required to confirm or rule out submucous cleft.

So instead of drawing definitive conclusions based on inspection, use the discretionary screening results to augment findings obtained during the routine inspection. The medical providers who serve the examinee generally find the superficial information that we provide useful when crafting an initial plan for assessment and care.

Consider Evidence From Discretionary Clinical Observation 16: Screening for Surplus Nasal Airflow During Speech

Clinical Question 33 (see Table 0–3) asks, "For individuals who will be referred for evaluation of the velum for structure or function, does the evidence strengthen a referral for more in-depth testing?" An affirmative response is noteworthy.

Normally, mirror condensation would not be observed during production of oral phonemes; if it does, this may indicate surplus nasal airflow, therefore mandating referral for medical evaluation, calling on the expertise of an otorhinolaryngologist, a neurologist, or a craniofacial team. That is, if a doctor-patient relationship has not yet been established and the examinee exhibits symptoms that imply compromised structural integrity (e.g., palatal or velar irregularity), refer to otorhinolaryngology. However, if the examinee presents a history of recent neurologic episode or exhibits other symptoms of neurologic involvement (e.g., muscle weakness or asymmetry), refer to neurology unless the medical relationship has already been established. Furthermore, for any child with surplus nasal airflow during speech, a craniofacial team referral may be the most effective means to ensure effective follow-up.

Consider Evidence From Discretionary Clinical Observation 17: Observations for Dysarthria

Oral-Facial Inspection Can Identify Symptoms of Dysarthria

Clinical Question 34 (see Table 0–3) asks, "When routine inspection reveals symptoms that imply dysarthria, does the evidence confirm or rule out a diagnosis?" An affirmative response is remarkable.

The oral-facial inspection is sensitive to symptoms of dysarthria. Therefore, the experienced clinician can confirm or rule out dysarthria using the evidence provided through the routine clinical observations.

Oral-Facial Inspection May Isolate Type of Dysarthria for Some

Clinical Question 35 (see Table 0–3) asks, "If evidence supports a diagnosis, does it provide enough data to reliably identify the type of dysarthria?" An affirmative response is noteworthy.

Although the oral-facial evaluation tool is not intended to be sensitive enough to differentially diagnose the type of dysarthria, some experienced clinicians may identify type of dysarthria through procedures provided herein. Less experienced clinicians are advised to seek expert input and follow up with more in-depth testing.

Additional Testing May Be Needed

Clinical Question 36 (see Table 0–3) asks, "If evidence does not support a diagnosis, does the evidence support a referral for more in-depth testing?" An affirmative response is remarkable.

Clinicians who do not regularly diagnose and treat motor-speech disorders are advised to use the dysarthria observations to confirm whether there is a need for referral to confirm or rule out dysarthria when findings are not readily apparent to them.

Consider Evidence From Discretionary Clinical Observation 18: Speech Sound Stimulability Screening

Clinical Question 37 (see Table 0–3) asks, "For individuals with atypical speech sound production, when clinical teaching opportunities are presented, does the examinee respond by improving or changing the speaking pattern?" A negative response is remarkable.

If the examinee responds to clinical teaching by making speech production improvements, that is a positive prognostic indicator for therapy. Furthermore, stimulable sounds may be considered low-hanging fruit when making decisions about where to begin a therapy protocol.

In cases where the oral-facial inspection identifies some structural differences that may or may not affect articulatory precision, stimulability testing can be extremely helpful. For example, if an examinee has a cathedral-like palatal arch and difficulty with palatal fricatives and affricates, it is possible that the palatal structure hinders precise articulation. However, some people with high palatal arch compensate well without benefit of clinical teaching, and others need a little help to achieve an effective compensatory strategy. If the person demonstrates stimulability for the error sounds, there is an excellent probability that the person is able to learn compensatory strategies for speech, leaving the error pattern behind after a period of successful treatment.

Consider the Evidence From Discretionary Clinical Observation 19: Screening for Laryngeal and Respiratory Efficiency (i.e., S:Z Ratio)

Clinical Question 38 (see Table 0–3) asks, "For examinees who exhibit symptoms of laryngeal or respiratory inefficiency, do S:Z ratio data provide additional information that strengthens a medical referral for more in-depth testing?" An affirmative response is remarkable.

Evidence Concerning Laryngeal Efficiency

Traditionally, an S:Z ratio of 1.2 or greater implies vocal inefficiency and may be indicative of vocal pathology (Prater & Swift, 1984; Shipley & McAfee, 2008; van der Meer, Ferreira, & Loock, 2010). However, this rule should be applied with caution, as others have found S:Z ratios for normal larynges to range from 0.46 to 1.57 (Gelfer & Pazera, 2006). Consequently, if audible symptoms suggest possible inefficient use of the larynx or possible laryngeal pathology, regardless of S:Z ratio, a referral to oto-rhinolaryngology is advised, and screening results should accompany the referral.

Evidence Concerning Respiratory Efficiency

Information on respiratory efficiency may be important for individuals whose breathing pattern calls attention to itself in conversational speech. As a general rule, the adult minimum for sustaining the /s/ and /z/ phonemes is 20 seconds, and the minimum expectation for children is 10 seconds. Duration of less than 20 seconds for adults and 10 seconds for children may have implications relative to breath support. Although duration data should not influence whether a medical referral is in order, these numbers may be included in the data sent to the physician who takes these data under advisement when responding to the referral.

Consider Evidence From Discretionary Clinical Observation 20: Gag Reflex Stimulation

Clinical Question 39 (see Table 0–3) asks, "For individuals who will be referred for neurologic or genetic evaluation, does response to gag reflex stimulation provide additional evidence to corroborate the referral?" An affirmative response is remarkable.

Results of gag reflex stimulation are generally inconclusive if taken out of context and are clearly irrelevant for individuals with no neurologic, craniofacial, or genetic concerns. Nevertheless, atypical or absent gag reflex can be associated with neurologic findings, genetic syndromes, dysphagia, or craniofacial anomaly; for that reason, atypical response to gag reflex stimulation is remarkable if it occurs in those who qualify for the procedure using the criteria provided. The findings may contribute to the data that partially support a referral to neurology or genetics.

Consider the Evidence From Discretionary Clinical Observation 21: Prompt for Dysphagia Screening

Clinical Question 40 (see Table 0–3) asks, "Does evidence support the need for dysphagia screening in aging adults?" An affirmative response is remarkable.

The purpose of this prompt is simply to identify clients who are not scheduled for routine dysphagia screening, who exhibit symptoms that place them at risk. Since all examinees with a recent history of neurologic episode or laryngectomy are customarily screened for dysphagia, there is no need to evoke this prompt for that type of client. However, individuals in other diagnostic categories can have dysphagia and should be screened if certain symptom patterns present.

When findings in this section are remarkable or inconclusive, temporarily discontinue oral feeding at once and recommend that dysphagia screening take place as soon as possible, before resuming a normal diet. Screening for dysphagia is within the scope of practice for speech-language pathologists as well as a few other health care professions, provided that the examiner has specialized training in dysphagia screening.

Consider Evidence From Discretionary Clinical Observation 22: Screening for Amblyopia

Clinical Question 41 (see Table 0–3) asks, "Does the young child examinee exhibit symptoms that suggest referral for amblyopia testing?" An affirmative response is remarkable.

Any child who does not pass the amblyopia screening as described in Chapter 4 is at risk for amblyopia, which is the leading cause of monocular vision and is usually preventable. Hope for successful medical treatment outcome diminishes at approximately age 6 years, at which time the condition tends to become permanent, although there are exceptions. Therefore, time is of the essence. A prompt referral to an ophthalmologist is advised.

Consider Evidence From Discretionary Clinical Observation 23: Screening for Primitive Reflexes in Young Children

Clinical Question 42 (see Table 0–3) asks, "For infants, toddlers, and some preschoolers suspected of having possible neurologic involvement, are primitive reflexes present and suppressed at developmentally appropriate ages?" A negative response is noteworthy.

Primitive reflexes begin in utero, are present at birth, and are gradually suppressed by emerging voluntary motor skills in infancy. Each primi-

tive reflex has a purpose. When absent or persisting past the normal age of suppression, this may be considered an indicator of compromised neurologic integrity. Furthermore, the persisting presence of primitive reflexes can interfere with normal motor development. Children who exhibit abnormal reflex patterns may be at risk for dysphagia, delayed speech, and even reading problems. Also, a connection between an imminent cerebral palsy diagnosis and persisting reflexes has been suggested (Capute, 1979; Jones, Morgan, Shelton, & Thorogood, 2007; Zafeiriou, 2004).

Only five primitive reflexes are selected for the screening, although there are more. Screening procedures for selected reflexes are simple and bear some relationship to oral movement, speech development, or feeding. Findings relative to primitive reflexes can meaningfully augment the basic information that we include when making a neurologic referral. Also, bear in mind that the neurologist who receives the referral will administer and interpret a full array of primitive reflex and postural response evaluations as a part of a comprehensive neurologic workup.

Consider Evidence From Discretionary Clinical Observation 24: Esophageal Speech Screening

Clinical Question 43 (see Table 0–3) asks, "For laryngectomized patients who plan to learn esophageal speech, does the evidence suggest candidacy for this type of alaryngeal speech?" A negative response is remarkable.

Since clinical teaching is involved when considering a person's candidacy for esophageal speech, the esophageal-speech screening procedures may be initiated during an oral-facial inspection, but completing the screening may continue over a period of several sessions. Although no person should be discouraged from learning esophageal speech based on the screening alone, resulting evidence may be a useful prognostic indicator, giving information about the person's readiness to begin esophageal speech work or even obstacles that the person may encounter when learning the skills required for fluid and intelligible esophageal speech.

CHAPTER 5

Deaf and Hard of Hearing

When inspecting the oral-facial region for deaf and hard-of-hearing clients, be alert to some potential patterns that may affect plan of care. Specifically, pay close attention to idiosyncrasies that affect breathing for speech, as well as articulation and voice (Lane & Perkell, 2005).

Also, bear in mind that when a deaf or hard-of-hearing person seeks speech-language pathology services, spoken language is or has recently become a communication goal for the person. Therefore, although we recognize that many Deaf individuals choose not to speak, those who seek services should be given the opportunity. The comments that follow assume that the deaf, Deaf, or hard-of-hearing examinee desires spoken communication.

Breathing for Speech

When evaluating deaf speakers, be alert to symptoms of habitual *improper use of inhalation and exhalation* for speech. That is, deaf and hard-of-hearing speakers who have not had the benefit of effective strategic listening practice may have learned to speak on residual air or on the inhalation phase of the breathing cycle. Notable features include stridor, glottal fry, low volume, short phrases, and inability to project the voice. Other breathing patterns may also be noteworthy in the deaf and hard of hearing. These may include *speaking on the expiratory reserve, inspiring insufficient lung volume* for free-flowing speech, or *large amounts of air expelled per syllable.*

Except in rare cases, difficulty coordinating breathing for speech occurs secondary to compromised auditory access to audible cues that are necessary for spoken-language learning. The habit can be changed with proper therapy that focuses on making the most of aided residual hearing for the purpose of effectively accessing spoken language. Success relies heavily on age, access to hearing through amplification, and motivation.

Articulation, Voice, and Resonance

Nasal-oral cognate confusion, imbalanced nasal-oral resonance, predominantly pharyngeal resonance, and cul-de-sac resonance may be detected in the deaf or hard-of-hearing speaker. In this population, this is not typically due to velar insufficiency, poor palatal integrity, or neurologic involvement. Instead, it inevitably results from incomplete or distorted access to the auditory signal.

Similarly, differences between voiced and voiceless cognates are not clearly available to the same group of examinees. Therefore, voice-voiceless confusion, breathy voice, or hoarse voice may also result, and normally it is attributable to incomplete auditory access as opposed to laryngeal malfunction or neurologic involvement.

Also, when considering articulation, consider that most speech sounds are ambiguous at best if the person relies on visual cues alone, placing the person at risk for articulation errors as well as comprehension confusions. For example, speech sounds in the bilabial viseme group (i.e., /b/, /p/, /m/, and /w/) can be seen but may be confused with one another; speech sounds in the labial-dental viseme group (i.e., /v/ and /f/) and the interdental viseme group (i.e., /ð/ and /θ/) are also visible but potentially confusing. All other consonants are not visible and absolutely visually ambiguous in connected speech. Furthermore, a similar set of problems occurs when attempting to interpret vowels visually. That is, all front vowels have the lips spread to some degree, all the back vowels have the lips somewhat rounded, and the mid-central vowels have the lips in a relatively neutral position that is neither spread nor rounded. These ambiguities affect access to spoken language for purposes of both spoken-language acquisition and verbal language comprehension.

History of Repaired Craniofacial Anomaly

Known History of Surgery

Typically, when performing an oral-facial inspection on a person with a history of repaired cleft, the examiner is made aware of the history at the time of referral; therefore, the door is already open for a relationship with the oral-facial surgeon and other members of the craniofacial team. In these cases, the team members responsible for surgical and medical decisions rely on the speech-language pathologist to provide relevant information that affects communication concerns.

It is possible that the person seeking additional assistance has reached maximum habilitation potential, and the clinician should be aware of this as early in the evaluation process as possible. Yet, it is also possible that the person is in a position to benefit from additional treatment.

One of the evaluation goals for a person with a history of craniofacial surgery is to ascertain the prognosis for additional progress with therapy. Stimulability testing can be helpful. Although the stimulability screening that is part of this protocol is limited to speech sound stimulability activities, the same stimulability principles can be applied to resonance and voice if the examiner is trained in that area and deems the screening appropriate.

Suspected Unreported History of Craniofacial Surgery

Rarely will an older child or adult with a history of craniofacial surgery appear for evaluation without disclosing the history at the front end. If one does, this situation establishes the need for seeking information about the surgical and speech therapy history to best understand the examinee's needs.

Mouth Breathers

Mouth breathers present a variation to the typical respiratory pathway, creating a detour that bypasses the nasal passages, so that air enters and exits through an oral egress. Although mouth breathing can be habitual, the pattern is more often due to an obstruction that prevents the free flow of respired air through the nasal passages. That is, nasal airflow obstructions can result in oral breathing.

Also, open-mouth posture, if co-occurring with hyponasal resonance, can be considered evidence supporting a screening for nasal cavity clearance.

If co-occurring with symptoms suggesting possible tongue-thrust swallow, it may lead to observations for that condition. And if co-occurring with poor muscle tone, open-mouth posture may indicate a need to observe for motor-speech disorder.

Mouth breathing should always be noted regardless of whether it interferes with speech production. Referral to a primary care physician, an otorhinolaryngologist, or an allergist is often appropriate.

Examinees at Risk for Dysphagia

An oral-facial evaluation, or some variation of it, is traditionally administered in patients who are screened or evaluated for dysphagia, regardless of whether speech symptoms are evident. Some (Leder, Suiter, Murray, & Rademaker, 2013) have found evidence that links both poor facial symmetry and reduced lingual range of motion to a high risk of aspiration in this population. For that reason, when inspecting a dysphagia patient's oral-facial mechanism, pay careful attention to symptoms of facial asymmetry (Routine Clinical Observation 1) and range of tongue excursion (Routine Clinical Observation 2). If irregularities are noted in either or both of these areas, terminate oral feeding immediately and do not resume oral feeding until dysphagia is either ruled out or the in process of being addressed.

Evaluating Evidence for Clinical Relevance

The topic of clinical relevance has been revisited at several turns throughout the manual. Overarching Clinical Question 4 (see Table 0–2) ensures that clinical relevance is considered for all noteworthy findings: Does evidence suggest a link between the identified anatomic or physiologic problem and the idiosyncratic speaking pattern?

Many remarkable physical features may be noted throughout the inspection. From a speech-language pathology perspective, however, physical symptoms are only clinically relevant if they can be linked to the examinee's speaking pattern. For example, a person's oral structure may include vaulted palatal arch; and although this feature may well be worthy of comment, in the absence of associated difficult palatal fricatives it has no clinical relevance to diagnosis or plan of care. On the other hand, a different person may have a similarly vaulted palatal arch accompanied by indistinct palatal fricatives, and for this person, the physical anomaly is considered clinically relevant.

Clinically relevant features typically influence the diagnosis, prognosis, or recommendations that follow the evaluation. This will be spoken to more directly in Chapter 6, which addresses documentation.

Furthermore, some features may not be considered clinically relevant from a speech-language perspective but warrant attention when making recommendations. For instance, dental decay has no known relationship to speech production errors but for health reasons merits referral to a dentist. Similarly, facial dysmorphia may not directly affect speech but can be associated with a syndrome or condition that deserves to be evaluated and diagnosed by a genetic specialist.

Diagnosis, Prognosis, and Recommendations

Every communication evaluation results in evidence that leads to clinical decisions, affecting plan of care. Universally relevant and fundamental clinical decisions include the assignment of a diagnosis, determining the prognosis, and making recommendations for follow-up. Although oral-facial inspection evidence may not contribute to these three clinical decisions in every case, oral-facial inspection evidence should always be evaluated with regard to whether it has clinical relevance to any of the three. They are discussed with that perspective in mind.

Diagnosis

Nearly every client or family member who participates in a communication evaluation wants to know: Is there a communication disorder? And if so, what is it? So ascertaining whether there is a disorder and

assigning a name (i.e., diagnosis) is fundamental to the diagnostic process. When considering this aspect of clinical decision making, assigning a diagnostic category is only a first step. Diagnosis requires that the examining clinician consider specific features that characterize the disorder, etiology or cause, and severity level.

Oral-facial inspection evidence can contribute to a person's diagnosis in a variety of ways by clarifying the parameters of the identified disorder. For example, as was said earlier, a lack of physical evidence overall gives support to the diagnosis of *functional communication disorder*, thereby defining the direction that plan of care takes.

Furthermore, if a physical trait is discovered through oral-facial evaluation and it is clearly linked to the speaking pattern, this adds defining information to each diagnostic parameter as well. That is, a diagnostic category can be determined based on certain oral-facial evidence (e.g., motor-speech disorder, speech production disorder, voice disorder, resonance disorder). Likewise, an etiology for speech symptoms may also become surmisable (e.g., poorly differentiated tongue movements, atypical palatal arch configuration, decreased intraoral space that limits tongue mobility). Oral-facial inspection evidence can also help to define the relevant features of the identified communication disorder (e.g., muscular weakness, difficulty with planning and programming articulatory movements, lingua-palatal fricative distortions). For severity level, the intelligibility rating that was assigned in the first oral-facial inspection procedure can also be diagnostically useful.

Prognosis

Once a family or client knows the diagnosis, the next set of questions on their mind is, "Will the condition improve? If so, how much? And can speech-language therapy benefit?" Thus, every communication evaluation should result in information that addresses these issues, and generally this is done through stating a prognosis.

Prognosis is defined as a statement of professional opinion based on evidence that speaks to whether the person is likely to improve either with or without therapy. Overall, the idea that the prognostic statement addresses is whether the person is *likely to improve*, either with or without therapy. Family members are typically quite interested in learning our response to this question.

Furthermore, a valid prognosis requires the clinical intuition and problem solving that an experienced *professional* brings to the table. Therefore, students and newer clinicians may rely on a mentor until confident with evaluating and implementing prognostic indicators effectively.

Since prognosis is a statement of *opinion*, it should never be viewed as a prediction of the future or a guarantee. However, the opinion should be reasonably reliable since it may be used to justify payment and is regarded as particularly meaningful to clients and their family members who want to know something of what the future holds. Therefore, clinical expertise is required to evaluate the evidence that is used to formulate the opinion.

A variety of prognostic indicators should be considered and recorded as *evidence* that supports the professional opinion. Evidence is weighed and measured to arrive at a statement of professional opinion with regard to anticipated expectations for progress.

Prognostic Indicators

Some prognostic indicators may be observed during the inspection; others become obvious during other parts of the evaluation process. For convenience, sample prognostic indicators that may become evident during oral-facial inspection are shown in Table 5–5.

Prognostic indicators, whether gleaned from oral-facial inspection or during some other part of the evaluation procedure, should be regarded as prognostic evidence. When considering the evidence from a professional point of view, these variables become foundational when formulating professional opinion that addresses whether the person is likely to improve.

Prognostic Categories

Five basic prognostic categories are useful. As stated above, the prognostic indicators observed during the inspection may contribute to the prognostic statement, but supporting evidence may come from other types of clinical observations as well.

Since oral-facial inspection yields evidence that meaningfully contributes to an examinee's prognosis, we are about to take a closer look at five prognostic options, as well as some prognostic indicators that can result from oral-facial inspection.

Prognosis: Likely to Improve Even Without Treatment. Some people receive a communication evaluation for a condition that is likely to resolve on its own, even without therapy. Examples include children who exhibit developmentally appropriate communication behaviors, children and adults who take medication that is known to negatively affect speech and can be discontinued or changed without harm to the patient, or individuals for whom targets are readily achievable through stimulability exercises and have made excellent progress on their own in the absence of intervention.

Prognosis: Likely to Benefit From Treatment. When all prognostic indicators suggest a positive response to treatment, the person can be described as *likely to benefit from treatment*. For example, if a young child who participates actively in clinical activities, enjoys a supportive family, responds positively to clinical teaching, and has no structural or functional anomaly that may interfere with progress, one may conclude that this person is likely to benefit from treatment.

Prognosis: Likely to Benefit From Treatment, With Reservations. Sometimes a number of prognostic indicators point to a positive outcome, whereas others cast doubt on whether progress is readily achievable. For instance, despite a plethora of positive prognostic indicators, if a physical anomaly stands in the way of speech accuracy, the potential for less than desirable results must be reflected when crafting the prognostic statement. Certainly, to pinpoint whether benefit is likely, potential barriers to progress mandate attention.

Prognosis: Unlikely to Improve Regardless of Whether Therapy Is Implemented. Unfortunately, some examinees with communication disorders are unlikely to benefit from speech-language pathology services. These may include people who have already reached the full capacity of their ability due to structural or cognitive limitations, people with

Table 5–5. Potential Prognostic Indicators That Oral-Facial Inspection May Yield

Prognostic Indicator	Potential for Impact on Prognosis
Age and years of practice using the speaking pattern	Younger age is typically a more positive prognostic indicator. However, this is relative. For instance, for a 15-year-old who continues to exhibit a /r→w/ substitution pattern, since the pattern is well established long after the normal age of suppression, this person's age is a negative prognostic indicator. On the contrary, for a person who experiences a cerebrovascular accident at age 35 years, the person's relatively young age has positive prognostic implications.
Attention, participation, and compliance	A person's ability to focus attention and comply can become apparent during the oral-facial evaluation. Obviously, a tendency to do these three things has a positive impact on prognosis, and the tendency to not do so has the opposite effect.
Comorbid concerns or physical limitations	As a general rule, concomitant disabilities and physical limitations have a tendency to affect prognosis in a negative way. Persons having only one isolated disability have a prognostic advantage over those who are multiply disabled.
Degenerative process	When a degenerative process is in operation, the therapy process may seem like an uphill battle. Judging prognosis may become more about whether the person is likely to respond to efforts that we make to improve quality of life. For example, an adult with amyotrophic lateral sclerosis should not be denied treatment because the person is facing guaranteed decline. Therefore, although prognosis for improvement may be poor, prognosis for benefit from services may be reasonably good.
Diagnosis or etiology	Diseases and conditions can become prognostic indicators in and of themselves. Each person's situation should be considered individually.
Health	Good health is a positive prognostic indicator. In some cases, poor health may be considered a negative one.
Motivation	Motivation is a positive prognostic indicator. Lack of motivation may interfere with progress in extreme cases.
Need for a concern to be addressed through referral or need for further testing	Sometimes the prognosis cannot be determined immediately following the evaluation because more information is needed
Severity	As a general rule, more severe symptoms can affect prognosis in a negative way
Support system	Persons with a strong family support system have prognostic advantage
Stimulability	Response to clinical teaching is an excellent prognostic indicator. Individuals who demonstrate stimulability have a prognostic advantage.

degenerative disease that promises deterioration over time, or even some who have a long-standing history of noncompliance.

Prognosis: Potential Response to Treatment Is Not Determinable. In very few cases, based on available evidence, prognosis for improvement is not readily apparent or not determinable. This may occur when a confounding variable such as guarded health condition or declining health obfuscates the clinician's ability to anticipate potential for therapy outcome. Also, when the examinee exhibits both positive and negative prognostic indicators, and neither materializes as having the greater impact on likely response to treatment, determining prognosis may become complicated.

Recommendations

Clinically relevant symptoms typically lead to recommendations and follow-up. Therapy, further testing, referral, and any combination of these three are all possible next steps in the process. This section addresses procedures for determining the most appropriate direction to take when responding to an examinee's needs.

How Prognosis Can Influence Whether Treatment Is Recommended

The prognostic statement can become pivotal evidence when addressing whether therapy should be recommended for the individual person. For the most part, there are three options with regard to addressing a therapy recommendation, and all are founded in the person's clinical prognosis. They are recommend therapy without reservation, recommend therapy for a trial period, and do not recommend therapy (Table 5–6).

Prognosis That Suggests a Recommendation for Therapy, Without Reservation. After considering the observed prognostic indicators, if it appears obvious that improvement is likely given opportunity for clinical intervention, therapy should be recommended. This circumstance applies to the majority of the clients that we serve.

Prognosis That Suggests a Recommendation for Therapy, With Reservations. For many individuals, several indicators point to a possible benefit from therapy, but at the same time, other observed indicators cast a shadow of doubt as to the likelihood or extent of progress. These clients may best be served by recommending trial therapy for a specified period of time, with careful monitoring of progress, and performance criteria clearly stated in advance.

When having reservations about whether to recommend therapy, the prognosis can be revised after giving the person the chance to show progress or after gathering more meaningful data about the person's response to treatment. This recommendation category applies to three prognostic groups: those who may possibly improve, those for whom progress is unlikely, and those for whom prognosis

Table 5–6. Relationship Between Prognosis and Treatment Recommendation

Prognosis	Treatment Recommendation
Patient is likely to improve even without therapy or patient does not need therapy	Treatment not recommended
Patient is likely to improve with therapy	Treatment recommended, no reservations
Patient is likely to improve with therapy, but there are some reservations	Recommend therapy, but address the potentially confounding variables in the treatment plan. Depending on the person's response to clinical teaching, this may lead to either continued therapy or discharge.
Patient is not likely to improve with therapy	
Whether the patient is likely to improve with therapy is difficult to determine	

is not determinable. The exact path that the recommendation takes may rely on the clinician's clinical problem-solving skills as well as patient-related circumstances surrounding a prognostic dilemma.

For some, many indicators point to *potential for a positive therapy outcome*, while a confounding variable or two has potential to hold back or hinder progress. Although a trial period of therapy may be recommended in this case, the confounding variable should be taken in hand as part of the treatment plan, and the prognosis should be reassessed after opportunity to respond to treatment. Confounding variables that may place prognosis at risk include exceedingly short attention span, persisting noncompliance, long-term illness, medication with relevant negative side effects, and physical limitation or anomaly, to name a few.

Making a decision about therapy when someone is *unlikely to make meaningful gains* can be a difficult one. Ideally, everyone deserves the opportunity to try. Consequently, recommending therapy for a trial period, with a concrete plan to respond to specific clinical criteria to be achieved within a specified time frame, can serve the client's best interest in many cases.

Moreover, considering the therapy needs of a person with a degenerative disease can be even more complicated and requires a large portion of clinical intuition and clinical problem solving. In some cases, the person may need compensatory communication strategies or a device that serves his or her needs even after intelligible speech is lost (e.g., amyotrophic lateral sclerosis). Promoting a reasonable quality of life for as long as possible begins to take precedence over meaningful spoken-language gains for this population.

On occasion, we encounter an examinee whose evidence contraindicates a recommendation for therapy. These may include people who have been making progress on their own and are likely to continue to make progress without intervention; this may also include people whose condition suggests that progress is not likely, despite our best clinical efforts to bring about progress.

Prognosis That Suggests a Recommendation for No Therapy. There is no need to recommend ther-

apy if prognostic indicators support the idea that adequate gains are highly likely to ensue without it. However, when therapy is not recommended for these reasons, recommending a recheck after a designated period of time is a good idea. For example, if a parent requests an evaluation due to concern about the child's speech development but the diagnostic findings suggest development near the lower end of normal limits, scheduling a recheck in 6 months or 1 year can be very useful to rule out the parental concerns or expose previously obscured data that support a recommendation for therapy. Under this circumstance, therapy can be recommended in some cases, but the issue of prognosis should be revisited within a designated reasonable time frame.

This category can also apply to examinees who are identified for evaluation but exhibit no need for treatment. For example, in some cases, parents request evaluation because they have concerns about their child's communication, but upon assessment, it becomes obvious that the child's perceived speech errors are developmental in nature. Although sometimes parental education is needed to ensure that they will not hold the child up to an unreasonable standard, a recommendation for therapy is not needed. In these cases, if the parent has lingering doubts about the child's communication development or if you judge the child's performance as borderline, the child can be seen for a trial period or be dismissed and scheduled to return for checkup after a designated period of time.

Also, on occasion, we refer an examinee for medical evaluation and follow-up, and when that individual returns for reassessment, the communication disorder was resolved through medical treatment. This may apply to someone whose medication had a negative side effect and for whom the physician was able to provide an alternative that did not provoke the same types of problems. It may also apply to a person who received treatment that completely eliminated both the physical symptoms and the communication disorder. No therapy is required for any individual for whom the communication disorder has been resolved satisfactorily.

Many factors can potentially indicate that a person is *not likely to improve, despite therapy*. One may be the *need for medical treatment* prior to embarking on a communication-focused plan of care. For example, we once examined a young adult with unintelligible hypernasal speech who was also lacking nearly all, if not all, of his visible velar tissue. Without medical intervention, the best of therapy efforts were not liable to improve resonance and articulation for this person. Therefore, instead of recommending therapy, a referral to otorhinolaryngology for evaluation and follow-up was set into motion, with a recommendation to reassess after anatomic issues were given medical consideration.

This category also applies to those with speaking concerns *who presently function to the best of their ability*, rendering treatment a laudable but potentially fruitless goal. An example may be an adult with a vaulted palatal arch who also distorts linguapalatal fricatives and demonstrates no change when presented with a variety of clinical teaching exercises over a period of time. Another example may be an adult with cognitive limitations whose speech, although not perfect, is judged as the person's best ability given restraints imposed by disability.

For a person in this category, although a short period of therapy can be recommended, specific concrete goals should be addressed and reasonable progress should be achieved to continue with therapy after the trial. This is done to ensure that the person receives maximum opportunity to respond to clinical teaching. If unequivocally certain that progress is unattainable for the individual, it is reasonable to withhold therapy entirely.

When Additional Testing Is Recommended

Once the decision about whether treatment should ensue has been formalized, the recommendations should also address any other follow-up that may be needed for an effective plan of care. In most cases, this includes two types of follow-up: within-discipline testing and external referrals. To ensure that the procedures are completed, they should appear in a formal list of recommendations.

Recommendations for Additional Within-Discipline Testing Outside the Scope of Oral-Facial Inspection. Sometimes the inspection leads to additional testing that can be completed by a speech-language pathologist but not within the context of the communication evaluation. It may be that the procedure extends beyond the realm of oral-facial inspection, or it may be that the procedure was not completed during the initial evaluation for some reason. Examples appear in Table 5–2.

Specialist Referrals. For some examinees, the oral-facial inspection leads to a recommendation that extends beyond the scope of speech-language pathology general practices. This may include testing that some speech-language pathologists are qualified to give under medical supervision (e.g., nasopharyngoscopy), or it may result from a need for information that requires an external referral, such as otorhinolaryngology, neurology, or genetics. Examples of specialist referrals are shown in Table 5–1.

Conclusion

Oral-facial inspections can yield a large amount of data that must be considered carefully and interpreted accurately so that the examining clinician can proceed to verbal and written communication with clients, their families, and other professionals. The information provided in this chapter is intended to serve as a convenient reference, supporting data interpretation for that purpose. Proceed to Chapter 6 for additional guidance that supports formal documentation.

CHAPTER 5

6

Documenting the Findings

Every communication evaluation culminates with documentation that becomes a critical piece of the examinee's clinical file. For that reason, the importance of professional report writing cannot be overemphasized. Yet, writing is an area of professional development that seriously challenges the majority of students, many newer clinicians, and even some who have years of practice behind them. In view of that, our final chapter gives attention to clinical report writing in a general way, while explicitly addressing how to document oral-facial findings and implications, highlighting them and embedding them into the appropriate report sections.

Documenting Oral-Facial Inspection: A Small Piece in a Large Puzzle

As stated in the front matter, evidence resulting from oral-facial inspection typically handles only one small piece in a relatively large puzzle that, when taken as a whole, sheds light on the examinee's idiosyncratic communication patterns (see Table 0–1). As a rule, the historical background and clinical findings, combined with observations, lead to an evidence-based and individualized diagnosis, prognosis, and list of recommendations. Competent professional report writing is required for documenting these matters in a way that is meaningful to consumers and their families, as well as colleagues and referral recipients.

To deliberate on how to meaningfully handle one report feature—that is, oral-facial findings and interpretations—it makes sense to consider that particular feature within the context of the full report. In view of that, a sample report format is shown in Table 6–1.

Headings and Subheadings That Apply When Reporting Oral-Facial Inspection Findings

Reporting Results of Testing

Note that Oral-Facial Inspection is one of many subheadings under Results of Testing; moreover, the chapter's primary focus is on reporting evidence that belongs in that section. Yet, consider that other report sections may appropriately cover certain aspects of the oral-facial findings. For instance, the subsection called Articulation is normally the best place to report results of speech sound stimulability screening or even the intelligibility judgment resulting from conversational speech sample. Likewise, when the conversational speech sample yields remarks relative to voice, fluency, or language, the commentary normally resides under a separate heading designating that particular aspect of speech or language.

Therefore, the chapter gives attention to a strategically selected assortment of subsections to demonstrate how inspection findings potentially affect various parts of the report. With regard to organization, much is left to professional discretion, while strongly cautioning less experienced writers to thoughtfully organize the evidence so that it flows logically, giving the reader a clear and orderly sense of the examinee's condition.

Table 6–1. Sample Format for Clinical Report Writing

Heading	Subheading(s)	Content
Identifying Information (using form-type format, not narrative)	None	Basic identifying data about the person precedes the narrative report. This may include but is not limited to: name, birth date, contact information, date of service, referral, names of significant others.
Diagnosis	None	Many find it helpful to provide a diagnostic statement on the front page of the clinical report, immediately following the identifying information
		Some clinicians omit this step
		A diagnostic statement on the front page can be extremely helpful to the next service provider for the purpose of orientating that person to the case
Introductory Paragraph	None	The introductory paragraph does not require a formal heading
		Purpose is to introduce the client to the reader
		Identifies the client by name, gender, and age
		Also states the type of service that is the subject of the clinical report (e.g., diagnostic evaluation), on what date the service was provided, and the names and relationships of any individuals who accompanied or provided information that is included in the report
		Preferred language, ethnicity, cultural orientation can be included in this section if relevant. The same applies for physical, cognitive, or sensory limitation if applicable
Statement of the Problem	None	The statement of the problem is a brief paragraph that reports the exact reason for the communication evaluation
		Often this section is best served by quoting the main informant who provided a reason for requesting services during the interview
Background Information	Birth/ Development	Generally, the case-history intake form that was completed prior to the evaluation session combined with results of the opening interview, yield information that is relevant to the assessment outcome. The subheadings that appear to the left are general subheadings that may be used either separately or in combination; the order of subheadings is determined by the magnitude of their contribution to the diagnosis and plan of care.
	Speech/ Language	
	Medical	
	Educational/ Vocational	Although a general statement of unremarkability may be made when no clinically relevant findings are noted in a particular area, there is no need to include every subheading or report on every topic.
	Social	
	Other	As to amount of detail, only milestones and events with potential for clinical relevance are reported, and only to the extent to which the information is clinically useful when ascertaining diagnosis, prognosis, and recommendations.

Table **6–1.** *continued*

Heading	Subheading(s)	Content
Results of Testing (includes standardized and informal testing)	Articulation/ Phonology	Similarly, the order of the subheadings shown on the left is determined by their relevance to the case; and subheadings with minor relevance or no noteworthy finding can be combined. For instance, if the client is being evaluated in the area of *voice*, that subheading would precede the others; and if no clinically relevant data emerge in articulation, language, and fluency, these three areas can be combined with a general statement of unremarkable findings in these areas.
	Language	
	Fluency	
	Voice	
	Hearing Screening	Typically however, the hearing screening and oral-facial inspection subheadings remain separate, and except in unusual circumstances, they appear last in the list of subheadings.
	Oral-Facial Inspection	
		It is in the subsections listed on the left that test scores, as well as all formal and informal observations, are recorded.
Clinical Impressions	None	The time spent with the client during the evaluation session often leads to observations that, if communicated, are likely to benefit the next service provider. Therefore, it is under this heading that the clinician shares information of that type. For instance, learning-style observations, extent to which the person participates in clinical work, sociability, physical or cognitive strengths or limitations, and areas of interest or preference are all examples of information that may be helpful when planning a therapy program or follow-up session.
		Clinical observations reported should begin with positive indicators, such as *engaging* or *attentive*. Most of what is reported in this section can be simply factual information, such as topic preferences or observations about learning style.
		If a clinical observation is made that indicates difficulty in a particular area, although this comment is needed, it should be carefully worded using family-friendly language. For example, if a child client demonstrates no interest in participation, then rather than stating that the child was *uncooperative* or *disinterested*, it may be better to state that *a clinical challenge exists in the area of finding topics and milieu that are likely to enhance participation* or that *the child frequently resisted clinician directed activities*.
		Unless there is virtually nothing positive to report or unless superficial features seem exceedingly relevant to the upcoming clinical decisions, clinicians should avoid comments on surface features such as grooming, whether eyewear is worn, or stature. Furthermore, these kinds of remarks do not typically reflect observations of a clinical type, and they may be perceived as condescending when read by the client or family.

continues

Table 6–1. *continued*

Heading	Subheading(s)	Content
Clinical Impressions *continued*	None	Bear in mind also, that some clinical observations may more appropriately be placed under other headings. For example, although commentary on response to clinical teaching may be helpful for the next clinician, it should have been reported when addressing stimulability and is again addressed under prognosis.
Summary (includes diagnosis)	None	The summary is most effective if it briefly highlights the preceding data that contributes to ascertaining the diagnosis, prognostic statement, and recommendations that follow. This section does not include test scores or specific data, as it is a summary only. Instead, it should make an interpretive statement that is based on concrete evidence.
		One way to end a summary paragraph is to write, *Therefore, Mr. Snow's diagnosis is . . . .* However, some prefer to begin the summary with the diagnostic statement, and allow the supporting evidence to follow. Either way, the summary should logically connect the outcome of the session with the person's diagnosis, even serving as rationale for it.
Prognosis	None	The prognosis is a statement of professional opinion based on evidence, and it addresses whether the client is likely to improve, either in response to treatment or in the absence of treatment. Supporting evidence for the prognosis should appear in the summary paragraph that precedes it.
		Prognostic indicators can be reported as part of the evidence, and they may include factors such as motivation, room for improvement, concerns about comorbidity, history of progress thus far, family support, sociability, or response to clinical teaching.
Recommendations	List of recommendations	A numbered list of recommendations generally appears in this section. Unless of course, there is only one recommendation, in which case a list is not needed. This circumstance is the exception rather than the rule.
		The recommendations section clearly defines the next steps to be taken in plan of care. Since most people seek the evaluation with the intention of beginning communication therapy, whether therapy is warranted is the first topic to be addressed under the heading of recommendations. Clearly the recommendation that addresses a treatment decision is connected to whether the prognostic statement supports the idea that the person is likely to benefit from treatment. Thus, the prognostic statement becomes a rationale for treatment. It is not necessary to repeat the prognostic statement since the information was highlighted directly above it.

Table 6–1. *continued*

Heading	Subheading(s)	Content
Recommendations *continued*	List of recommendations	Recommendations can also include the directive to perform specific diagnostic therapy activities. They may include referral(s) for additional work outside of the speech-language pathologist's scope of practice. The rationale can be found in the summary paragraph, and can be repeated so that it stands out from the other information reported in the summary.
		One should consider carefully whether a particular follow-up activity is optional before placing it on the recommendations list. This is because the word recommendation mandates a need for follow-up. If the type of follow-up that you have in mind is merely a suggestion and not required, these ideas may be separated out and called clinical suggestions.
Closing statement	None	A well-written report ends with a closing statement that immediately follows the recommendations. A subheading may or may not separate this from the recommendations.
		Essentially the purpose of the closing statement is to end on a positive note, and invite the client or family to initiate if more communication is needed. For example, one might say: *It was our pleasure to evaluate Dr. Garcia's communication needs. Please contact us if you have any questions.*
Signature lines	None	Signature lines are important. They testify to the credentials of the person who either oversaw the session or completed it independently. Underneath each signature line, a typed line should make clear the name of the person, highest degree earned (e.g., M.S., M.A., Ph.D., Ed.D), and clinical credential (e.g., CCC-SLP). The line may also state the person's position in the agency or institution, such as speech-language pathologist, clinical supervisor, or professorial rank.
		All signatures should be dated.

CHAPTER 6

When Findings Affect Clinical Implications and Plan of Care

Furthermore, beyond reporting results, oral-facial inspection findings have potential to affect sections that address clinical implications and plan of care (e.g., Summary, Prognosis, Recommendations). Sometimes, this comes in the form of ruling out physical cause, but on occasion, the inspection can add evidence of physical idiosyncrasy that contributes to the communication disorder and perhaps even requires attention in the plan of care.

Thus, depending on the nature of the findings, at the very minimum, inspection findings are briefly encapsulated in the Summary section. In addition, when inspection findings are clinically relevant or more complex, their influence may also seep into the diagnostic statement, the prognosis, or even the list of recommendations. Evidence from the inspection finds its way to these sections only if they contribute meaningfully to the message that the section conveys.

Basic Report Writing Guidelines

Fundamental writing guidelines affect all aspects of clinical reporting. Consequently, clinicians should familiarize themselves with both discipline-specific and general resources that are dedicated to professional and scientific writing. Some examples include Burrus and Willis (2013); Goldfarb and Serpanos (2009); Hegde (2010); Pannbacker, Middleton, Vekovius, and Sanders (2001); Stein-Rubin and Fabus (2012); Strunk and White (1999); and Zinsser (2006).

For convenience, Box 6–1 provides a set of quick-reference guidelines. These parameters are not intended to substitute for as-needed consultation with dedicated resources.

Box 6–1. Report Writing Guidelines: A Quick Reference Resource

Organization and Content

An effective clinical report builds a case that logically leads up to the Summary, including all relevant findings and only the relevant findings. The Summary then leads to the diagnostic statement, Prognosis, and Recommendations. Comments on organization and content that follow support this objective.

Eliminate Unnecessary Information

Before deciding to include any specific evidence in any report section, evaluate whether that particular detail is needed to prepare the reader for the Summary, Prognosis, and Recommendations. This guideline can eliminate superfluous information that, although perhaps interesting, is not relevant to clinical decisions that ultimately define the case.

State Each Idea Once and State It Under the Correct Heading

Having reduced the data down to essentials, decide which report section rightfully and meaningfully houses each critical piece. Doing this before beginning to write can diminish the tendency to repeat the same commentary in multiple sections; it can also eliminate an inclination to ramble.

The only report section that is permitted to repeat previously stated information is the Summary. Yet, even the Summary should not simply restate ideas but rather integrate them with evidence gathered throughout the session, creating an overall picture. Each report section includes information that prepares the reader for the Summary, while the Summary also prepares the reader for the diagnostic statement, prognosis, and recommendations. Repetition is permitted only to the extent that it serves this purpose.

Keep Words to a Minimum

Eliminate all unnecessary words and statements. Complying with the guidelines set forth in this box should be helpful in reducing report length.

Ideally, a well-written, single-spaced report does not exceed four pages. Certainly, there are exceptions to this guideline, depending on case complexity, types of tests administered, and results of testing. However, wordy reports may not be taken seriously in the professional community; therefore, the goal of having a four-page maximum should be considered reasonable. Since student-generated reports present an opportunity to prepare future colleagues for realistic professional practice, clinical practicum exercises are not exempt from this guideline.

Divide Content Appropriately

Headings and subheadings are meaningful dividers (see Table 6–1) that separate content, thereby facilitating the reader's understanding. When complex evidence emerges as a result of testing in a particular area, deciding exactly how to effectively present the findings within a section can be challenging. As a general rule, effective reports succinctly summarize unremarkable information first and then tackle the more complex set of atypical findings, grouping like information together. This avoids the problem of jumping back and forth between normal and atypical observations within the same section. It also requires separating typical from atypical findings when organizing the data.

In addition, paragraph divisions should be used as frequently as necessary. Each paragraph should cover one topic only. Initiate a new paragraph to mark even subtle shifts in topic.

Avoid Single-Sentence Paragraphs

Avoid single-sentence paragraphs whenever possible. When faced with what seems like an unavoidable single-sentence paragraph, dividing a longer sentence in two or even allowing an occasional single-sentence paragraph is preferred to attaching an unrelated idea to an otherwise cohesive paragraph.

Use Tables

Whenever data do not lend themselves to free-flowing narrative, consider presenting them in tabular form. This gives the reader at-a-glance access to complex data that, if written out, would be awkward or confusing, requiring much mental effort to process.

Tables are particularly useful when reporting results of testing in certain areas. Examples include but are not limited to numerical results of multi-subtest evaluation tools, lists of multiple articulation errors organized according to word position or difficulty level, responses to a series of pure tones by frequency, and phonological processes with examples organized according to type.

Be Specific and Concrete

Well-written reports leave no doubt in the reader's mind with regard to activities, findings, and clinical implications. One way to ensure that this happens is to use specific, concrete meaningful language.

Avoid Judging the Client's Ability. Many times, we request that a client perform an act, and the person responds by either not doing the act or making an unsuccessful attempt at compliance. When this happens, some may report that the person is *unable* to accomplish the act. However, using the word *unable* may not be entirely accurate, since some clients do not demonstrate every capability during clinical testing. Commenting on ability therefore becomes a tenuous practice and should be avoided.

There are a few ways to handle documentation when a person does not demonstrate a skill during testing. One option is to state that the person *did not demonstrate the ability* to perform the act. Another way is to simply describe the request and state what the person *did not do* in response to it.

Avoid Discussing Your Feelings. When making clinical judgments, phrases like *the clinician felt . . . or the clinician feels . . .* seem to creep into some reports. This may result from an effort to avoid definitively stating that the client is *unable* to do something, as it often appears in statements such as the following: *The clinician* feels *that the client is* unable *to perform the activity.*

Nevertheless, commenting on how we *feel* is not appropriate in clinical reports. Again, it is best to say what the person did or did not do, allowing that information to stand for itself.

Professional Jargon. Since the report is a professional document, professional jargon cannot be avoided entirely. However, it should be used with discretion, keeping in mind that the report is only useful to the recipient if the language is comprehensible to that person or entity. So, whenever using terms that are not familiar to people outside the profession, these terms should be defined parenthetically or by way of footnote, using everyday language.

Active Voice. Use active voice, avoiding passive voice whenever possible. Active voice gives the impression of being more direct. However, we recognize that there are times when passive voice is inescapable.

An avoidable example of passive voice is the following: *The oral-facial inspection* was completed by *the clinician in order to* . . . We can easily replace this sentence with a more direct statement, such as: *The inspection's purpose was to* . . . , *The inspection revealed* . . . , or even *We [or the clinician] completed the inspection so as to* . . . .

Avoid Euphemisms and Other Vague Language. Stay away from euphemisms, while taking care to also use family-friendly wording and steer clear of overstepping professional boundaries. For example, suppose a child client demonstrates a *high level of distractibility and activity throughout the session that sometimes interfered with productivity and concentration;* that statement can be made as stated here since it is accurate and concrete. Furthermore, it expresses the concerns in a way that is respectful to both the family and other professionals.

An example of euphemism expressing the same idea may be a reference to the child as *energetic* or *active*, with no mention of distractibility and performance consequences. This euphemistic description is too vague since it leaves out important information in what seems to be an attempt to spare the parents' feelings.

Avoid Terms Reserved for Other Professions. Another improper way to report a behavior similar to that described immediately prior is to label the child's intense activity level as *hyperactive*. *Hyperactivity* is a medical diagnosis that lies outside the scope of practice for speech-language pathologists. Although many practitioners have extensive experience with the behaviors associated with the condition, speech-language pathologists do not have authority to label or diagnose hyperactivity; therefore, the term becomes ambiguous in our hands, unless authorized by a formal diagnosis from the appropriate service provider. The better choice is to simply describe the behavior, as was done in the previous section.

Avoid Clichés and Colloquialisms. Colloquial language and clichés have no place in clinical report writing. For example, in an earlier section, a child was described as having a *high level of distractibility and activity throughout the session that sometimes interfered with productivity and concentration*. It is not appropriate to describe this child using a cliché or colloquial expression, such as *bouncing off the walls*, *jacked up*, or *out of control*.

Support Every Clinical Decision With a Rationale

Rationale is defined as *a reasoned exposition, especially one defining the fundamental reasons for a course of action*. Clinical decisions generally include courses of action such as test selection, assigning a diagnosis and prognosis, and prescribing recommendations. Expressing the reasoning behind clinical decisions is therefore essential to competent report writing. That is, as succinctly as possible, put into writing the reason for each course of action taken during or as a result of the evaluation.

Clinical rationale can come in a variety of forms. That is, in most cases, rationale reflects clinical evidence obtained during the diagnostic session, combined with the clinician's expertise. For instance, the summary of findings is the rationale for the diagnosis, and the prognosis is the rationale for the recommendation that addresses a decision about treatment.

In some cases, it is also possible that a rationale may come in the form of scientific information that relates to similar cases found in the literature. For example, if a particular treatment program is recommended, the supporting rationale may quote a research-based statement that reports on the effectiveness of the program relative to other individuals with similar symptoms. On the occasions that this is necessary, a short bibliography is needed for the report.

The concept of *rationale*, as it relates to clinical decision making, is covered in the body of the chapter. Refer to it for more information and for clinical examples.

Only Recommend What You Are Authorized to Recommend

When writing the Recommendations section, take care to stay within scope of practice boundaries. For example, speech-language pathologists are competent to recommend therapy, no therapy, an additional procedure by name if the procedure is within professional practice boundaries, and referrals to specialists and other professionals. Speech-language pathologists can also make suggestions with regard to specific types of speech-language procedures or treatment programs.

On the other hand, be aware of professional boundaries when making referrals. That is, it is entirely appropriate to solicit medical evaluation for the purpose of answering specific clinical questions and to accompany that request with an appeal for follow-up communication. It is not appropriate, however, to recommend that a specialist perform a particular procedure. For instance, if noting that the examinee has dental crowding that hinders hygiene, you may recommend a visit to the orthodontist requesting evaluation of dental alignment specifically as it relates to hygiene, but you may not recommend orthodonture or any other specific treatment for the condition. Similarly, if noting a short frenum that is judged to restrict lingual movement, you may recommend a visit to the oral surgeon for evaluation and follow-up, but you may not recommend surgery.

Grammar, Lexicon, and Other Details

Parallel Use of Tense

Erroneous tense switching within a section is a cardinal report writing mistake. Yet many struggle with it, even to the extent of shifting tense improperly within a sentence.

As a rule, historical data including clinical results require simple past tense. Thus, as a rule, past tense is suitable throughout the sections called Background Information, Results of Testing, and Summary, up to but not usually including the diagnostic statement (see Table 6–1).

When introducing the client in the introductory paragraph and Statement of the Problem, however, the present tense is more often the tense of choice. Similarly, the diagnostic statement (which is part of the Summary), Prognosis, and Recommendations usually employ simple present tense.

There are exceptions to these rules. For example, if using the past tense gives the impression that a living person has died, present tense should be substituted. Furthermore, at times, background information reports an ongoing state, giving present tense an appropriate place in that section.

Simple Verb Forms

Helping verbs and complex verbs forms are generally not needed and therefore potentially distracting. For example, when reporting a child's response to the request to open the mouth for viewing the oral interior, simply report that the child *opened the mouth* or *did not open the mouth*.

Reporting that the child *was opening the mouth, would open the mouth, did open the mouth,* or *will open the mouth* demonstrates poor writing technique. Furthermore, the practice adds unnecessary words to the report.

Noun-Verb Agreement

Word-processing programs consistently call attention to noun-verb disagreement when a writer makes an error of that type. Yet, some clinicians overlook the computer's guidance in this area, and this not recommended.

Noun-verb disagreement can be particularly challenging when using longer sentences with embedded clauses. So, shorter, simpler sentences can prevent the problem.

Shorter Sentences Preferred

Shorter sentences tend to be clearer, are more reader friendly, and support the clinician's effort to conform to other standards of report writing. Always divide run-on sentences into smaller units.

Pronouns

Pronouns should have a clear point of reference. That is, if using the word *he* or *she* in reference to the client, for clarity, the person's name should appear previously in the same paragraph. Otherwise, the point of reference for the pronoun can be unclear. Furthermore, if reporting information that involves two people of the same gender, names are preferred over pronouns to avoid confusion.

Moreover, incorrect use of the reflexive pronoun has become popular in the vernacular and is completely unacceptable in any type of professional communication. The reflexive pronouns are *myself, ourselves, yourself, yourselves, himself, herself, itself,* and *themselves.* If used, these words occur in the predicate of the sentence and refer back to the subjective case of a noun or pronoun. For example, it is improper to say, *The parent and myself agree . . .* since the word *myself* has no place in the subject of the sentence. Instead, the same idea can be expressed correctly by saying, *We agree with the parent . . . .*

An example of correctly using a reflexive pronoun is, *When given markers, Johnny drew on himself.* In this sentence, the word *himself* refers back to *Johnny.* (Note: The subjective referent may actually appear in the sentence, or it may be understood using the context of the sentence. For example, it is permissible to say, *When talking about yourself,* even though the word *you* does not appear in the subject. That is because the word *you* is understood, with the more complete sentence being *When you are talking about yourself.*)

Also, with regard to pronouns, using the editorial *we* (i.e., first-person plural) is permissible in formal writing. For example, it is permissible to say *we administered the test,* even if the word *we* refers to only one person. Conversely, though, it is not permissible to say *I administered the test,* since first-person singular is not acceptable in this type of formal writing. The editorial *we* can be an occasional refreshing change from the habit of constantly referring to yourself as *the clinician* or *the examiner.*

Sentences Do Not End in Prepositions

Any sentence that ends in a preposition is grammatically incorrect and has no place in the professional report. If noting a sentence that ends in a preposition while proofreading, rework the grammar to eliminate the problem.

Referring to Clients and Family Members

When referring to a child, use the full name when presenting the person in the introductory paragraph. If the child is also the client, use the full name again in the first sentence of the Summary, and refer to the child by first name only throughout all other parts of the report.

For an adult, refer to the person by full name, including title (e.g., Ms. Daisy Culpepper), when introducing the person in the introduction. If the adult is also the client, use the full name again in the first sentence of the Summary, and refer to the adult using title and last name only (e.g., Ms. Culpepper) throughout all other parts of the report.

Some prefer to substitute *the client* or *the child* for the person's name throughout the report, never referring to the person by name. However, this is neither a client-friendly nor a family-friendly writing technique; therefore, we suggest using the person's name and pronouns that have a clear point of reference throughout the report. Rare references to the person as *the client* or *the child* are permissible, but the report should not give the impression that the writer does not know the client's name or is avoiding reference to the person by name.

Acronyms

Clinical reports can require the use of acronyms, especially since acronyms apply to many of the evaluation tools we use. When using a test's acronym, refer to the test by its full name the first time, with the acronym in parentheses and to the right, and then refer to the test by its acronym every time after that.

Parallel Form for Bulleted Lists

Bulleted lists are often a part of a clinical report. Specifically, the recommendations appear in the form of a bulleted or numbered list that is preceded by a carrier phrase.

For example, a report may say, *As a result of the evaluation, we recommend: [followed by a bulleted list].* Each entry should then be an obvious sequitur that is grammatically consistent with the carrier phrase and grammatically parallel to the other items on the list.

Use of Quotations

If used, quotations should be short and meaningful. Often the statement of the problem includes a short quotation that captures the reason for the evaluation in the client or informant's own words. This is a meaningful use of a quotation. Lengthy or frequent quotations are not appropriate in clinical reports.

Never begin a sentence with a quotation. Instead, lead into the quotation by saying, *When asked to share the reason for seeking an evaluation, Mr. Maxwell replied . . . "[quotation]."*

Furthermore, since the quotation represents another person's idea as expressed through his or her own words, it is not necessary for the quotation to be grammatically correct. More important, the quotation should accurately represent the person's idea.

Punctuation

Rules for using periods, commas, colons, semicolons, hyphens, and dashes may be more complex than what can be covered in a quick-reference guide. Therefore, readers are encouraged to refer to dedicated publications for more information. A few essentials are included here for convenience.

Periods. Use a period to denote the end of a sentence. A sentence expresses a complete thought, having at least a verb and usually a subjective noun.

Periods can also appear at the end of each item in a numbered or bulleted list, but this is not required. For consistency, if the period is included at all, it needs to be included for all items in all lists in the document.

Commas. Commas are useful for separating items in a series of three or more and for separating the parts of a compound predicate. In some cases, a conjunction, such as *and*, substitutes for a comma; in that case, both conjunction and comma are not needed.

Colons. Colons often precede a group of like items that appear in sequence; they can also be considered the mathematical or grammatical notation to represent ratios (e.g., S:Z) and can be used to express a person's age in years and months (e.g., three years two months can be expressed as 3:2). Colons are also used when dividing a title into two meaningful parts, with the main idea preceding the colon and the modifier following it.

Semicolons. Semicolons divide two parallel independent clauses (e.g., *The oral-facial inspection identified generous anterior diastema that coincided with distorted sibilant production; therefore, the articulation disorder is judged to be secondary to dental misalignment.*). Semicolons are also used to separate items in a list if smaller units are separated by commas (e.g., *Elia is diagnosed with a moderate articulation disorder, secondary to oral-structural anomalies; mild language disorder, characterized by age-inappropriate syntax errors; and fluency disorder.*).

Dashes. Dashes can be useful for interrupting the flow of a sentence in order to interject a related idea. However, they are not particularly desirable in formal writing. A better way to handle a situation that seems to call for a dash is to reword the sentence so that the dash is not needed (e.g., *Mr. Small reported that his problems with his voice started immediately after a cold about 6 months ago—became more severe—and the symptoms have been fairly stable ever since.* The sentence can be rewritten to eliminate the use of dashes: *Mr. Small reported that his problems with his voice began with cold symptoms about 6 months ago. Although the symptoms worsened at first, they have been relatively stable for several months.*).

Hyphens. Hyphens are generally used within a word or compound word. They can separate double vowels (e.g., co-occur). In addition, they can appear between two modifiers when both modify the same noun (e.g., motor-speech disorder).

Apostrophes. Apostrophes express possessive forms as well as contractions. Contractions are not permitted in professional reports. We only address the possessive use of apostrophe, since it may possibly occur in a report.

For singular possessive, place the apostrophe before the possessive *s* marker; unless the word ends in *s*, then place it after the last letter of the word (i.e., *s*), but do not add another *s* or the letters *es*. For example: *Mary*'s *book*; *Morris*' *book*.

For regular plural possessive, place the apostrophe after the plural *s*. For example: *the siblings' ages*.

For irregular plural possessive, add *'s*, much as you would for singular possessive. For example: *the children's playroom*.

Some incorrectly use an apostrophe to denote the plural form of a surname ending in the letter *s*. For example, if a family's surname is *Woods*, refer to them as the *Woods family*, as the *Woods*, or even as the *Woodses*, but do not refer to them as the *Woods'*. Apostrophes are not used to denote plurality in any context.

Expressing Numbers

Use the following rules for expressing numbers:

- For cardinal and ordinal forms of the numbers *zero* through *nine*, spell out the word.
- Use numerals for numbers 10 and above, negative numbers, decimals, dates, fractions, addresses, numbers denoting list items, numbers that are part of a test name or procedure, and test scores appearing in a table. This list is not exhaustive.
- When beginning a sentence with a number, spell out the word, overriding any other rule for that number (e.g., *Eleven* family members attended the session.).
- When expressing decimals, the ones column should always have a placeholder, even if no whole number is associated with the notation. That is, *0.1* is correct decimal notation, whereas *.1* is not.

Dated, Legible, Appropriately Signed

Report Date

The date of the clinical service appears on the front page of the report and in the paragraph that introduces the client to the reader. It may also appear in the Summary, but it should not be repeated randomly throughout the report.

The date that the report is approved and signed is often different from the date of service. It appears beside the signature that authorizes the report. If additional signatures are obtained (e.g., student clinician or assistant), they should also be dated.

Report Legibility

Word processing has all but eliminated potential for illegible reports finding their way to client files or the hands of other service providers. Handwritten reports and poor printer quality are generally the causes of illegibility when it occurs. Therefore, do not create handwritten reports, and change printer cartridges as needed.

Report Signatures

The signature of a fully credentialed speech-language pathologist appears immediately following the report content, and exact credentials are specified directly below the signature line. Student signature lines may also appear on the signature page.

Basic Guidelines That Apply to Most Reports, Regardless of Complexity

Certain principles apply to most reports regardless of type or complexity of findings. In this section, a clinical example sheds light on these reporting fundamentals. For the sake of simplicity, the example intentionally lacks any hint of complexity.

For convenience, the sample case findings are itemized in Tables 6–2A and 6–2B. Then, Box 6–2 displays a completed sample report using the data shown in the tables. The parts of the report that directly pertain to the oral-facial inspection are highlighted using italic type.

Written Rationale for Clinical Decisions

As stated in Box 6–1, clinical decisions require a clearly stated rationale. Leading examples of clinical decisions include test selection, assigning a diagnosis, assigning a prognosis, and prescribing a plan of care. For that reason, the concept of clinical rationale permeates the discussion that follows.

Reporting the Decision to Perform Oral-Facial Inspection or Any Other Procedure

A comment stating that a particular test was performed precedes any documentation of findings that result from that test. Furthermore, since selecting to perform a specific test is a clinical decision, a statement of rationale points out the reasoning behind administering the specific procedure, also before reporting results.

The oral-facial evaluation's ubiquitous presence in the diagnostic protocol does not exempt one from ascertaining and stating the rationale for it. That is, the reasoning behind any customary practice is clearly stated when declaring that the procedure was administered, even if the procedure or one like it is universally performed. Table 6–2A and Box 6–2 display rationale statements for the four clinical procedures reported in the example.

Reporting Results

Immediately following the statement that a test was given, with its rationale, results of each test are then reported. Since reporting results entails stating qualitative and quantitative evidence learned through planned observations, no clinical decision requiring a rationale is involved. Only the data that result from the procedure are needed, reserving comments on implications and follow-up for the sections called Summary, Prognosis, and Recommendations.

See Table 6–2A and Box 6–2 for examples showing how results pertaining to the clinical case are reported in the example. Note that not every piece of data finds its way to the report since the report is generally reserved for noteworthy findings, and the order of testing does not determine sequencing in the report. That is, the formal report organizes topics according to meaningful subheadings, then within each subheading briefly comments on unremarkable findings first, and after that describes clinically relevant concerns, grouping similar information together.

Summary and Diagnosis

Summary Section

The Summary section's purpose is to bring together all noteworthy findings that affect the client's

Table 6–2A. Highlights for Simplest Clinical Example: Data Collection

Name: Damon Bellows

Age: 8:0

Referral: Third-grade teacher

Statement of the Problem: Damon noticed that his speech is different from peers.

	Clinical Decision	Rationale	Data
Background Information	No		Developmental milestones achieved as expected
			Certain words were always difficult to say (e.g., soup, zoo, Bellows)
Articulation Test	Administered the *Photo Articulation Test* (*PAT*) (Lippke, Dickey, Selmar, & Soder, 1997)	. . . to identify speech sound production errors in various word positions and contexts	/s→θ/, /z→ð/ in all positions and all contexts, *including connected speech*
Conversational Speech Sample	*According to Oral-Facial Evaluation for Speech-Language Pathologists (OFESLP)*	*. . . to ascertain impact on connected speech*	
Speech Sound Stimulability Screening	*Performed speech sound stimulability screening for /s/ and /z/ phonemes, targeting these sounds in the onset position of CV syllables, according to OFESLP*	*. . . This was done to ascertain Damon's response to clinical teaching relative to error sounds*	*Damon responded by closely approximating the targets*
Hearing Screening	Presented pure tones at 20 dB for frequencies 1K, 2K, and 4K Hz . . .	. . . to rule out or confirm the need for audiometric testing	Responded to all tones
Oral-Facial Inspection	*Administered the OFESLP*	*. . . to ascertain whether all parts necessary for speech were present, intact, and functioning*	*The oral-facial mechanism was found to be adequate for speech*
Clinical Impressions	No		Cooperated fully throughout
			Demonstrated motivation

diagnosis, prognosis, and recommendations. This includes oral-facial inspection observations as well as all other remarkable findings and observations. Relevant data to be included in the summary statement for the first sample case appear in Table 6–2B, and the full narrative Summary can be found in Box 6–2.

Table 6–2B. Highlights from Simplest Clinical Example: Clinical Implications

Name: Damon Bellows

Age: 8:0

Referral: Third-grade teacher

Statement of the Problem: Damon noticed that his speech is different from peers.

	Clinical Decision	Rationale/Evidence Information found in this column should appear in the report summary
Summary Note: Rationale for diagnosis comprises the information that appears in the report summary	Diagnosis: mild *functional* articulation disorder . . .	Frontal lisp characterized by /s→θ/ and /z→ð/; occurs in all word positions and in *all contexts*
		Oral-facial evaluation revealed no physical barriers that would prevent modifying the speaking pattern
		Responded to clinical teaching by approximating the identified targets in the onset position of CV syllables
Prognosis	Damon is likely to benefit from speech therapy . . .	Demonstrates room for improvement
		Cooperates during clinical activities
		Modifies his behavior when presented with clinical teaching opportunities
Recommendations	As a result of the evaluation, we recommend speech therapy to occur three times weekly for 30-minute sessions	(The rationale for the therapy recommendations is the prognosis statement, directly above. It does not need to be restated due to its close proximity to the diagnosis.)

CHAPTER 6

The summary paragraphs include observations that support each topic that follows them: diagnosis, prognosis, and plan of care. In fact, any report recipient should find the rationale for any of these three fundamental decisions within the context of the summary paragraphs. Thus, when writing the Summary, briefly condense all findings that support diagnosis, prognosis, and recommendations, and as a general rule, be careful to exclude any information that does not directly affect these three clinical decisions.

Also, the diagnosis appears immediately after the summary paragraphs and within the same section. Essentially, the summary states the evidence that leads to the diagnosis, is considered the rationale for it, and finds its logical conclusion in the diagnostic statement.

Assigning a Prognosis

The summary section also prepares the way for assigning a prognosis by giving information that potentially projects how the client may respond to treatment. Evidence that supports the prognostic statement for the example appears in Table 6–2B, and the full prognostic statement with rationale appears in Box 6–2.

Prescribing Recommendations

As a rule, the recommendations clearly and concretely define the next steps. In the first sample case, however, an effort is made to simplify; for that reason, only one recommendation applies.

Since the recommendation is a clinical decision, a rationale is needed. For the one recommendation that appears in Table 6–2B and Box 6–2, the prognostic statement serves as a rationale. As noted in examples that follow, more complex recommendations, such as those that call for further testing and referrals, reflecting back on the summary paragraphs, may more accurately serve the purpose of establishing a rationale for some recommendations. The clinical examples that follow frame opportunities for presenting recommendation rationales under a variety of circumstances.

Box 6–2. Clinical Report: Simplest Example

Identifying Information

Name: Damon Bellows

Date of Clinical Service: [date]

Mother's Name: Henrietta Bellows

Primary Language: English

Referral: Third-grade teacher

Diagnosis: Mild *functional* articulation disorder

Date of Birth: [date]

Age: 8:0

Father's Name: Haley Bellows

Secondary Language: None

Damon Bellows is an 8-year-old male who received a communication evaluation on [date]. Damon's mother, Ms. Henrietta Bellows, accompanied him to the session and served as primary informant via case history intake form as well as interview. Damon also participated in the interview.

Statement of the Problem

Damon requested the evaluation. When asked to comment on his reasons, he said, "I noticed the way I say some words is different from my friends."

Background Information

Speech and language milestones were achieved at expected ages. However, Damon's speech seemed different from his peers, and he has had difficulty pronouncing certain words (e.g., soup, zoo, Bellows).

Other background information for Damon is chiefly unremarkable. That is, he achieved developmental milestones at expected ages, has consistently performed at or above grade level in school since kindergarten, enjoys social activities with his friends, and reports no history of noteworthy medical concerns.

Results of Testing

The diagnostic protocol included the following procedures.

- *Photo Articulation Test (PAT)*
- Hearing screening
- *Oral-Facial Evaluation for Speech-Language Pathologists* (OFESLP)

Articulation Results

We administered the *PAT* to identify speech sound errors in words and sentences. Damon committed the following speech sound errors in all contexts: /s→θ/, /z→ð/.

Damon also participated in a speech sound stimulability screening as part of the OFESLP in an effort to judge response to clinical teaching. The phonemes /s/ and /z/ were targeted in the onset position of CV syllables. Damon consistently responded to clinical teaching by more closely approximating the target phoneme.

Intelligibility, Voice, Fluency, and Language

We engaged Damon in conversational speech according to the OFESLP so as to judge his overall intelligibility, fluency, voice, and language. Fluency, voice, and language were judged appropriate for Damon's age and gender. Furthermore, his overall intelligibility was judged as good. However, speech sound substitution errors in connected speech were consistent with those identified through the PAT.

Hearing Screening

Pure tones were presented at 20 dB for 1K, 2K, and 4K Hz to rule out or identify a need for audiometric testing. Damon responded to all tones bilaterally.

Oral-Facial Evaluation

We administered the OFESLP to ascertain whether all parts needed for speech were present, intact, and functioning. The oral-facial mechanism was judged adequate for speech.

Clinical Impressions

Damon participated in the clinical activities throughout the session, demonstrating both motivation and perseverance. Furthermore, he demonstrated awareness by noticing that his speech was different and by requesting help.

Summary

Damon Bellows is an 8-year-old male who requested a communication evaluation because of concerns with the way he pronounces some words. The evaluation took place on [date] at [name of clinic or agency]. Damon cooperated fully throughout the session, demonstrating both perseverance and motivation to improve.

CHAPTER 6

Articulation testing and *conversational speech* sample revealed features of a frontal lisp characterized by /s→θ/ and /z→ð/ sound substitutions in all positions of words *and in conversational speech. Oral-facial evaluation revealed no physical barriers preventing success in speech therapy, and he responded to clinical teaching by approximating the two target phonemes.*

As a result of the evaluation, Damon is diagnosed with a mild *functional* articulation disorder that affects the /s/ and /z/ consonants only.

Prognosis

Damon is likely to benefit from speech therapy. He demonstrates room for improvement, *positive response to clinical teaching,* cooperation, motivation, error awareness, and perseverance.

Recommendations

As a result of the communication evaluation, we recommend speech therapy for three 30-minute sessions weekly.

It has been a pleasure working with Damon. If we can be of any further assistance, please contact us directly.

Barbara Ann Johnson-Root, PhD, CCC-SLP
Professor and Speech-Language Pathologist

[Date of signature]

Handling Report Writing Challenges

When Inspection Reveals Idiosyncrasies That Do Not Contribute to the Communication Disorder

Occasionally, oral-facial inspection can uncover physical idiosyncrasies that have no identifiable impact on the person's speech but nevertheless deserve documentation. For instance, a person may adeptly compensate for a physical difference that has potential to result in speech production errors for some people, or the observation may potentially affect the examinee's health or well-being.

Reporting Physical Idiosyncrasies for Which the Person Compensates

The second clinical example illustrates a way to document a noteworthy physical difference that does not appear to influence speech production errors. Specific data relevant to the case appear in Tables 6–3A and 6–3B, while the sample report is shown in Box 6–3. Italics highlight notes and commentary that relate to oral-facial inspection.

The oral-facial inspection is sensitive enough to identify physical anomalies that, although they may potentially affect speech for some people, in the sample case they do not. For instance, the examinee exhibits a high palatal arch configuration for which there is no apparent link to speech production errors.

Table 6–3A. Highlights for Clinical Example With Physical Idiosyncrasies That Do Not Contribute to Speech Production Errors: Data Collection

Name: Whitney Jarvis

Age: 6:11

Statement of the Problem: Whitney's speech seems to interfere with social development and learning to read

	Clinical Decision	Rationale	Data
Background Information	No		Feeding difficulties in infancy; resolved by first birthday
			Gross and fine motor development, as expected
			First word (baby) emerged at 15 months
			Two-word sentences (more cookie) emerged at 21 months
Articulation Test (supplement with conversational speech sample)	Administered the *Clinical Assessment of Articulation and Phonology* (*CAAP*) (Secord & Donohue, 2002)	. . . to identify speech-sound production errors in various word positions and contexts	/s→θ/, /z→ð/ /r→w/, /l→j/ in all positions and all contexts
	Conversational speech sample according to Oral-Facial Evaluation for Speech-Language Pathologists (OFESLP)	*. . . to ascertain impact on connected speech*	*Same errors in connected speech*
			Usually intelligible
			Easier to understand once familiar with her speaking pattern
Speech Sound Stimulability Screening	*Performed speech sound stimulability screening for /s/, /z/, /r/, and /l/ phonemes, according to OFESLP, targeting these sounds in the onset position of CV syllables . . .*	*. . . This was done to ascertain Whitney's response to clinical teaching relative to error sounds*	*Responded to clinical teaching by increasing loudness but not by improving articulation*
Hearing Screening	Presented pure tones at 20 dB for frequencies 1K, 2K, and 4K Hz . . .	. . . to rule out or confirm the need for audiometric testing	Responded to all tones

continues

CHAPTER 6

183

Table 6–3A. *continued*

	Clinical Decision	Rationale	Data
Oral-Facial Inspection	*Performed OFESLP*	*. . . to ascertain whether all parts necessary for speech were present, intact, and functioning*	*All parts were found to be present, intact, and functioning*
			Palatal arch configuration was observed to be remarkably high and narrow
			Pervasive dental decay
Clinical Impressions	No		Pleasant child
			Enjoys playing games
			Easily distracted from task, which interfered with ability to focus

Since this is merely a sample case, high palatal arch is only one possible feature that could have been chosen to illustrate an anomaly that may or may not affect speech. Other examples include dental misalignment, malocclusion, and poorly differentiated tongue movements, to name only a few.

Since the aberrant physical feature, high palatal arch in this case, is noted during the inspection and since it has potential to be identified at a later time by other professionals, documenting it in the report is appropriate for the sake of the record. Stating its lack of relevance to communication is equally necessary.

Reporting a Single Physical Idiosyncrasy Not Affecting Speech, With Medical or Health Care Significance

Another type of physical difference that does not affect speech that may be noteworthy is one that has significance to overall health or medical care. The examinee's dental decay does not seem to directly affect speech but poses a threat to health and well-being. Other examples of features that may not affect speech but call for medical attention could include enflamed tonsils, tissue discoloration, allergy symptoms, malocclusion, or dental misalignment. These types of observations require attention in the report since follow-up is generally required.

Since medical or specialist attention is needed, although this information does not affect speech production, the documentation appears under Oral-Facial Examination in the Results of Testing section. Furthermore, a succinct statement is included in the Summary, logically leading to a recommendation for follow-up, as shown in Table 6–3.

Handling Multiple Recommendations

In the first clinical example, there was no opportunity to look at techniques for prescribing a complex plan of care. Yet, in most cases, the plan of care includes multiple recommendations. The second example provides opportunity to discuss this aspect of diagnostic report writing.

Box 6–3 illustrates a report having three recommendations. Note that a lead-in statement precedes the three recommendations, the recommendations appear in a numbered list, each recommendation completes the lead-in sentence and is grammatically consistent with it, and the three recommendations use grammatically parallel syntax. Furthermore, each of

Table 6–3B. Highlights From Clinical Example With Physical Idiosyncrasies That Do Not Contribute to Speech-Production Errors: Clinical Implications

Name: Whitney Jarvis		
Age: 6:11		
Statement of the Problem: Whitney's speech seems to interfere with social development and learning to read		

	Clinical Decision	Rationale/Evidence Information found in this column should appear in the report summary
Summary (with diagnosis)	Diagnosis: mild *functional* articulation disorder . . .	Articulation errors occur in all word positions and in all contexts: /s→θ/, /z→ð/ /r→w/, /l→j/
		Conversational intelligibility slightly compromised
		Oral-facial evaluation revealed high palatal arch that is not believed to prevent modifying the speaking pattern
Prognosis	Whitney is likely to improve . . .	Demonstrates room for improvement
		Enjoys playing games
		Pleasant child
	Progress may be slow . . .	*Responds to clinical teaching by increasing loudness but not by changing the articulatory pattern*
		Easily distracted from task, which interferes with ability to focus
Recommendations: As a result of the evaluation, we recommend . . .	. . . speech therapy to occur three times weekly for 30-minute sessions . . .	(The prognostic statement should serve as rationale for a therapy recommendation. It does not need to be restated.)
	Referral for educational testing to identify or rule out difficulties with attention	Easily distracted from task, which interferes with ability to focus
	Referral to dentist for evaluation and hygiene education	*Pervasive dental decay*

the three recommendations has a rationale that can be found in the Summary section. Due to the Summary's proximity to the Recommendations, the specific ratio-nale is not repeated, although there is nothing that prevents a clinician from repeating the rationale if doing so enhances report readability or clarity.

Box 6–3. Clinical Report: Clinical Example With Observations That Do Not Contribute to Speech Production Errors

Identifying Information

Name: Whitney Jarvis

Date of Birth: [date]

Date of Clinical Service: [date]

Age: 6:11

Mother's Name: Amanda Holcolm

Father's Name: Nathan Jarvis

Primary Language: English

Secondary Language: None

Referral: First-grade teacher

Diagnosis: Mild *functional* articulation disorder

Whitney Jarvis is a 6-year, 11-month-old female who received a communication evaluation on [date]. Whitney's parents, Ms. Amanda Holcomb and Mr. Nathan Jarvis, accompanied her to the session. Ms. Holcomb served as primary informant via interview as well as case history intake form; Mr. Jarvis also participated, adding information that supported Ms. Holcomb's remarks.

Statement of the Problem

Ms. Holcomb requested the communication evaluation because, "Whitney's teacher says my daughter's speech is causing her problems with learning to read and with making friends at school."

Background Information

Speech-Language Development

Although not all speech-language milestones were recalled, parents expressed that there has been concern with Whitney's speech since she was about 18 months old, when they first noticed that her speech development seemed to lag behind that of her peers. For example, Whitney said her first intelligible word at the age of 15 months (i.e., baby), and she said her first two-word sentence at the age of 21 months (i.e., more cookie). Vocabulary development and sentence structure quickly caught up, but she continued to demonstrate difficulty pronouncing some words (e.g., lamp →/jæmp/, yellow →/ˈjɛ jo/, red →/wɛd/).

Motor Development

All fine and gross motor developmental milestones reportedly emerged at expected ages. For example, Whitney sat at 7 months, walked at 12 months, was potty trained at 25 months, and presently successfully participates in gymnastics and ballet classes. Ms. Holcomb and Mr. Jarvis expressed no concerns with Whitney's motor development.

Medical History

As a newborn, Whitney experienced feeding difficulties that resolved before her first birthday. Otherwise, her medical history was unremarkable.

Social and Educational Histories

Whitney is enrolled in first grade. She has been experiencing difficulties with both academic progress and social development.

Results of Testing

The diagnostic protocol included the following procedures.

- *Clinical Assessment of Articulation and Phonology (CAAP)*
- Hearing screening
- *Oral-Facial Evaluation for Speech-Language Pathologists (OFESLP)*

Articulation Results

We administered Consonant Inventory and School-Age Sentences of the *CAAP* to identify speech sound errors in words and sentences. Whitney made the following speech sound errors in all contexts: /s→θ/, /z→ð/, /r→w/, /l→j/.

Whitney also participated in a speech sound stimulability screening as part of the OFESLP in an effort to judge response to clinical teaching. The phonemes /s/, /z/, /r/, and /l/ were targeted in the onset position of CV syllables. Whitney responded to clinical teaching by increasing loudness but not by approximating target phonemes.

Intelligibility, Language, Voice, and Fluency

We engaged Whitney in conversational speech according to the OFESLP so as to judge intelligibility, language, fluency, and voice. Fluency, voice, and language were judged as appropriate for Whitney's age and gender.

Intelligibility was judged as good when the context was known but otherwise somewhat compromised. Furthermore, intelligibility improved with continued exposure to Whitney's predictable speech pattern.

Hearing Screening

Pure tones were presented at 20 dB for 1K, 2K, and 4K Hz to rule out or identify a need for audiometric testing. Whitney responded to all tones bilaterally.

Oral-Facial Evaluation

The OFESLP was used to ascertain whether all parts needed for speech were present, intact, and functioning. Oral-facial mechanism was judged adequate for speech; however, some idiosyncrasies were noted. That is, the inspection identified an exceedingly high palatal arch configuration and dental decay. Although we judged both features as unrelated to the articulation errors noted, they were considered noteworthy.

CHAPTER 6

Clinical Impressions

Whitney enjoyed playing clinical games that the clinicians presented, and overall, she was a pleasant child throughout the testing. However, it was apparent that Whitney became distracted easily, and this interfered with focus during several activities.

Summary

Whitney Jarvis is a 6-year, 11-month-old child who participated in a communication evaluation on [date] because of concerns with the way she pronounces some words and the impact that her speech may have on social development and literacy. She demonstrated that she enjoyed the clinical activities and games throughout the session but occasionally became distracted and lost focus.

Articulation testing and *conversational speech* sample revealed four sound substitutions that occurred in all positions of words and in conversational speech. *Whitney did not demonstrate stimulability for any of the error phonemes. Oral-facial evaluation revealed no physical barriers that prevent modifying the identified speech pattern. Furthermore, the procedure revealed high palatal arch configuration and dental decay that are judged clinically insignificant relative to speech.*

As a result of the communication evaluation, Whitney is diagnosed with a mild *functional* articulation disorder that affects the /s/, /z/, /r/, and /l/ consonants only.

Prognosis

Whitney is likely to benefit from speech therapy, but progress may be slow. That is, she demonstrates room for improvement and interest in clinical activities. However, she also demonstrates distractibility that interferes with focus and *does not modify her speech pattern when presented with clinical teaching.*

Recommendations

As a result of the communication evaluation, we recommend:

1. Speech therapy for three 30-minute sessions weekly
2. Referral for educational testing to explore options that may improve focus during clinical and academic work
3. *Referral to a dentist for evaluation, as well as hygiene education*

We enjoyed working with Whitney. If we can be of any further assistance, please contact us directly.

_____   _____
Barbara Ann Johnson-Root, PhD, CCC-SLP   [Date of signature]
Professor and Speech-Language Pathologist

When Inspection Reveals Idiosyncrasies That Contribute to the Communication Disorder

Symptom Cluster Leading to Medical Referral

The oral-facial inspection presents an opportunity to critically observe a person's craniofacial structure; therefore, a symptom cluster may be discovered that deserves genetic or otorhinolaryngology evalu-ation. Although in many cases, symptom clusters call attention to themselves during infancy and early development, when developmental delay, cognitive limitations, or craniofacial anomaly are not involved, features may not call attention to themselves until the child is older.

A third clinical example is presented to illustrate how one might handle noting a symptom cluster, regardless of the client's age or history. Tables 6–4A and 6–4B provide the data, and Box 6–4 compiles relevant data into a sample clinical report.

Table 6–4A. Highlights for Clinical Example With Symptom Cluster Noted: Data Collection

Name: Abner Lyon

Age: 6:3

Referral: Dr. [name], Otorhinolaryngologist

Medical diagnosis: Functional dysphonia, per referring physician

Statement of the Problem: Abner's voice is much higher than other children his age. We want to help him lower his voice.

	Clinical Decision	Rationale	Data
Background Information	No		Early feeding problems and failure to thrive; no sucking reflex; resolved with lactation coaching
			Speech development: unremarkable
			Walked late (15 months); parents express no concerns with motor development
			Does well in school; at grade level
			Does not like physical education class; does not enjoy games requiring physical activity or coordination
Speech and Language	Administered the *Fluharty Preschool Speech and Language Screening Test–2nd Edition (Fluharty-2)* (Fluharty, 2001)	. . . to identify or rule out speech or language concerns that may need complete evaluation, since the present evaluation's focus is voice	Receptive Language Quotient (RLQ) raw score = 23 (age equivalent >6:9) Expressive Language Quotient (RLQ) raw score = 18 (age equivalent of 6:9) No need for further testing in areas tested

continues

Table 6–4A. *continued*

	Clinical Decision	Rationale	Data
Voice (otorhino-laryngology testing completed prior)	Qualitative judgments . . .	. . . to supplement scientific data sent from Dr. [name of physician], Otorhinolaryngologist	High pitch
			Low vocal loudness (occasionally interferes with intelligibility)
			Reduced range of pitch and loudness
			Did not change voice in response to clinical teaching
Conversational Speech Sample	*According to Oral-Facial Evaluation for Speech-Language Pathologists (OFESLP)*	*. . . to judge all aspects of speech production in connected speech*	*Speech sound production, language, and fluency were all judged appropriate for age and gender*
			Vocal pitch was judged as high; vocal loudness was judged as low
			Low vocal loudness occasionally affected intelligibility
Hearing Screening	Presented pure tones at 20 dB for frequencies 1K, 2K, and 4K Hz . . .	. . . to rule out or confirm the need for audiometric testing	Responded to all tones
Oral-Facial Inspection	*Performed the OFESLP*	*. . . to ascertain whether all parts necessary for speech were present, intact, and functioning*	*All parts were found to be present, intact, and functioning*
			Micrognathia with retrognathia
			Low-set ears
			Depressed nasal tip
			Anteverted nares
			Incomplete dentition
			High palatal arch
Clinical Impressions	No		Friendly
			Intelligent
			Cooperative
			Socially awkward

Table 6–4B. Highlights From Clinical Example With Symptom Cluster: Clinical Implications

Name: Abner Lyon

Age: 6:3

Referral: Dr. [name], Otorhinolaryngologist

Medical diagnosis: Functional dysphonia

Statement of the Problem: Abner's voice is much higher than other children his age. We want to help him lower his voice.

	Clinical Decision	Rationale/Evidence Information in this column should appear in the report summary.
Summary (with diagnosis)	Diagnosis: voice disorder; genetic syndrome not ruled out	Intelligent
		Cooperative
		Articulation, fluency, and language all judged to be appropriate for age
		High vocal pitch
		Low vocal volume that interferes with intelligibility
		Does not change vocal pitch when presented with clinical teaching
		All anatomic parts needed for speech were found to be present, intact, and functioning
		Micrognathia with retrognathia
		Low-set ears
		Depressed nasal tip
		Anteverted nares
		Incomplete dentition
		High palatal arch
Prognosis	Abner may improve . . .	Demonstrates room for improvement
		Intelligent
		Cooperative
	Extent of progress is difficult to determine . . .	*Does not modify voice in response to clinical teaching*
		Questions remain as to origin of the problem
Recommendations: As a result of the evaluation, we recommend . . .	. . . speech therapy to occur three times weekly for 30-minute sessions. Impact of therapy will be reassessed after 6 weeks.	(The prognostic statement should serve as rationale for a therapy recommendation. It does not need to be restated.)
	Referral to genetics specialist to explore the identified symptom patterns . . .	*Cluster of physical symptoms, concomitant to unexplained voice disorder*

Box 6–4. Clinical Report: Example Illustrating Symptom Cluster

Identifying Information

Name: Abner Lyon

Date of Clinical Service: [date]

Mother's Name: Josephina Lyon

Primary Language: English

Date of Birth: [date]

Age: 6:3

Father's Name: Abner Lyon

Secondary Language: None

Referral: Dr. [name of physician], Otorhinolaryngologist

Diagnosis: Functional dysphonia (per Dr. [name of referring physician]); *genetic syndrome not ruled out.*

Abner Lyon is a 6-year, 3-month-old male child who participated in a communication evaluation at the [name of clinic] on [date]. His parents, Mr. and Mrs. Abner and Josephina Lyon, accompanied him to the session. Unless otherwise indicated, Mrs. Lyon served as informant with regard to the historical information that appears in this report.

Statement of the Problem

According to Mr. Lyon, "Abner's voice is really high. We want to help him find a voice that is easier to listen to."

Background Information

Speech-Language Development

Abner achieved speech and language milestones at expected ages. His parents expressed no concern in the area of language development.

Medical History

Abner experienced feeding problems and failure to thrive as a young infant. At the age of 1 month, his pediatrician, Dr. [name of doctor], discovered that he lacked the sucking reflex and referred the family for lactation consultation at the [name of clinic]. Feeding problems resolved within 6 months.

Dr. [name of physician], an otorhinolaryngologist, evaluated Abner for his atypical voice on [date] and referred Abner to the [name of clinic] with a diagnosis of functional dysphonia, characterized by "high pitch and monotone."

Abner's measured fundamental frequency in connected speech was 305 Hz, with a range of 185 to 405 Hz, which is somewhat high for his age and gender. Dr. [name of physician] reported that visual inspection of the larynx revealed no evidence of vocal pathology.

Educational History, Social History, and Motor Development

Abner attends first grade at the [name of school] Elementary School, where he is performing at grade level. He enjoys reading and math but refrains from many social activities. His best friend is his cousin, who attends kindergarten at the same school.

When asked about school, Abner commented that he "hates PE class." Furthermore, he stated that he does not enjoy playing games that require physical activity and coordination. Although Abner walked later than his peers (i.e., 15 months), his parents reported no concerns with gross or fine motor development.

Results of Testing

The diagnostic protocol included the following procedures:

- Subjectively judge voice quality, pitch, loudness, resonance, and impact on intelligibility
- *Fluharty Preschool Speech and Language Screening Test–2nd Edition (Fluharty-2)*
- Hearing screening
- *Oral-Facial Evaluation for Speech-Language Pathologists (OFESLP)*

Voice

In conversational speech, Abner's voice quality and resonance were judged to be within normal limits for age and gender. However, voice was judged as high-pitched with low volume and characterized by little variation in pitch and loudness. When given opportunities to modify pitch and loudness through clinical teaching, although he put in a heroic effort, Abner's pitch and loudness did not change.

Intelligibility

Abner's intelligibility in connected speech was judged as good, with some burden placed on the listener due to inadequate volume.

Articulation, Language, and Fluency

The *Fluharty-2* was administered to rule out or identify areas of communication development that may require comprehensive evaluation, in addition to voice. The screening tool revealed Receptive and Expressive Language Quotients at or above age level. Furthermore, based on a conversational speech sample, articulation, language, and fluency were judged to be within normal limits for Abner's age and gender.

Hearing Screening

Pure tones were presented at 20 dB for 1K, 2K, and 4K Hz to rule out or identify a need for audiometric testing. Abner responded to all tones bilaterally.

Oral-Facial Evaluation

Upon inspection, the oral-facial mechanism was judged adequate for speech production. However, we noted a cluster of craniofacial idiosyncrasies that, although not relevant to speech, may be significant when considering Abner's overall condition. They include high-palatal arch, micrognathia with retrognathia, low-set ears, depressed nasal tip, anteverted nares, and incomplete dentition.

Clinical Impressions

Abner cooperated fully throughout the evaluation session. Although at times he seemed socially awkward, he demonstrated a friendly demeanor and an interest in pleasing the clinician.

Summary

Abner Lyon is a 6-year, 3-month-old male child who participated in communication evaluation on [date] in order to respond to a referral from otorhinolaryngology. Abner arrived with a medical diagnosis of functional dysphonia, characterized by "high pitch and monotone."

Abner cooperated fully throughout the session and put a tremendous amount of effort into the clinical teaching activities. Speech production, language, and fluency were all judged to be within normal limits for Abner's age and gender.

However, Abner's voice was judged to be high-pitched, with decreased loudness, and characterized by minimal pitch and inflection. His response was minimal when attempts were made to modify his pitch and loudness through clinical teaching. At times, Abner's decreased loudness interfered with intelligibility.

Oral-facial inspection revealed a cluster of craniofacial symptoms that may imply a possible genetic syndrome that, if diagnosed, has potential to shed light on issues relevant to plan of care. More information is needed in this area.

Our findings corroborate the diagnosis of functional voice disorder with high pitch, low volume, and reduced inflection. Furthermore, *a cluster of craniofacial symptoms* suggests that more information is needed to rule out or confirm a genetic etiology.

Prognosis

It is likely that Abner will benefit from voice therapy. He has room for improvement, cooperates with clinical activities, and makes a noteworthy effort to adjust his voice when given opportunity to do so.

However, it is difficult to determine the extent to which Abner will benefit from therapy at this point. That is, he does not change his voice when given clinical teaching opportunities, and some questions remain as to whether a concomitant diagnosis is yet to be determined.

Recommendations

As a result of the communication evaluation, we recommend the following:

1. Voice therapy twice weekly for 45-minute sessions
2. Assess progress in 6 weeks to evaluate whether treatment is effective
3. *Genetic evaluation to explore whether the cluster of craniofacial symptoms is significant to Abner's plan of care. Follow-up communication is requested.*

Barbara Ann Johnson-Root, PhD, CCC-SLP
Professor and Speech-Language Pathologist

[Date of signature]

When Anomaly or Idiosyncrasy Is First Noticed Through Oral-Facial Evaluation

Whenever evaluating a person with speech production disorder, discovering organic explanation through oral-facial inspection always remains a possibility. It is because of this fact that oral-facial inspection is a standard part of every communication evaluation protocol.

When inspection exposes a single anomaly that is not previously identified, and the idiosyncrasy indisputably contributes to the identified communication disorder, the documentation can be quite simple. Yet, clinically significant findings are often somewhat convoluted, with documentation requiring complex organization and problem solving to clearly and concisely interpret and communicate the concerns noted.

The next case example illustrates unanticipated findings that are complex. When this happens, organization and planning are fundamentally important to drawing conclusions and writing a meaningful report. Findings and implications appear in Tables 6–5A and 6–5B. The resulting diagnostic report occupies Box 6–5, with oral-facial related information italicized.

Table 6–5A. Highlights for Complex Clinical Example: Data Collection

Name: Ms. Maribel Guerra

Age: 22 years

Informant: Self

Reported Dominant Language: English; Reported Nondominant Language: Spanish

Statement of the Problem: Ms. Guerra is a theater student whose atypical speech prevents her from obtaining acting roles that she desires. Her acting professor referred her.

	Clinical Decision	Rationale	Data
Background Information	No		Late talker: was told she began talking at 2 years
			History of speech therapy from age 2 years through sixth grade; discharged because she no longer qualified for services
			As a child, language of the home was Spanish; language in school and the community was English; prefers English
			Reported same problems with speaking Spanish
Articulation Test (supplement with conversational speech sample)	Administered the *Photo Articulation Test (PAT)* (Lippke et al., 1997)	. . . to identify speech sound production errors in various word positions and contexts	Slight speech sound distortions affecting lingua-alveolar and linga-palatal fricatives, and affricates in all positions and all contexts: /s/, /z/, /ʃ/, /ʒ/, /tʃ/, /dʒ/
	Conversational speech sample according to Oral-Facial Evaluation for Speech-Language Pathologists (OFESLP)	*. . . to ascertain impact on connected speech*	*Speech sound errors were consistent with those identified through PAT.* *Other random errors were also noted, particularly when speech rate increased.*
Speech Sound Stimulability Screening	*Performed speech sound stimulability screening for /s/, /z/, /ʃ/, /ʒ/, /tʃ/, and /dʒ/ phonemes, according to OFESLP, targeting these sounds in the onset position of CV syllables . . .*	*. . . This was done to ascertain Ms. Guerra's response to clinical teaching relative to error sounds*	*Ms. Guerra put much effort into the clinical teaching activity, with little success. Although productions changed, they did not approximate the targets.*

Table 6–5A. *continued*

	Clinical Decision	Rationale	Data
Hearing Screening	Presented pure tones at 25 dB for frequencies 1K, 2K, and 4K Hz . . .	. . . to rule out or confirm the need for audiometric testing	Responded to all tones
Oral-Facial Inspection	*Performed OFESLP*	*. . . to ascertain whether all parts necessary for speech were present, intact, and functioning*	*All parts necessary for speech: present and intact, with some noteworthy performance idiosyncrasies*
			Tongue movements: poorly differentiated from jaw movements
			Verbal diadochokinetic rate: judged as slow for speech-alternating motion (i.e., three to four syllables per second)
			Verbal diadochokinetic coordination: speech-sequential motion resulted in speech sound transpositions and substitutions
Clinical Impressions	No		Engaging
			Demonstrated motivation by the *effort she put into the activities, especially speech sound stimulability*
			Enjoys acting
			Animated

Table 6–5B. Highlights From Complex Clinical Example: Clinical Implications

Name: Ms. Maribel Guerra

Age: 22 years

Reported Dominant Language: English; Reported Nondominant Language: Spanish

Statement of the Problem: Ms. Guerra is a theater student whose atypical speech prevents her from obtaining acting roles that she desires. Her acting professor referred her.

	Clinical Decision	Rationale/Evidence Information found in this column should appear in the report summary.
Summary (with diagnosis)	Diagnosis: mild articulation disorder; motor-speech disorder not ruled out	Consistent mild distortions of /s/, /z/, /ʃ/, /ʒ/, /tʃ/, /dʒ/ in all contexts
		Random articulation errors noted in connected speech, particularly when rate increased
		Ms. Guerra put in much effort but accomplished little change in her speech production when presented with clinical teaching
		Poorly differentiated tongue movements
		Slow verbal diadochokinetic rate (speech-alternating motion and speech-sequential motion)
		Speech-sequential motion resulted in speech sound transpositions and substitutions
Prognosis	Mr. Guerra is likely to improve . . .	Demonstrates room for improvement
		Demonstrates motivation and works hard at activities presented
	Progress may be slow . . .	*Simple clinical teaching activity did not result in speech changes*
		Possible motor-speech disorder
Recommendations	Speech therapy to occur three times weekly for 50-minute sessions . . .	(The prognostic statement should serve as rationale for a therapy recommendation. It does not need to be restated.)
	More in-depth testing to clarify whether symptoms are secondary to a motor-speech disorder	*Oral-facial symptoms*
		Articulation deteriorated with increased rate in connected speech

Box 6–5. Clinical Report: Complex Example: Complex Findings With No A Priori Knowledge

Identifying Information

Name: Ms. Maribel Guerra

Date of Clinical Service: [date]

Primary Language: English

Referral: Acting Professor

Diagnosis: Mild articulation disorder

Date of Birth: [date]

Age: 22 years

Secondary Language: None

Ms. Maribel Guerra is a 22-year-old bilingual woman who considers English her dominant language but is also fluent in Spanish since childhood. Ms. Guerra served as her own informant by completing a case history intake form with input from her mother and by participating in an interview. Although her friend, Mr. Eric Sjoblad, accompanied her to the session, he provided no information and did not participate in the interview.

Statement of the Problem

Ms. Guerra requested the communication evaluation because, "My [acting] professor told me that it is my speech that keeps me from getting the parts that I want."

Background Information

Ms. Guerra reported speech difficulties since childhood. Therefore, we sought information on her overall development, focusing on communication.

As a child, the language of Ms. Guerra's home was Spanish. She began to learn English when she entered a Head Start program at the age of 4 years and considers English her primary language at present.

Ms. Guerra was a late talker who did not speak at all until age 2 years and recalled that people had difficulty understanding her until about second grade. She participated in speech therapy from age 2 years until she completed the sixth grade, at which time she was discharged because she no longer qualified for services in the public education system. Ms. Guerra recalled that her problems with learning to speak occurred in both English and Spanish and that her speech therapy focused primarily on English.

Social and Educational Histories

Ms. Guerra graduated from [name of high school] with honors 3 years ago. Presently, she studies acting at [name of college]. She enjoys school and the many social activities that are available on her campus.

CHAPTER 6

Results of Testing

The diagnostic protocol included the following procedures.

- *Photo Articulation Test (PAT)*
- Hearing screening
- *Oral-Facial Evaluation for Speech-Language Pathologists (OFESLP)*

Articulation Results

We administered the *PAT* so as to identify speech sound production errors in various word positions and contexts. The results exposed slight speech sound distortions affecting lingua-alveolar and lingua-palatal fricatives and affricates in all positions and all contexts.

Ms. Guerra also participated in a speech sound stimulability screening as part of the OFESLP in an effort to judge response to clinical teaching. Ms. Guerra put much effort into the clinical teaching activity, with little success. Although speech sound productions changed, she did not successfully approximate the targets.

Intelligibility, Language, Voice, and Fluency

We engaged Ms. Guerra in conversational speech according to OFESLP so as to ascertain impact on connected speech. Fluency, voice, and language were judged appropriate for Ms. Guerra's age and gender. Although intelligibility was judged as reasonably good, additional random articulation errors not recorded on the PAT were also apparent, especially when Ms. Guerra spoke at an increased rate.

Hearing Screening

Pure tones were presented at 25 dB for 1K, 2K, and 4K Hz to rule out or identify a need for audiometric testing. Ms. Guerra responded to all tones bilaterally.

Oral-Facial Evaluation

The OFESLP was used to ascertain whether all parts needed for speech were present, intact, and functioning. All parts necessary for speech were found to be present and intact; however, some functional idiosyncrasies were noted. That is, tongue movements were poorly differentiated from jaw movements, verbal diadochokinetic rate for speech-alternating motion was judged as slow (i.e., three to four syllables per second), and speech-sequential motion resulted in speech sound transpositions as well as slow rate.

Clinical Impressions

Ms. Guerra demonstrated skill as an *engaging and animated conversationalist*. She also displayed exceptional motivation to improve, based on the *effort that she put into the activities, particularly those that required response to clinical teaching.*

Summary

Ms. Maribel Guerra is a 22-year-old bilingual woman who participated in communication evaluation on [date]. She engaged in conversation easily and *demonstrated deep commitment to improving her communication skills* so as to make progress in her chosen career of acting. Ms. Guerra presents a history of delayed speech development, unintelligible speech in childhood, and long-term speech therapy through elementary school.

Articulation testing revealed consistent consonant distortions affecting lingua-alveolar and lingua-palatal fricatives in all contexts. The *same mild distortions were noted in conversational speech, but additionally, conversation revealed random articulation errors that seemed more prevalent when speech rate increased.* Although Ms. Guerra put *much effort into the speech sound stimulability activity, her speech sound productions did not improve with clinical teaching.*

The *oral-facial inspection revealed some idiosyncrasies that may contribute to the speech production pattern. They include poorly differentiated tongue movements, slow rate for speech-alternating motion and speech-sequential motion, and consonant transpositions for speech-sequential motion.*

As a result of these findings, Ms. Guerra is diagnosed with a mild articulation disorder. Due to her speech development history and *apparent difficulties with programing for articulation,* neurologic etiology resulting in previously undiagnosed developmental apraxia of speech has not been ruled out.

Prognosis

Due to her strong motivation, room for improvement, and engaging nature, we judge that Ms. Guerra is likely to make progress in speech therapy. However, progress may be slow due to a *weak response to clinical teaching*, a long-term history of speech therapy with minimal progress, and *possible motor-speech disorder*. Furthermore, whether Ms. Guerra will achieve her goal of achieving articulatory precision that adequately supports a successful acting career is yet to be determined.

Recommendations

As a result of the communication evaluation, we recommend the following:

1. Speech therapy for three 45-minute sessions weekly
2. *Referral to a specialist for more in-depth testing to clarify whether symptoms are secondary to motor-speech disorder and to seek input with regard to plan of care*

It was our pleasure to evaluate Ms. Guerra's communication needs. If there are any questions or if we can offer additional help, we trust that you will contact us.

Barbara Ann Johnson-Root, PhD, CCC-SLP   [Date of signature]
Professor and Speech-Language Pathologist

CHAPTER 6

When There Is A Priori Knowledge of Organic Pathology

Frequently, when craniofacial or neurogenic anomalies cause or contribute to a communication disorder, the condition is known prior to the oral-facial inspection. That is, the examining speech-language pathologist would hardly be first to notice a cleft lip or palate, acquired neurogenic disorder resulting from a neurologic incident, laryngectomy, or well-known syndrome such as trisomy 21 or fragile X. Under these circumstances of a priori knowledge of organic pathology, the oral-facial evaluation and its documentation take on a completely different character compared to the inspection for individuals whose physical idiosyncrasy is first discovered through the inspection process.

When a person with a known physical anomaly is referred for oral-facial inspection, although the clinical questions (see Tables 0–2 and 0–3) are still relevant, portions are essentially addressed prior to the session. That is, the examining clinician already knows that certain parts are not present, intact, or functioning; is at least partially aware of which parts; has some information about what has gone awry; and is cognizant of the physical anomaly's impact on speech symptoms. The goal then becomes adding to what is already known and thereby shedding light on strengths and challenges that the available physical mechanism poses for the person.

Also, the historical sections take a more prominent position in the report since they are likely to include information that may otherwise appear as a discovery under Results of Testing. For example, if a breach in palatal integrity is already a known feature, this knowledge should appear under Background Information, along with the official source. Oral-facial inspection, then, does not identify the feature but instead focuses on discovering how the feature affects communication for the individual.

The sample case for this section is a child with an undiagnosed multiple anomaly syndrome, for whom a host of aberrancies are known prior to testing. The data collection and clinical implications are shown in Tables 6–6A and 6–6B. A sample clinical report follows in Box 6–6.

Table 6–6A. Highlights for Clinical Example With A Priori Knowledge of Anomaly: Data Collection

Name: Ethan Walters

Age: 2:9

Informant: Foster parent: Ms. Jenny Dobson

Statement of the Problem: Ethan's speech is really behind other children his age.

	Clinical Decision	Rationale	Data
Background Information	No		Birth: full-term, 7 lbs, 3 oz, 19 inches
			NICU 14 days, due to heart defect
			Eyelid ptosis
			Heart failure at 6 weeks; two heart catheterizations in first year
			Genetics ruled out velocardiofacial syndrome at 2 months
			Myringotomy tubes: secondary to chronic otitis media
			Frequent hospitalizations for croup, pneumonia, and high fever; classified medically fragile
			Failure to thrive: removed from family of origin at 11 months
			Walked with a walker at 22 months, independently at 27 months
			Presently walks with an awkward gait, poor depth perception
			Did not babble
			First word: more → /mo/ at 23 months; present vocabulary: more → /mo/, doggy → /'dɑ di/, mama, and eat
			Beginning to make syntactic connections through gesture: "Mama" + sign for drive + point at picture of a car

continues

Table 6–6A. *continued*

	Clinical Decision	Rationale	Data
Background Information *continued*			Service providers who follow Ethan: • Primary care • Cardiology • Genetics • Otorhinolaryngology • Hematology • Neurology • Gastroenterology • Ophthalmology • Early intervention since 1 month of age: physical therapy, speech therapy, occupational therapy, special instruction, social work therapy
Speech and Language Screening	*Preschool Language Scales–5 (PLS-5)* (Zimmerman, Steiner, & Pond, 2011)	. . . to determine level of functioning, identify strengths and challenges, and facilitate plan of care	
Speech Sound Stimulability Screening	*According to Oral-Facial Evaluation for Speech-Language Pathologists (OFESLP)*	*. . . to ascertain Ethan's response to clinical teaching for two highly visible phonemes: /b/ and /p/*	*Ethan did not change speech in response to clinical teaching*
Hearing Screening	Attempted free-field hearing screening using voice at 25 dB . . .	. . . to judge whether hearing is adequate for spoken language learning	Ethan responded to free-field testing by looking at the right and left speakers appropriately
Oral-Facial Inspection	*Administered OFESLP*	*. . . to identify whether all parts needed for speech production are present, intact, and functioning*	*High palatal arch*
			Missing lateral incisor
			Bifid uvula
			Lingual asymmetry in motion
			Labial asymmetry in motion
			Depressed nasal tip
			Eyelid ptosis
			Facial asymmetry at rest
Clinical Impressions			Sociable; enjoys social attention
			Short attention span
			Resistant to clinician-directed activities
			Enjoys play
			Imitates gestures

Table 6–6B. Highlights for Clinical Example With A Priori Knowledge of Anomaly: Clinical Implications

Name: Ethan Walters

Age: 2:9

Informant: Foster parent: Ms. Jenny Dobson

Statement of the Problem: Ethan's speech is really behind other children his age.

	Clinical Decision	Rationale/Evidence Information found in this column should appear in the report summary.
Summary (with diagnosis)	Diagnosis: global speech-language delay secondary to global developmental delay; motor-speech disorder not ruled out; genetic etiology not ruled out	Sociable, enjoys play, imitates gestures
		History of many complex medical problems, including failure to thrive, heart defect, chronic otitis media, history of seizures
		Developmental delay
		Language development at approximately 1 year level; possible hypernasal speech
		High palatal arch, bifid uvula, facial asymmetry, eyelid ptosis
		Not stimulable for bilabial consonants
		Receives all therapy services and followed by many physicians and specialists; enrolled in early intervention
Prognosis	Ethan may improve with therapy . . .	Room for improvement
		Sociable, enjoys play, enjoys social attention
		Imitates gestures
		Creatively combines modalities to create syntax
	Progress may be slow and the extent of progress cannot be determined	*Not stimulable for speech*
		Serious health problems
		Concerns with structure and function of speech mechanism
		Motor-speech disorder not ruled out
		Genetic etiology not ruled out
Recommendations	Continue with speech therapy	See prognosis
	Refer to craniofacial team	*Coordinate services; evaluate adequacy of speech mechanism*
	Refer to developmental specialist	Identify strengths and challenges to enhance plan of care

Box 6–6. Clinical Report: A Priori Knowledge of Anomaly

Identifying Information

Name: Ethan Walters

Date of Clinical Service: [date]

Primary Language: English

Referral: Pediatrician

Date of Birth: [date]

Age: 2:9

Secondary Language: None

Diagnosis: Severe language and speech delay, secondary to global delay in all developmental areas.

Ethan Walters is a 2-year, 9-month-old male child who was seen for communication evaluation on [date]. Ethan's foster-care parent, Ms. Jenny Dobson, brought him to the session and served as primary informant. Additional information was also obtained from Ethan's pediatrician, Dr. [name of doctor]. Unless otherwise stated, the information in this report was obtained through the case history intake form that Ms. Dobson provided as well as her responses to questions during the interview.

Statement of the Problem

Ethan's pediatrician referred him for a comprehensive communication evaluation to gain a "more complete picture relative to Ethan's communication development."

Background Information

Birth and Medical Histories

Ethan was born at full term by way of caesarian section, weighing 7 pounds, 3 ounces and 19 inches in length. Immediately he was rushed by ambulance to the neonatal intensive care unit (NICU) at [name of hospital] in [city] so that he could receive treatment for a cardiac condition. He remained in the NICU for 14 days.

At birth, a relationship was immediately established with a pediatric cardiologist, Dr. [name of physician], who sees Ethan for follow-up twice yearly. Ethan experienced an episode of heart failure at 6 weeks and underwent heart catheterization for aortic stenosis twice in his first year.

A relationship was also established with a genetics specialist, Dr. [name of specialist], at birth. Dr. [name of specialist] sees Ethan once yearly for follow-up. Dr. [name of specialist] ruled out velocardiofacial syndrome during Ethan's first year; however, as symptoms develop, other syndromes may be explored.

Ethan was born with physical symptoms indicating neurologic involvement. They include sacral dimple, eyelid ptosis, and Marcus Gunn jaw wink. Ethan also experienced several episodes of seizures shortly after his second birthday. Pediatric neurologist, Dr. [name of specialist], follows Ethan on an annual basis and as needed.

Chronic otitis media necessitated myrigotomy tubes on [date]. Otorhinolaryngologist, Dr. [name of specialist], also follows Ethan annually and on an as-needed basis.

Due to Marcus Gunn jaw wink and eyelid ptosis, Ethan is at risk for amblyopia and other vision problems. Therefore, he visits the ophthalmologist, Dr. [name of specialist], twice yearly.

Early Physical Development

As an infant, Ethan did not grow and develop normally. Following two episodes of failure to thrive, he was removed from his family of origin at age 11 months and placed in foster care. At that time, he weighed 12 pounds and measured 21 inches. Although he did not sit unsupported and did not visually track at that time, Ethan responded to social play by laughing and giggling.

Since in foster care, Ethan has gained 10 pounds. He began sitting independently and pulling himself up to stand at 18 months of age. He began to walk using a metal walker at 22 months, and he took his first independent steps at the age of 27 months. Presently, Ethan walks independently using an unsteady gait. He has not learned to climb or run. He has not yet begun toilet training.

Ethan has received physical therapy since 1 month of age. He has also received speech therapy, occupational therapy, social work therapy, and special instruction since 13 months of age. These services have been provided through [name of county] County Early Intervention.

Language Development

Ethan was a quiet baby and did not babble. His first word was more →/mo/ at 23 months.

He has not yet put two words together and does not initiate verbal communication. However, it is Ms. Dobson's impression that Ethan comprehends simple sentences.

Ethan's speech-language pathologist, [name of service provider], reports that Ethan has not shown an interest in speaking and that most of the work has been focused on helping Ethan become a safe eater.

Results of Testing

The diagnostic protocol included the following procedures:

- *Preschool Language Scale* (5th ed.) *(PLS-5)*
- Hearing screening
- *Oral-Facial Evaluation for Speech-Language Pathologists (OFESLP)*

Language and Speech Results

The *PLS-5* was administered to determine level of functioning, identify strengths and challenges, and facilitate plan of care.

Receptively, Ethan was judged to function at the 1:0 to 1:5 age level. That is, he consistently stopped to look when his name was called, looked at a person or object when it was named, and responded to the word *no*. However, he did not demonstrate functional play, relational play, or self-directed play.

CHAPTER 6

Expressively, he seemed to function at the 0:6 to 0:11 age level and is in the process of transitioning to the 1:0 to 1:5 level. That is, he demonstrated reciprocal social smiles, vocalized using distinctly different kinds of sounds for happy and sad, moved his arms and legs when socially engaged, pushed objects away that he did not want, and imitated funny faces. Although he did not seek adult attention and did not take social turns by imitating speech sounds, he produced a few CV syllables and participated in a game of peek-a-boo.

Informal social interaction with Ethan also provided useful information. Presently, Ethan's vocabulary comprises only a few words: more →/mo/, doggy →/ˈdɑ dɪ/, mommy →/ˈmɑ mə/, daddy →/ˈdɑ dɪ/. He makes animal sounds to denote some animals: cow →/mu/, cat →/ˈmi ə/. He uses manual communication for some words, such as eat, doggy, daddy, mommy. Furthermore, Ethan's phonetic repertoire includes only /m/, /d/, /ɑ/, /ə/, /o/, /ɪ/, /i/, and /u/. The same sounds also comprise his phonemic repertoire. In addition, Ethan substitutes some nonspeech sounds, such as popping and clicking, in his attempts to label objects that begin with bilabials or velars, respectively.

With the exception of a few words, speech intelligibility is judged as poor.

In an attempt to judge Ethan's response to clinical teaching, we provided him with stimulability opportunities prompting bilabials /p/ and /b/ using the OFESLP. Ethan responded by producing the same bilabial pop that he used spontaneously for the same sounds during informal play.

Voice and Resonance

Ethan's voice is judged as hypernasal, with a quality that is more typical of a younger child.

Fluency

Judging Ethan's fluency in connected speech will be revisited when he begins to produce sentences.

Hearing Screening

Ethan participated a free-field audiometric screening so as to ascertain whether a full audiologic evaluation was needed. At 25 dB, he consistently responded to voice by looking at the sound source bilaterally. Ethan did not demonstrate the ability to respond to a pure-tone screening.

Oral-Facial Evaluation

The OFESLP was performed so as to more completely describe the impact that physical limitations impose on Ethan's speech development. Although all parts were present, some idiosyncrasies were noted relative to structure and function.

As for the external face, asymmetry was noted at rest. This included eyelid ptosis as well as minor structural differences between the left and right sides. During vocalization and other oral movements, lips and tongue were observed to move asymmetrically.

Due to young age, combined with developmental delay, Ethan was not asked to complete the oral exercises involving lips and tongue. He opened his mouth briefly for a cursory inspection, and the following features were noted: small orifice, missing right maxillary lateral incisor, exceedingly high palatal arch, and bifid uvula.

Velar movement was observed during crying but not during /ɑ/ phonation. Movement was asymmetrical.

Surplus nasal airflow screening was performed. Mirror condensation while saying /ˈda di/ indicates that there may be surplus nasal airflow during speech.

Furthermore, Ethan was judged to be at risk for developmental apraxia of speech. This judgment is based on parental responses to questions relative to speech-motor development.

Clinical Impressions

During the session, Ethan demonstrated a keen interest in human interaction and receiving social attention. Although he participated in some clinician directed activities, he demonstrated a short attention span and distractibility. Eye contact during interaction was infrequent.

Summary

Ethan Walters is a 2-year, 9-month-old male child who received a communication evaluation on [date]. He is a friendly child who enjoys social interaction but occasionally resists clinician-directed activities.

Ethan has a diagnosis of developmental delay and a cardiac condition concomitant to a number of additional health-related concerns. Due to failure to thrive, Ethan has been in foster care since infancy.

With regard to speech and language, Ethan appears to be functioning just above the 1-year age level for receptive skills and approaching the 1-year age level for expressive skills. He has only a few phonemes in his repertoire, including a few vowels and the consonants /d/ and /m/. Ethan substitutes a popping sound for bilabials /p/ and /b/ and a clicking sound for velars /k/ and /g/, and he *does not demonstrate change when presented with clinical teaching.*

Oral-facial findings indicate a number of structural anomalies. Furthermore, submucous cleft is not ruled out.

As a result of the evaluation, Ethan is diagnosed with a global communication delay that appears to be secondary to global developmental delay. Motor-speech disorder, submucous cleft, and genetic syndrome are not ruled out.

Prognosis

Ethan is likely to benefit from speech therapy since he has room for improvement, responds well to social activity, and enjoys play. However, a number of factors may hinder progress. They are various serious medical and health concerns, developmental delay, possibility of undiagnosed genetic syndrome, possibility of motor-speech disorder, possibility of submucous cleft or craniofacial anomaly, and domestic instability due to foster-care placement.

Recommendations

As a result of the evaluation, we recommend the following:

1. Speech therapy, three times weekly for 30 minutes per session
2. Speech-language pathology follow-up to evaluate for motor-speech disorder and augment the plan of care
3. *Referral to craniofacial team to explore genetic and/or craniofacial concerns, hypernasality, and difficulty with pressure consonants*

CHAPTER 6

It was our pleasure to meet this very friendly child and to interact with him. As his plan of care continues to develop, please continue to keep us informed.

_____   _____

Barbara Ann Johnson-Root, PhD, CCC-SLP   [Date of signature]
Professor and Speech-Language Pathologist

Summary

The scope of Chapter 6 extends somewhat beyond the oral-facial evaluation in that it addresses documentation in the context of comprehensive communication evaluation for a sampling of conceivable clinical scenarios. Certainly, the full extent of possibilities extends well beyond this chapter's content. However, the principles and practices presented herein should serve useful when documenting oral-facial inspection findings and when embedding them in the context of the full clinical report.

APPENDIX A

Recording Forms

Seven different recording forms reside in Appendix A. Their purpose is to facilitate gathering various types of client-focused evidence so that it can be arranged it in such a way that it leads to effective analysis and interpretation, thereby contributing to both meaningful outcomes and valid clinical decisions.

A recording form for general use appears first. Consider it the default form as it is applicable for examinees who require no modification or accommodation. Then consider the remaining six forms *special* in that they apply when special needs obligate substantial change in type, extent, or method of documentation.

The full array of forms appears in this appendix and online. Photocopying is permitted.

1. Recording Form: General Use (Appropriate for Most Examinees)
2. Special Recording Form: Preverbal Children (Infants)
3. Special Recording Form: Children With Limited Language (Toddlers)
4. Special Recording Form: Preschoolers (Age 4 Years to School Age)
5. Special Recording Form: Adults With History of Neurologic Episode
6. Special Recording Form: Preoperative Laryngectomy
7. Special Recording Form: Postoperative Laryngectomy

Rationale for Using Checklists and Descriptive Entries Instead of Numeric Scores

Recording forms associated with this tool rely on descriptive entries and checklists, not numeric scores. This is unlike norm-referenced evaluation tools that lend themselves to numeric ratings and lead to an overall score that quantitatively distinguishes between normal and atypical findings or may even classify disorders.

Instead, the clinical tool more closely resembles a criterion-referenced protocol. That is, since the inspection is intended to ascertain whether any physical anomaly could potentially hinder speech production, it is the discovery of the anomaly and its contribution to the speaking pattern that are relevant, not the sum of numeric ratings for a series of observations. Therefore, with regard to oral-facial inspection, the goal of achieving a meaningful outcome is better served by checklists and descriptive entries.

Instructions for Using the Recording Forms

The recording forms correspond to the procedural instructions shown in Chapters 2 through 4. They provide a framework for completing a checklist and for providing brief descriptions.

As described in the preceding chapters:

- Regardless of which form best suits the examinee, complete routine clinical observations first. With few exceptions, routine procedures are found in Chapter 2. However, a few discretionary procedures should be performed routinely for certain special populations, and they are located in Chapters 3 and 4, depending on whether they are classified as simply discretionary or discretionary and special.
- Then, use decision boxes to flag procedures that may be needed for some individuals, and administer the appropriate discretionary clinical observations. Discretionary procedures are located in Chapter 3, with few exceptions. That is, some of the special procedures found in Chapter 4, although routine for some populations, can be considered discretionary for others.
- Identify any additional testing that is needed, either within or outside the scope of practice for speech-language pathologists.
- Refer to Chapter 5 to identify clinical implications based on the unique findings that apply to the examinee under consideration. As a result, flag physical features or symptoms that are suspected of contributing to a speech production disorder and incorporate these findings into the individualized plan of care.

Oral-Facial Evaluation for Speech-Language Pathologists
Barbara Ann Johnson-Root, PhD, CCC-SLP

Recording Form: General Use (Appropriate for Most Examinees)

Intake Information	
Client name:	Date of evaluation:
Date of birth:	Age:
Examiner:	Agency or facility:
Reason for evaluation:	
Relevant history:	
Comments:	

APPENDIX A

Prepare the Work Area for Testing (instructions in manual, Chapter 1)
Checklist
Place a check mark in the column to the left after completing each preparatory step in the list below.
Inventory equipment and supplies listed Table 1–2 and described in Appendix B.
Check batteries that power battery-operated equipment. Replace weak or dead batteries.
Verify that all cords and strings were removed from equipment. If not, remove and dispose of them.
Sanitize the work area, and unwrap equipment as instructed in Chapter 1.
Wash hands thoroughly.
Put on examination gloves, using procedures provided in Chapter 1.
Arrange equipment as shown in Figure 1–1.

Instruct the Examinee (and Significant Other if Appropriate)

Use your own words and developmentally appropriate language to communicate the following talking points before you begin.

- The oral-facial evaluation is a customary part of every speech-language evaluation.
- It involves inspecting all observable body parts necessary for speaking so that we may ascertain whether all parts are present, complete, and working properly.
- This is done to look into whether there is a physical explanation for the speech problem that brought you here or if there is any physical problem that we should address in order to help you.
- None of the procedures are painful or harmful.
- A few items situated on the table may not be needed.
- For some people, oral-facial evaluation findings may lead to more detailed testing or possibly referral to another professional, although this is not the case for everyone.
- You may ask questions before we begin or at any time. Do you have any questions now? (If *yes*, either answer briefly or diplomatically table the question for a more appropriate time. If *no*, move on.)
- Are you ready? Let's get started!

Routine Clinical Observations

As a matter of course, complete the eight routine clinical observations that are described in Chapter 2. If you believe there is a reason to omit one or more of the routine procedures, consider that perhaps one of the special forms may be appropriate for the examinee. If after considering special forms you are certain that they do not apply and the identified routine procedure should be deleted, clearly mark the rationale for your decision on the recording form and proceed with the testing as you deem appropriate.

	Routine Clinical Observation 1(A): Conversational Speech Sample (instructions in manual, Chapter 2)
	Rate intelligibility. Check the one that applies.
	Place a check mark in the corresponding column to the left if intelligibility is judged as "good." For all intelligibility ratings that are less than "good," place a minus sign (−) in the corresponding column.
	Good: Completely or nearly completely intelligible.
	Slightly Compromised: Intelligible more than half the time.
	Fair: Intelligible about half of the time.
	Poor: Intelligible less than half of the time.
	Unintelligible: Completely unintelligible (or nearly so).
	Comment on age appropriateness for speech intelligibility.

Area(s) Noted as Difficult During Conversational Speech	
Use a minus sign (−) to mark areas identified as possibly deficient during conversational speech.	
Articulation/phonology.	Fluency.
Language.	Resonance.
Voice.	Motor-speech.
Describe speech difficulty.	

APPENDIX A

Routine Clinical Observations 1(B): Facial Region Inspection (instruction in manual, Chapter 2)		
Use a minus sign (−) to mark all features noted during facial region inspection. If multiple options appear on the same line, circle those that apply.		
Resting	**Speaking or Vocalizing**	**Feature**
		Facial or oral asymmetry, drooping, tremor, fasciculation, spasm.
		Poor saliva management (as compared to others of similar age and development).
		Scarring.
		Thin upper lip, cleft lip.
		Micrognathia, macrognathia, retrognathic jaw, prognathic jaw.
		Hypoplastic midface, flat philtrum, epicanthal folds.
		Malformed ears, low-set ears.
		Eyelid ptosis, strabismus, wandering eye.
		Wide-set eyes.
		Forward tongue posture.
		Cranial asymmetry, prominent forehead, microcephaly, macrocephaly.
		Other dysmorphic features:
After completing above checklist, place minus sign (−) in column for any applicable condition.		
	Facial features suggest need for referral to genetics, neurology, or otorhinolaryngology if doctor-patient relationship has not yet been established.	
	Facial features appear to possibly contribute to atypical speaking pattern. Specify.	

Routine Clinical Observation 1(C): Breathing Observations (instructions in manual, Chapter 2)	
Does the examinee's daily life require vocal projection? If yes, place a check mark in the box and circle the role that demands vocal projection. If the examinee has vocal projection needs not included in the list, write that information in the space provided.	
	Teacher, singer, actor, attorney, clergy, public speaker.

Identify the type of breathing noted. For all examinees, *nasal* and *diaphragmatic* breathing are optimal. *Lower thoracic* breathing is acceptable for examinees whose life does not require vocal projection.

For the list on the left, place a check mark in the far-left column for all that apply. If any pattern described in the column on the right is observed, place a minus sign (−) to its left, since this is an atypical pattern. Also, where multiple options occupy the same line, circle those that apply.

Type of Breathing			
	Nasal.		Oral.
	Diaphragmatic.		Upper thoracic, clavicular.
	Lower thoracic.		Noisy, evidence of respiratory distress or struggle.

Describe.

APPENDIX A

	Routine Clinical Observation 2: Lip and Tongue Mobility and Strength (instruction in manual, Chapter 2)		
	Place a check mark in the column to the left if the examinee performs the act smoothly, accurately, completely, and in a timely manner. Place a minus sign (−) in the column if noting any other response, and use the space below to provide additional descriptive data.		
	**Action**		
	Pucker.		Quick repetitions of /b/ or /p/.
	Spread.		Smack the lips.
	Sustain exaggerated /u/.		
	Describe atypical responses; comment on possible relationship to speech concern.		

	Lip Strength and Seal		
	Place a check mark in the box to the left if the act is judged to be within normal limits. Place a minus sign (−) in the column if noting any other response, and use the space below to provide additional descriptive data.		
	**Action**		
	Seal.		Resistance.
	Describe atypical responses; comment on possible relationship to speech concern.		

	Tongue Mobility		
	Place a check mark in the column to the left of each action if examinee performs the act smoothly, accurately, completely, and in a timely manner. Place a minus sign (−) in the column if noting any other response, and use the space below to provide additional descriptive data.		
	**Action**		
	Protrusion.		Wiggle to the left and to the right.
	Elevation.		Rotation.
	Lateralization.		

Describe atypical responses; comment on possible relationship to speech concern.

Other Tongue Observations

Place a check mark in box to the left if feature is observed to be within normal limits. Place a minus sign (−) in the column if noting any other response, and use the space below to provide additional descriptive data.

Feature	
Shape of tongue tip.	Lingual frenum length.

Describe atypical features; comment on possible relationship to speech concern.

Tongue Strength

Place a check mark in the column on the left if the act is judged to be within normal limits. Place a minus sign (−) in the column if noting any other response, and use the space below to provide additional descriptive data.

Action
Resistance.

Describe atypical responses; comment on possible relationship to speech concern.

APPENDIX A

Routine Clinical Observation 3: Dental Bite and Alignment
(instruction in manual Chapter 2)

Dental Bite

For examinees with unremarkable bite pattern, place a check mark in the column to the left corresponding to the word *normal*. If any other bite pattern is noted, place a minus sign (–) in the column that resides directly to the left of the term that best describes the person's bite. (Typically one applies; there are exceptions.)

Bite

	Normal.		Edge-to-edge bite.		Overjet.
	Open bite.		Underbite.		Flared bite.
	Closed bite.		Cross bite.		

Add descriptive information if needed; describe relationship to speech, if any.

Alignment and Condition of Teeth

Mark age-appropriate dental chart below to indicate dental alignment concerns noted.

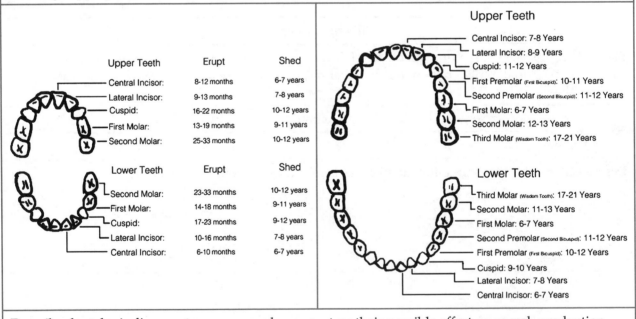

Describe dental misalignment concerns, and comment on their possible effect on speech production, if any.

Routine Clinical Observation 4: Dental Occlusion (instruction in manual, Chapter 2)
Dental Occlusion
For examinees with neutroclussion, place a check mark in the column that resides directly to the left of that term. For examinees with distoclusion or mesioclusion, place a minus sign (−) in the column that corresponds to that classification.
Dental Occlusion Classification

	Neutroclusion (typical).		Distoclusion.		Mesioclusion.

Describe occlusal relationship. Comment on any possible relationship to speech production.

APPENDIX A

Routine Clinical Observation 5: Oral Interior (instructions in manual, Chapter 2)	
Response to Request to Open the Mouth: **Freedom of Mandibular Movement and Response to Resistance**	
Place a minus sign (–) in the column to the left, corresponding to any statements that apply.	
Activity	
	Difficulty with opening the mouth adequately for observing oral interior.
	Pain or other sensation reported when opening the mouth for oral inspection.
	Mandible deviates to left or right when lowered.
	Extraneous mandibular movements at rest or in motion.
	Not successful in resisting examiner's attempt to prevent mandibular movement.
Place a minus sign (–) in the column to the left of any statements that describe examinee's condition.	
	Symptoms suggest *possible* temporomandibular joint disorder.
	Symptoms suggest evidence of muscle weakness, asymmetry, discoordination, or difficulty with motor planning.
Describe additional concerns.	

Tongue Surface, Size, and Shape	
Place a check mark in the column to the left if the feature is judged to be within normal limits. Place a minus sign (–) in the column if noting any atypical trait, and use the space below to provide additional descriptive data.	
Feature	

	Texture.		Shape.
	Size.		Other noteworthy feature:

Describe concern with the feature noted particularly as it may or may not relate to speech production.

Hard Palate	
Place a check mark in the column to the left if the feature is judged to be within normal limits. Place a minus sign (−) in the column if noting any atypical trait, and use the space below to provide additional descriptive data.	

Feature	
Alveolar ridge.	Posterior nasal spine.
Palatal arch.	Foveae palate.
Median raphe.	Scarring.
Mucous membrane.	Coloring.

Describe concerns; comment on possible relationship to speech pattern.

Posterior Soft Tissue	
Place a check mark in the column to the left if the feature is judged to be within normal limits. Place a minus sign (−) in the column if noting any atypical trait, and use the space below to provide additional descriptive data.	

Feature	
Velum (structure only).	Palatine tonsils.
Uvula.	Posterior pharyngeal wall.
Faucial pillars.	

Describe concern. Comment on possible relationship to speech problem.

APPENDIX A

Routine Clinical Observation 6: Velar Movement (instructions in manual, Chapter 2)	
Velar Movement	
Place a check mark beside "velum moves up and back symmetrically on /ɑ/ phonation" if that is the case. Place a minus sign (–) in the columns corresponding to any other trait noted; use the space below to provide additional descriptive data.	
Velar response to /ɑ/ phonation	
	Velum moves up and back symmetrically on /ɑ/ phonation.
	Velum moves up and back asymmetrically on /ɑ/ phonation.
	Velum moves sluggishly on /ɑ/ phonation.
	Velum is not observed to move on /ɑ/ phonation.
	Misplaced velar dimple noted on /ɑ/ phonation.
Describe concerns. Comment on possible relationship to speech pattern.	

Routine Clinical Observation 7: Verbal Diadochokinesis (instructions in manual, Chapter 2)					
Speech-Alternating Motion: Rate					
Record syllables produced per second in the column that appears to the left of each syllable designation.					
Syllables/Second	Syllable	Syllables/Second	Syllable	Syllables/Second	Syllable
	/pə/		/tə/		/kə/

Speech-Alternating Motion: Perceptual Evaluation	
Place a minus sign (–) in the box on the left for all that apply.	
	Fewer than five syllables/second; specify consonants:
	Reduced range of motion for the articulators (i.e., jaw, tongue, lips).
	Arrhythmic or unsteady performance.
	Poor articulatory precision; specify consonants:
	Rate, precision, or volume decreased over time; specify:
Describe concerns. Comment on possible relevance to speech pattern.	

Speech-Sequential Motion: Rate	
Syllables/Second	Syllables
	/pə tə kə/

Speech-Sequential Motion: Perceptual Evaluation	
Place a minus sign (–) in the column to the left for all that apply.	
	Fewer than five syllables/second.
	Difficulty rapidly sequencing the three distinctively different syllables in succession (i.e., syllable transpositions, perseveration across syllable boundaries).
	Decrease in rate, precision, or volume over time.
Describe concerns. Comment on possible relevance to speech pattern.	

APPENDIX A

Routine Clinical Observation 8: Vowel Prolongation (instructions in manual, Chapter 2)		
Vowel Prolongation: Duration		
Measure vowel duration according to instructions in the Chapter 2. Write results for each of three trials in the designated column. Circle the longest duration.		

	Trial 1	Trial 2	Trial 3
/ɑ/			

Vowel Prolongation: Subjective Evaluation	
Place a minus sign (–) in column to the left for all that apply.	
	Adult sustains /ɑ/ for fewer than 20 seconds, or child sustains /ɑ/ for fewer than 10 seconds.
	Decrease in duration across three trials.
	Voice quality or volume deteriorates.
	Atypical resonance.
	Atypical vocal quality or pitch.
Describe concern. Comment on relevance to speech.	

Identifying and Completing Appropriate Discretionary Clinical Observations

Although in most cases, the inspection ends with routine clinical observations, once routine procedures are complete, the next step is to determine whether the evidence indicates a need for any discretionary clinical observations. For the sake of convenience, a series of decision boxes provides structure that can facilitate identifying discretionary clinical observations that should be considered.

Bear in mind that none of the decision boxes is intended to prompt a perfunctory decision that results in a discretionary procedure. Certainly, an understanding of the examinee's overall symptom pattern, combined with a rich bank of clinical experience and intuition, should also contribute, albeit such intangibles are highly individualized and therefore difficult to place on a form. Even so, strategically considering tangible client-centered evidence, as recorded on the form, can contribute to a good decision relative to proceeding with a discretionary clinical observation, and that is the intended purpose of the decision boxes.

Once a decision box is evaluated, if it flags the corresponding discretionary clinical observation, the inspection can proceed to that discretionary observation if the examining clinician deems it appropriate. Generally, no more than three discretionary observations are flagged for an individual; however, there are exceptions.

Decision Box for Nasal Cavity Clearance Screening: Discretionary Clinical Observation 9	
Place a minus sign (–) in the column to the left if noting any of the following indicators. Proceed to nasal cavity clearance screening (i.e., Discretionary Clinical Observation 9) if indicators are noted.	

	Symptom	Clinical Observation Noted
	Hyponasal resonance detected during any speech or vocalization event.	
	Nasal asymmetry.	1
	Visible or audible symptoms of congestion[a] (including mouth breathing).	

[a]May table the procedure if the person exhibits symptoms of temporary obstruction such as a cold or allergy.

Discretionary Clinical Observation 9: Nasal Cavity Clearance Screening (instructions in manual, Chapter 3)	
Screening for Nasal Cavity Clearance	
Place a minus sign (–) in column to left for all symptoms that apply.	
	Nasal asymmetry.
	Nasal obstruction due to mucosal swelling, deviated septum, hypertrophied conchae, excess mucous.
	Difficulty admitting or discharging air via the nasal passages.
	Difficulty expelling air through either nare when the other is occluded.
	Difficulty with prolonging /m/: /m→/.
Describe concerns. Comment on potential relevance to speech.	

APPENDIX A

Decision Box for Facial Dimension Estimates: Discretionary Clinical Observation 10	
Place a minus sign (−) in left column if noting any of the following indicators. Proceed to facial dimension estimates (i.e., Discretionary Clinical Observation 10) if indicators are present.	

	Symptom	Clinical Observation Noted
	Facial profile appears disproportionate and the person is likely to be referred for follow-up (e.g., genetics or otorhinolaryngology).	1
	Malocclusion.	4
	Tongue tip does not line up with alveolar ridge.	5

Discretionary Clinical Observation 10: Facial Dimension Estimates
(instructions in manual, Chapter 3)

Facial Dimension Estimates

Place a minus sign (−) to left for all that apply. If a minus sign (−) is placed in the left column in the first three rows, measure distances in millimeters and record the measurements in the divided mm column on right. Then calculate percentage for each measurement and record it in the % column on far right. Any minus sign (−) on the left should be reported to the referral recipient.

			mm	%
	Overall Facial Dimension: Distances between (1) hairline and glabella, (2) glabella and subnasale, and (3) subnasale and pogonion are not segments of approximate equal length.	1		
		2		
		3		
	Dimensions for Lower Third of Face: Distances between (1) subnasale and stomian, (2) stomian and supramentale, and (3) supramentale and pogonion are not segments of approximate equal length.	1		
		2		
		3		
	Size and Spacing of Eyes: (1) Length of palpebral fissures and (2) distance between eyes are not segments of approximate equal length.	1		
		2		
	Facial Angle: Facial angle deviates grossly from 90° or misses subnasale plane completely.			
	Frankfurt Horizontal Plane: Tragion is lower than ipsilateral lid-cheek junction.			
Describe concerns.				

Decision Box for Temporomandibular Joint Disorder Screening: Discretionary Clinical Observation 11		
Place a minus sign (−) in the column to the left if noting any of the following indicators. Proceed to screening for temporomandibular joint disorder (i.e., Discretionary Clinical Observation 11) if indicators are present.		
	Symptom	Clinical Observation Noted
	Limited mandibular excursion during speech activities.	1
	Limited mandibular excursion during nonspeech activities.	5
	Reported sensation of localized or referred pain when moving the jaw.	

Discretionary Clinical Observation 11: Temporomandibular Joint Disorder Screening (instructions in manual, Chapter 3)
Screening for Temporomandibular Joint Disorder
Place a minus sign (−) in the box to the left for all that apply.
Maximum opening height of oral orifice is less than 40 mm.
Range of side-to-side jaw movement is less than 7 mm.
Range of motion for jaw protrusion is less than 6 mm.
Popping, clicking, grinding of temporomandibular joint is palpable during rapid opening and closing of jaw or while moving jaw from side-to-side.
Examinee reports sensation of popping, snapping, or grinding during opening and closing of jaw or while moving jaw from side-to-side.
Examinee reports pain in jaw, ear, or lower molar during opening and closing of the jaw or while moving jaw from side-to-side and rates pain at 2 to 5 on 5-point scale.
Describe concerns.

APPENDIX A

Decision Box for Tongue-Thrust Swallow Observations: Discretionary Clinical Observation 12		
Place a minus sign (–) in the column to the left if noting any of the following indicators. Proceed to tongue-thrust swallow observation (i.e., Discretionary Clinical Observation 12) if indicators are present.		
	Symptom	Clinical Observation Noted
	Age-inappropriate oral habits, bruxism, sleep apnea, allergies.	Case history intake
	Interdental lisp.	1
	Forward tongue posturing.	
	Mouth-open posture.	
	Habitual oral breathing.	
	Chronic chapped lips.	
	Unilateral lip or cheek biting.	
	Tongue sucking.	
	Tongue or lip resting posture idiosyncrasies.	
	Poor saliva management.	
	Deviated septum.	
	Restricted upper lip movement.	2
	Short lingual frenum.	
	Open bite, flared bite, cross bite, deep overbite.	3
	Any of the following, if associated with forward tongue posture:	5
	Extra-large palatine tonsils.	
	Small pharyngeal orifice.	
	Shallow or vaulted hard palate.	
	Incomplete eruption of anterior dentition.	
	Restricted lingual frenum.	
	Palatal asymmetry.	
	Suspected temporomandibular joint disorder.	

Discretionary Clinical Observation 12: Observation for Tongue-Thrust Swallow
(instructions in manual, Chapter 3)

Observation for Tongue-Thrust Swallow

Place a minus sign (–) in box to the left for all that are observed during the swallow procedure.	
	Tongue visibly protrudes between the incisors, involuntarily and forcefully.
	Lips close, and either seal or attempt to seal, involuntarily and forcefully.

Describe concerns.

Obligatory or Habitual Tongue Thrust?
Proceed if tongue-thrust swallow is noted.

Place a minus sign (–) in the column to the left for any feature noticed.

Features may potentially obligate tongue-thrust swallow.

	Nasal obstruction.		Shallow or vaulted palatal arch.
	Enlarged palatine tonsils.		Symptoms indicate possible temporomandibular joint disorder.
	Small pharyngeal orifice.		

Describe concerns.

APPENDIX A

	Decision Box for Developmental Apraxia of Speech Observations: Discretionary Clinical Observation 13	
	Place a minus sign (–) in the column to the left if noting any of the following indicators in a child. Proceed to developmental apraxia of speech observations (i.e., Discretionary Clinical Observation 13) if indicators are present.

	Symptom	Clinical Observation Noted
	History of speech production problems in the family, or history of speech therapy in family.	Case history intake
	Delayed speech development.	
	Did not engage in canonical babbling between the ages of 5 and 10 months.	
	Persisting unintelligible speech, not explained by phonological disorder or organic pathology.	1
	Difficulty with multisyllabic words.	
	Sound transpositions (i.e., metathetic errors).	
	Perseveration across word boundaries.	
	Apparent disfluency or choppiness, not consistent with stuttering or cluttering.	
	Difficulty with volitional tongue or lip movements in the absence of difficulty with automatic tongue or lip movements. (Symptom may be indicative or oral apraxia, which although is not the same as verbal apraxia, can co-occur with it.)	2
	Difficulty with sequencing movements for volitional speech.	7

Discretionary Clinical Observation 13: Developmental Apraxia of Speech Observation (instructions in manual, Chapter 3)

Observations for Preverbal or Limited Language Children

Place a minus sign (–) in the column to the left for all that apply. Parental reports are a good source for some of this information.

	Child did not engage in canonical babble between the ages of 5 and 10 months.
	Child was an unusually quiet infant.
	Child is 18 months or older and prefers to communicate using gesture.
	Child is 18 months or older and single-word utterances that are frequently holophrastic or supported by gesture dominate.
	Child frequently supplements unintelligible speech with gestures and environmental sounds.
	Child makes unusual speech sound production errors (e.g., vowel distortions, consonant insertions, voicing confusions, metathetic errors, perseveration across word boundaries, nonspeech sounds).

Describe concerns.

Observations for Verbal Children

Place a check mark in the column to the left of each word if the child makes any of the following error types when saying the words and sentences below: manner-type substitutions, additions, prolongations, repetitions, nonphonemic productions, voicing and nasality errors, vowel and diphthong errors, difficulty with sequencing phonemes in syllables, inconsistent errors, articulatory groping, silent posturing, unusual prosodic patterns, dysfluency, or choppiness.

	Alligator.		Eucalyptus.		Macaroni.
	Buttercup.		Elephant.		Vegetable.
	Cucumber.		Hippopotamus.		Washing machine.

My hippopotamus' name is Buttercup.
An alligator eats macaroni and eucalyptus every day.

Describe concerns.

APPENDIX A

Decision Box for Acquired Apraxia of Speech Observation: Discretionary Clinical Observation 14		
Place a minus sign (–) in the column to the left if noting any of the following indicators in a person who has experienced a neurologic episode postlingually or is suspected as such. Proceed to acquired apraxia of speech observation (i.e., Discretionary Clinical Observation 14) if indicators are present.		
	Symptom	Clinical Observation Noted
	Difficulty with multisyllabic words or words of increased length and complexity.	1
	Sound transpositions (or metathetic errors).	
	Perseveration across word boundaries.	
	Apparent disfluency or choppiness.	
	Difficulty with volitional tongue or lip movements in the absence of difficulty with automatic tongue or lip movements. (Symptom may be indicative of oral apraxia, which although is not the same as verbal apraxia, can co-occur with it.)	2
	Difficulty with sequencing movements for volitional speech.	7

Discretionary Clinical Observation 14: Acquired Apraxia of Speech Observation
(instructions in manual, Chapter 3)

Observations for Acquired Apraxia of Speech

Observations for Oral Apraxia

Place a minus sign (−) in the column to the left for any behavior for which the examinee exhibits difficulty performing volitionally.

	Cough.			Bite the lower lip.
	Click the tongue.			Puff the cheeks.
	Blow.			

Describe concerns.

Observations for Acquired Apraxia of Speech

Place a check mark in the box to the left for all that apply.

	Marked difference in the fluidity of speech for counting to five compared to naming numbers one to five on command, with counting being the more fluid of the two.
	Marked difference between fluidity of speech when counting backward from 20 to 11 compared to counting backward from 10 to 1, with the 10-to-1 countdown sequence being the more fluid.
	Marked difference between saying the word *November* in series, compared to saying the same word in response to a question, with saying the word in series being more fluid.
	Increasing difficulty with words of increased length and complexity. Place a minus sign (−) to the left of the triad(s) with increasing difficulty:
	But . . . Butter . . . Buttercup.
	Wash . . . Washing . . . Washing machine.
	Lead . . . Leader . . . Leadership.
	You . . . You call . . . Eucalyptus.
	Chalk... Chocolate . . . Chocolate cake.
	Straw . . . Strawberry . . . Strawberry shortcake.

Describe concerns.

APPENDIX A

Decision Box for Submucous Cleft Screening: Discretionary Clinical Observation 15		
Place a minus sign (−) in the column to the left if noting any of the following indicators. Proceed to screening for submucous cleft (i.e., Discretionary Clinical Observation 15) if indicators are noted.		
	Symptom	Clinical Observation Noted
	Hypernasal resonance.	1
	Difficulty with pressure consonants (i.e., plosives, stops, affricates, fricatives; particularly voiceless).	
	History of otitis media with effusion or nasal reflux.	
	Posterior or superior leakage of air during labial seal activity.	2
	Palatal asymmetry.	5
	Dark or bluish shading at palatal midline (i.e., median palatal raphe).	
	Palatal translucency.	
	Bifid uvula.	
	Anterior or posterior placement of velar dimple.	
	Notch in posterior hard palate, implying absence of nasal spine.	
	Hypernasality or difficulty with pressure consonants during verbal diadochokinesis.	7
	Hypernasal resonance during sustained vowel.	8

Discretionary Clinical Observation 15: Submucous Cleft Screening (instructions in manual, Chapter 3)	
Screening for Submucous Cleft	
Place a minus sign (−) in the box to the left for all that apply.	
	Notch is noted instead of nasal spine.
	Any area palpated was noted to have decreased tactile resistance. Identify the area to which this applies:
	Palatal torus noted.
Describe concerns.	

Decision Box for Surplus Nasal Airflow Screening: Discretionary Clinical Observation 16	
Place a minus sign (–) in the column to the left if noting any of the following indicators. Proceed to surplus nasal airflow screening (i.e., Discretionary Clinical Observation 16) if indicators are present.	
Symptom	Clinical Observation Noted
Perception of any of the following during speech or vocalization event.	1
Hypernasal resonance.	
Audible nasal airflow.	
Short utterance length.	
Difficulty with obstruent consonants with or without hypernasality.	
Atypical voice.	
Compensatory articulation substitutions for obstruents (i.e., plosives, stops, affricates, fricatives; particularly voiceless):	
Glottal stops.	
Pharyngeal stops, fricatives, or affricates.	
Velar fricatives.	
Posterior nasal fricative (i.e., nasal snort).	
Anterior nasal fricative (i.e., facial grimace).	
Posterior or superior air leakage during labial seal activity.	2
Velar movement on /ɑ/ phonation is asymmetrical, weak, or absent.	6
Localized velar contractions on /ɑ/ phonation.	7
Hypernasal resonance during sustained vowel.	8

Discretionary Clinical Observation 16: Surplus Nasal Airflow Screening (instructions in manual, Chapter 3)
Screening for Surplus Nasal Airflow During Speech.
Place a minus sign (–) in the column to the left if the following applies.
Mirror condensation noted for oral consonants during speech.
Describe concerns.

APPENDIX A

Decision Box for Dysarthria Observation: Discretionary Clinical Observation 17		
Place a minus sign (–) in the column to the left if noting any of the following indicators. Proceed to dysarthria observations (i.e., Discretionary Clinical Observation 17) if indicators are noted.		
	Symptom	Clinical Observation Noted
	Imprecise consonants or slurred speech.	1
	Hypernasality.	
	Mixed resonance.	
	Jaw hangs in open position when at rest, mandible deviates to the right or left at rest or in motion.	
	Oral asymmetry at rest or in motion, fasciculations in perioral area.	
	Atypical voice (e.g., breathy, harsh, strained-strangled).	
	Labial asymmetry at rest or in motion, unilateral or bilateral labial seal weakness.	2
	Tongue: Extraneous movements at rest or in motion, deviation at rest or in motion, weakness, imprecise movements, reduced range of motion, fatigue.	
	Mandible: Deviates to right or left when lowered, weak resistance, extraneous movements at rest or in motion.	5
	Tongue: Asymmetry, deviations, signs of atrophy, fasciculations, extraneous movements at rest or in motion.	
	Velum: Asymmetry at rest or in motion, rhythmic or arrhythmic movements at rest or in motion, unilateral or bilateral weakness.	
	Weak, absent, or asymmetrical velar movement on /ɑ/ phonation.	6
	Motion activities: Imprecise consonants, reduced range of motion for articulators, decreasing rate or precision, slow rate, evidence of fatigue.	7
	Evidence of hypernasality or fatigue on /ɑ/ phonation.	8

Discretionary Clinical Observation 17: Dysarthria Observation (instructions in manual, Chapter 3)			
Dysarthria Observation			
Place a minus sign (–) in the column to the left that is marked "S" for all symptoms noted during spontaneous speech. Place a minus sign (–) in the column marked "R" for all symptoms noted during reading.			

S	R	Symptoms	
		Imprecise articulation.	Articulation
		Intermittent, sudden, or unpredictable articulation breakdown.	
		Difficulty initiating articulation.	
		Unpredictable vowel distortions.	
		Hypernasal resonance with nasal airflow emissions.	Resonance
		Hypernasal resonance without nasal airflow emissions.	
		Mixed resonance.	
		Low pitch.	Voice
		Irregular pitch.	
		Sudden elevation of pitch.	
		Reduced variation in pitch and loudness.	
		Sudden bursts of loudness, irregular loudness.	
		Increased loudness overall.	
		Reduced loudness or inaudible voice.	
		Harsh, hoarse, or strained-strangled quality.	
		Breathy quality.	
		Unpredictable interruptions in speech flow (e.g., variations in pitch and loudness).	Prosody
		Monotone.	
		Slow rate.	
		Short distorted phrases.	
		Dysrhythmia.	
		Sound prolongations.	
		Equal syllable stress.	

continues

APPENDIX A

Discretionary Clinical Observation 17: Dysarthria Observation *continued*

S	R	Symptoms	
		Prolonged intervals between syllables and words.	Prosody
		Seemingly measured pace.	
		Reduced vocal emphasis.	
		Pitch peaks and valleys.	
		Loudness variability that flattens to a monotone.	
		Short rushes of speech with illogically placed pauses.	
		Variable or accelerated rate.	
		Inappropriate silences.	
		Repetitions of initial sounds.	
		Audible inspiration.	Respiration
		Breathy exhalation.	
		Sudden gusts of exhaled air.	
		Altered breathing cycle.	
		Much effort required for speech.	Overall
		Muscular weakness.	
		Extraneous movements.	
		Imprecise movements.	

Describe concerns.

Decision Box for Speech Sound Stimulability Screening: Discretionary Clinical Observation 18
Place a minus sign (–) in the column to the left if noting any of the following indicators. Proceed to speech sound stimulability screening (i.e., Discretionary Clinical Observation 18) if indicators are present.

	Symptom	Clinical Observation Noted
	Speech sound errors are not fully attributable to organic anomaly; stimulability testing was not completed earlier.	Any routine clinical observation.

Discretionary Clinical Observation 18: Speech Sound Stimulability Screening
(instructions in manual, Chapter 3)
Speech Sound Stimulability Screening
List selected speech sound stimulability targets in the columns marked "target 1," "target 2," "target 3," and "target 4." In the column to the left of each target, write "HS" for highly stimulable targets, "S" for stimulable targets, and "NS" for not-stimulable targets.

	Target 1		Target 2		Target 3		Target 4

Describe concerns.

APPENDIX A

Decision Box for Respiratory and Laryngeal Efficiency Screening: Discretionary Clinical Observation 19		
Place a minus sign (–) in the column to the left if noting any of the following indicators. Proceed to respiratory and laryngeal efficiency screening (i.e., Discretionary Clinical Observation 19) if indicators are present.		
	Symptom	Clinical Observation Noted
	Evidence of respiratory inefficiency or distress during any speech or nonspeech activity.	1, 7, 8
	Voice quality that indicates possible inefficient use of the larynx (e.g., breathiness, harshness, hoarseness, or strained quality).	
	Failure to sustain the vowel /ɑ/ for at least 20 seconds for adults and 10 seconds for children.	8

Discretionary Clinical Observation 19: Screening for Laryngeal and Respiratory Efficiency (instructions in manual, Chapter 3)	
Screening for Laryngeal and Respiratory Efficiency (i.e., S:Z ratio)	
Place a minus sign (–) in column to the left for any symptom noted.	
	For adult examinee, measured duration was less than 20 seconds. For child examinee, measured duration was less than 10 seconds.
	Audible symptoms of vocal pathology.
	Duration decreased with consecutive trials.
	S:Z ratio was calculated as 1.2 or greater.
Describe concerns.	

Decision Box for Gag Reflex Stimulation: Discretionary Clinical Observation 20	
Place a minus sign (–) in the column to the left if noting any of the following indicators. Proceed to gag reflex stimulation (i.e., Discretionary Clinical Observation 20) if indicators are present.	
Note: If gag reflex is stimulated, in most cases it should be the last activity of the evaluation since it is somewhat invasive and may negatively affect compliance in some cases, particularly for younger examinees.	

	Symptom	Clinical Observation Noted
	Hypernasal resonance during speech.	1
	Difficulty with obstruent sounds.	
	Any symptoms suggesting possible neurologic involvement.	
	Any craniofacial symptom leading to a genetic referral.	
	Possible inadequate velar movement.	6
	Any symptom leading to observations for motor-speech disorder (e.g., developmental apraxia of speech, acquired apraxia of speech, dysarthria).	7
	Hypernasal resonance during sustained vowel.	8
	Any symptom suggesting a need for neurologic referral.	1–8

Discretionary Clinical Observation 20: Gag Reflex Stimulation (instructions in manual, Chapter 3)	
Gag Reflex Stimulation	
Place a minus sign (–) in the column to the left for any that apply.	
	Absent gag reflex: no response.
	Hypoactive gag reflex: weak response.
	Hyperactive gag reflex: forceful response.
	Premature gag reflex: response prior to touching the pharyngeal wall.
	Delayed or latent gag reflex: delay between stimulating pharyngeal wall and the reflexive response.
Describe concerns.	

Decision Box for Dysphagia Screening Prompt: Discretionary Clinical Observation 21	
Regulations require that all poststroke patients should be screened for dysphagia as soon as the acute phase of the illness has passed and before returning to an oral diet. However, stroke is not the only etiology resulting in dysphagia. Recently laryngectomized patients and aging nonstroke patients should also be considered for dysphagia referral if experiencing any of the following symptoms.	
Place a minus sign (−) in the column to the left for any symptom noted.	

	Symptom	Occasion Noted
	Older adult.	Case history intake.
	Patient reports difficulty with feeding or swallowing.	

Discretionary Clinical Observation 21: Dysphagia Screening Prompt (instructions in manual, Chapter 3)	
Dysphagia Screening Prompt	
Place a minus sign (−) in the column to the left if any of the following apply. Proceed to dysphagia screening if two or more symptoms are noted or if the person has a history of recent neurologic incident. If in doubt, refer to screening.	
	Recent history or cerebrovascular accident, neurologic incident or disease, or laryngectomy (required dysphagia screening).
	Cough after swallow.
	Voice change after swallow.
	Reduced lingual range of motion (Routine Clinical Observation 2) or incomplete facial symmetry (Routine Clinical Observation 1).
	Patient is flagged to be observed for any motor-speech disorders procedure (Discretionary Clinical Observations 15, 16, and 17).
	Abnormal volitional cough.
	Abnormal gag reflex.
Describe concerns.	

Summarize the Findings and Make Recommendations

Summarize the Findings: General Form		
Review the evidence collected. Note minus signs (−) and descriptions of concerns. Record evidence of structural or performance anomaly that has potential to negatively influence speech production or result in a need for clinical follow-up. Use additional space provided at bottom if needed.		
Anomaly Was Noted When Evaluating:	**Anomaly Observed**	**Comment on Performance**
Facial region.		
Respiration.		
Lip/tongue strength/mobility.		
Dental alignment or bite.		
Dental occlusion.		
Oral interior.		
Velar movement.		
Verbal diadochokinesis.		
Vowel prolongation.		
Nasal cavity clearance.		
Facial dimensions.		
Temporomandibular joint.		
Tongue-thrust swallow.		
Childhood apraxia of speech.		
Acquired apraxia of speech.		
Submucous cleft.		
Surplus nasal airflow.		
Dysarthria.		
Speech sound stimulability.		
Laryngeal/respiratory efficiency.		
Gag reflex stimulation.		
Amblyopia screening.		
Screening for primitive reflexes.		

continues

Summarize the Findings: General Form *continued*

Prompt for dysphagia screening.		
Other.		

Recommendations for Individualized Plan of Care
Place a check mark in the column to the left for all that apply. Supply descriptive information as suggested.

	Clinical Implications
	Result of oral-facial inspection is unremarkable. No impact on speech production is suspected. No follow-up is needed.
	Oral-facial inspection yields evidence that may support a particular diagnosis or plan of care. If so, specify evidence and suspected diagnosis:
	Oral-facial inspection yields evidence that clearly supports a particular diagnosis or plan of care. If so, specify evidence and diagnosis:

Plan of Care			
	Next Step	Rationale Circle all that apply.	Responsible Party Circle all that apply
	Additional testing is needed.	• Part of oral-facial inspection that was not yet completed requires more time or clinical teaching to perform. • Testing that is beyond the scope of oral-facial inspection is identified as needed. • Other (specify).	• Examiner, follow-up. • Speech-language pathologist receiving case for therapy. • Specialist speech-language pathologist referral. • Health care provider outside speech-language pathology referral. • Other (specify).
	Recommend that therapy plan include objectives/procedures designed to address concerns identified through inspection.	Specify:	Specify:

Oral-Facial Evaluation for Speech-Language Pathologists
Barbara Ann Johnson-Root, PhD, CCC-SLP

Special Recording Form: Preverbal Children (Infants)

Intake Information	
Client name:	Date of evaluation:
Date of birth:	Age:
Examiner:	Agency or facility:
Reason for evaluation:	
Relevant history:	
Comments:	

Prepare the Work Area for Testing, Adapted for Young Children (instructions in manual, Chapters 1 and 4)
Checklist Place a check mark in the column to the left after completing each preparatory step in the list below.

	Inventory equipment and supplies listed in Table 1–2 and described in Appendix B.
	Check batteries that power battery-operated equipment. Replace weak or dead batteries.
	Verify that all cords and strings were removed. If not, remove and dispose of them.
	Sanitize the work area and unwrapped equipment as instructed in Chapter 1.
	Wash hands thoroughly.
	Put on examination gloves, using procedures provided in Chapter 1.
	Arrange equipment in a small plastic box.

Instruct the Examinee (and Guardian if Appropriate)

Use your own words and developmentally appropriate language to communicate the following talking points before you begin.

- The oral-facial evaluation is a customary part of every speech-language evaluation.
- It involves inspecting all observable body parts necessary for speaking so that we can learn whether all parts are present, complete, and working properly.
- This is done to look into whether there is a physical explanation for the speech problem that brought you here or if there is any physical problem that we should address while we are helping you.
- None of the procedures are painful or harmful.
- For some people, oral-facial evaluation findings may lead to more detailed testing or possibly referral to another professional, although this is not the case for everyone.
- You may ask questions before we begin or at any time. Do you have any questions now? (If *yes*, either answer briefly or diplomatically table the question for a more appropriate time. If *no*, move on.)
- Are you ready? Let's get started!

Routine Clinical Observations

Routinely complete the following six clinical observations for all infants.

- Routine Clinical Observation 1: Social Interchange (A), Facial Region Inspection (B), and Breathing Observations (B) for Infants
- Routine Clinical Observation 2: Condition of Tongue Screening for Infants
- Routine Clinical Observation 5: Oral Interior Screening for Infants
- Routine Clinical Observation 6: Spontaneous Velar Movement Screening for Infants
- Discretionary Clinical Observation 22: Amblyopia Screening (routine for this population)
- Discretionary Clinical Observation 23: Screening for Selected Primitive Reflexes (routine for this population)

Routine Clinical Observation 1(A): Social Interchange, Adapted for Infant or Preverbal Child (instructions in manual, Chapters 2 and 4)	
Rate comprehensibility for child's use of gestures, vocalizations, and other nonverbal methods. Check the one that applies.	
	Consistent communication success.
	Communication success more than half the time.
	Communication success about half of the time.
	Communication success less than half of the time.
	Communication success achieved rarely if ever.
Clinical judgment of age appropriateness as a communicator.	
Place a minus sign (–) to the left of any feature noted as atypical during vocalization.	
Check all that apply.	
Voice.	Resonance.
Describe concerns.	

Identify stage of babbling. Place a check mark to the left of the stage that dominates vocalizations.

	Prebabbling.		Marginal.		Canonical.		Variegated.

Describe noteworthy features.

If prebabbling is identified, describe vocalizations, volubility, type of sounds in repertoire, and any other noteworthy feature.

APPENDIX A

		Routine Clinical Observations 1(B): Facial Region Inspection (instruction in manual, Chapter 2)
Use a minus sign (−) to mark all features noted during facial region inspection. If multiple options appear on the same line, circle those that apply.		
Resting	**Speaking or Vocalizing**	**Feature**
		Facial or oral asymmetry, drooping, tremor, fasciculation, spasm.
		Poor saliva management (as compared to others of similar age and development).
		Scarring.
		Thin upper lip, cleft lip.
		Micrognathia, macrognathia, retrognathic jaw, prognathic jaw.
		Hypoplastic midface, flat philtrum, epicanthal folds.
		Malformed ears, low-set ears.
		Eyelid ptosis, strabismus, wandering eye.
		Wide-set eyes.
		Forward tongue posture.
		Cranial asymmetry, prominent forehead, microcephaly, macrocephaly.
		Other dysmorphic features:
After completing above checklist, place minus sign (−) in column for any applicable condition.		
	Facial features suggest need for referral to genetics, neurology, or otorhinolaryngology if doctor-patient relationship has not yet been established.	
	Facial features appear to possibly contribute to atypical speaking pattern. Specify.	

Routine Clinical Observation 1(C): Breathing Observations, Adapted for Young Child
(instructions in manual, Chapters 2 and 4)

Identify the type of breathing noted upon observation. For all examinees, *nasal* and *diaphragmatic* breathing are optimal; upper thoracic breathing is acceptable.

Place a check mark in the far-left column if any of the features on the left apply. For the features on the right, place a minus sign (−) in the corresponding column if any are noted.

Type of Breathing

	Nasal.		Oral.
	Diaphragmatic.		Upper thoracic, clavicular.
	Lower thoracic.		Noisy, evidence of respiratory distress or struggle.

Describe concerns.

Routine Clinical Observation 2: Condition of Tongue, Amended for Preverbal Child or Infant
(instructions in manual, Chapters 2 and 4)

Tongue Observations

Place a minus sign (−) in the column that corresponds to the feature if it is observed to be atypical.

Feature

	Shape of tongue tip.		Lingual frenum length.

Describe atypical features; comment on potential for impact on speech.

Routine Clinical Observation 5: Oral Interior, Amended for Preverbal Child or Infant
(instructions in manual, Chapters 2 and 4)

Dentition

Use the dental chart to mark erupted dentition by circling the teeth that have erupted.

Upper Teeth	Erupt	Shed
Central Incisor:	8–12 months	6–7 years
Lateral Incisor:	9–13 months	7–8 years
Cuspid:	16–22 months	10–12 years
First Molar:	13–19 months	9–11 years
Second Molar:	25–33 months	10–12 years

Lower Teeth	Erupt	Shed
Second Molar:	23–33 months	10–12 years
First Molar:	14–18 months	9–11 years
Cuspid:	17–23 months	9–12 years
Lateral Incisor:	10–16 months	7–8 years
Central Incisor:	6–10 months	6–7 years

Describe concerns, if any.

Tongue Surface, Size, and Shape

Place a check mark in the column to the left if the feature is judged within normal limits. Place a minus sign (−) in the column if noting any atypical trait. Write *N.O.* (not observed) in the column if unable to observe. Use the space below to provide additional descriptive data.

Feature			
	Texture.		Shape.
	Size.		Other noteworthy feature:

Describe concern with the feature noted.

	Hard Palate		
	Place a check mark in the column to the left if the feature is judged to be within normal limits. Place a minus sign (−) in the column if noting any atypical trait. Write *N.O.* (not observed) in the column if unable to observe. Use the space below to provide additional descriptive data.

	Feature		
	Alveolar ridge.		Posterior nasal spine.
	Palatal arch.		Foveae palate.
	Median raphe.		Scarring.
	Mucous membrane.		Coloring.

Describe concerns.

	Posterior Soft Tissue		
	Place a check mark in the column to the left if the feature is judged to be within normal limits. Place a minus sign (−) in the column if noting any atypical trait. Write *N.O.* (not observed) in the column if unable to observe. Use the space below to provide additional descriptive data.

	Feature		
	Velum (structure only).		Palatine tonsils.
	Uvula.		Posterior pharyngeal wall.
	Faucial pillars.		

Describe concerns.

APPENDIX A

	Routine Clinical Observation 6: Spontaneous Velar Movement, Amended for Preverbal Child or Infant (instructions in manual, Chapters 2 and 4)		
	Velar Movement		
	Place a check mark in the first box on the left if "velum moves up and back symmetrically" or if able to observe normal velar movement in any context. Write *N.O.* (not observed) in the second box on the left if "did not observe velar movement" applies. For features listed on the right, if observed, place a minus sign (–) in the corresponding column. Use space below to provide additional descriptive data.		
	Subjective Judgment of Observed Velar Movement		
	Velum moves up and back symmetrically.		Velum moves up and back asymmetrically.
	Did not observe velar movement.		Velum moves sluggishly.
Describe concerns.			

	Discretionary Clinical Observation 22: Amblyopia Screening (instructions in manual, Chapter 4)	
	Amblyopia screening is considered a discretionary procedure since it is only administered to select examinees. For children younger than 6 years, however, it is considered a routine part of the inspection.	
	Place a check mark in the "L" column that corresponds to "no change" for children who exhibit no negative response to covering the left eye, and place a check mark in the "R" column that corresponds to "no change" for children who exhibit no negative response to covering the right eye. Place a minus sign (–) in "L" or "R" column if the "child makes a determined attempt to see around the eye test paddle or exhibits signs of distress" when either eye is covered.	

L	R	Response to Covering One Eye During Conversation or Visual Activity
		No change.
		Child makes determined effort to see around the eye test paddle or exhibited signs of distress.
		Place a minus sign (–) in the column to the left if the child tries to peer around the paddle or shows signs of distress when either eye is covered. Refer to ophthalmologist.

	Discretionary Clinical Observation 23: Screening for Selected Primitive Reflexes (instructions in manual, Chapter 4)	

Place a check mark in the column to the left for reflexes that are found to be present within the appropriate age boundaries. Place a minus sign (−) in the column to the left for reflexes that are found to be absent during the developmental period identified as appropriate for the reflex to occur. Place an arrow (→) in the column to the left for reflexes that persist beyond the age of normal suppression for that reflex.

	Reflex	Age Boundaries for Response
	Rooting.	Present at birth; inhibited between ages of 6 and 12 months.
	Sucking.	Present at birth; inhibited between ages of 2 and 3 months.
	Palmar grasp.	Present at birth; normal up to 6 months.
	Tongue-thrust reflex (not to be confused with tongue-thrust swallow).	Present at birth; normal up to 6 months.
	Babinski.	Always abnormal.

Comments.

If you believe there is a reason to omit one or more of the procedures that are listed as routine for this age group, clearly write the rationale for your decision on the recording form. Then proceed with the inspection.

Identifying and Completing Appropriate Discretionary Clinical Observations

In most cases, the inspection ends with routine clinical observations. Yet once routine procedures are complete, the next step is to determine whether the evidence indicates a need for any discretionary clinical observations. For the sake of convenience, a series of decision boxes provides structure that can facilitate identifying discretionary clinical observations that should be considered.

Only four discretionary clinical observations are relevant for this age group:

- Discretionary Clinical Observation 9: Nasal Cavity Clearance Screening for Infants
- Discretionary Clinical Observation 10: Facial Dimension Estimates
- Discretionary Clinical Observation 15: Screening for Submucous Cleft
- Discretionary Clinical Observation 20: Gag Reflex Stimulation

APPENDIX A

Bear in mind that none of the decision boxes is intended to prompt a perfunctory decision that results in a discretionary procedure. Certainly, an understanding of the examinee's overall symptom pattern combined with a rich bank of clinical experience and intuition should also contribute, albeit such intangibles are highly individualized and therefore difficult to place on a form. Even so, strategically considering tangible client-centered evidence as it is arranged on the form can contribute to a good decision relative to proceeding with a discretionary clinical observation, and that is the intended purpose of the decision boxes.

Once a decision box is evaluated, if it flags the corresponding discretionary clinical observation, the inspection can proceed to that discretionary observation if the examining clinician deems it appropriate. Generally, no more than three discretionary observations are flagged for one individual. However, there are exceptions, especially when working with children who present multiple anomaly conditions.

Decision Box for Nasal Cavity Clearance Screening: Discretionary Clinical Observation 9	
Place a minus sign (−) in the column to the left if noting any of the following indicators. Proceed to nasal cavity clearance screening (i.e., Discretionary Clinical Observation 9) if indicators are noted.	
Symptom	Clinical Observation Noted
Hyponasal resonance detected during any speech or vocalization event.	1
Nasal asymmetry.	
Visible or audible symptoms of congestion[a] (including mouth breathing).	

[a]May table the procedure if the person exhibits symptoms of temporary obstruction such as a cold or allergy.

Discretionary Clinical Observation 9: Nasal Cavity Clearance Screening, Amended for Infant (instructions in manual, Chapters 3 and 4)	
Screening for Nasal Cavity Clearance	
Place a check mark in the box to left for all that apply.	Describe concerns. Comment on relevance to speech.
Nasal asymmetry.	
Nasal obstruction due to mucosal swelling, deviated septum, hypertrophied conchae, excess mucus.	
Difficulty admitting or discharging air via the nasal passages.	

Decision Box for Facial Dimension Estimates: Discretionary Clinical Observation 10

Place a minus sign (–) in the left column if noting any of the following indicators. Proceed to facial dimension estimates (i.e., Discretionary Clinical Observation 10) if indicators are present.

Symptom	Clinical Observation Noted
Facial profile appears disproportionate and the person is likely to be referred for follow-up (e.g., genetics or otorhinolaryngology).	1
Malocclusion.	4
Tongue tip does not line up with alveolar ridge.	5

Discretionary Clinical Observation 10: Facial Dimension Estimates (instructions in manual, Chapter 3)
Facial Dimension Estimates

Place a minus sign (–) to left for all that apply. If a minus sign (–) is placed in the left column in the first three rows, measure distances in millimeters and record the measurements in the divided mm column on right. Then calculate percentage for each measurement and record it in the % column on far right. Any minus sign (–) on the left should be reported to the referral recipient.

			mm	%
	Overall Facial Dimension: Distances between (1) hairline and glabella, (2) glabella and subnasale, and (3) subnasale and pogonion are not segments of approximate equal length.	1		
		2		
		3		
	Dimensions for Lower Third of Face: Distances between (1) subnasale and stomian, (2) stomian and supramentale, and (3) supramentale and pogonion are not segments of approximate equal length.	1		
		2		
		3		
	Size and Spacing of Eyes: (1) Length of palpebral fissures and (2) distance between eyes are not segments of approximate equal length.	1		
		2		
	Facial Angle: Facial angle deviates grossly from 90° or misses subnasale plane completely.			
	Frankfurt Horizontal Plane: Tragion is lower than ipsilateral lid-cheek junction.			

Describe concerns.

APPENDIX A

Decision Box for Submucous Cleft Screening: Discretionary Clinical Observation 15, Amended for Preverbal Child or Infant	
If any of the following indicators is noted, plan to proceed with screening for submucous cleft (i.e., Discretionary Clinical Observation 15). Instructions are found in Chapter 3.	
Symptom	Clinical Observation Noted
Hypernasal resonance.	1
History of middle ear effusion and nasal reflux.	
Palatal asymmetry.	5
Dark or bluish shading at palatal midline (i.e., median palatal raphe).	
Palatal translucency.	
Bifid uvula.	
Anterior or posterior placement of velar dimple.	

Discretionary Clinical Observation 15: Submucous Cleft Screening (instructions in manual, Chapter 3)	
Screening for Submucous Cleft	
Place a minus sign (−) in the box to the left for all that apply.	
	Notch is noted instead of nasal spine.
	Any area palpated was noted to have decreased tactile resistance. Identify the area to which this applies:
	Palatal torus noted.
Describe concerns.	

Decision Box for Gag Reflex Stimulation: Discretionary Clinical Observation 20, Amended for Infant or Toddler
If any of the following indicators is noted, plan to stimulate gag reflex (i.e., Discretionary Clinical Observation 20). Instructions are found in Chapter 3.
If gag reflex is stimulated, in most cases it should be the last activity of the evaluation since it is somewhat invasive and may negatively affect compliance in some cases, particularly for younger examinees.

Symptom	Clinical Observation Noted
Any craniofacial symptom leading to a genetic referral.	1
Suspected inadequate velar movement.	6
Any symptom suggesting a need for neurologic referral.	1–8

Discretionary Clinical Observation 20: Gag Reflex Stimulation (instructions in manual, Chapter 3)
Gag Reflex Stimulation
Place a minus sign (−) in the column to the left for any that apply.

	Absent gag reflex: no response.
	Hypoactive gag reflex: weak response.
	Hyperactive gag reflex: forceful response.
	Premature gag reflex: response prior to touching the pharyngeal wall.
	Delayed or latent gag reflex: delay between stimulating pharyngeal wall and the reflexive response.
Describe concerns.	

APPENDIX A

Summarize the Findings and Make Recommendations

Summarize the Findings: Infant or Toddler		
Review the evidence collected. Note minus signs (–) and descriptions of concerns. Record evidence of structural or performance anomaly that has potential to negatively influence speech production or result in a need for clinical follow-up. Use additional space provided at bottom if needed.		
Anomaly Was Noted When Evaluating:	Anomaly Observed	Comment on Performance
Facial region.		
Respiration.		
Lip/tongue strength/mobility.		
Emerging dentition.		
Oral interior.		
Spontaneous velar movement.		
Amblyopia screening.		
Primitive reflexes.		
Nasal cavity clearance.		
Facial dimensions.		
Submucous cleft.		
Gag reflex stimulation.		

	Recommendations for Individualized Plan of Care

Place a check mark in the column to the left for all that apply. Supply descriptive information as suggested.

	Clinical Implications
	Result of oral-facial inspection is unremarkable. No impact on speech production is suspected. No follow-up is needed.
	Oral-facial inspection yields evidence that may support a particular diagnosis or plan of care. If so, specify evidence and suspected diagnosis:
	Oral-facial inspection yields evidence that clearly supports a particular diagnosis or plan of care. If so, specify evidence and diagnosis:

Plan of Care		
Next Step	Rationale Circle all that apply.	Responsible Party Circle all that apply
Additional testing is needed.	• Part of oral-facial inspection that was not yet completed requires more time or clinical teaching to perform. • Testing that is beyond the scope of oral-facial inspection is identified as needed. • Other (specify).	• Examiner, follow-up. • Speech-language pathologist receiving case for therapy. • Specialist speech-language pathologist referral. • Health care provider outside speech-language pathology referral. • Other (specify).
Recommend that therapy plan include objectives/procedures designed to address concerns identified through inspection.	Specify:	Specify:

APPENDIX A

Oral-Facial Evaluation for Speech-Language Pathologists
Barbara Ann Johnson-Root, PhD, CCC-SLP

Special Recording Form: Children With Limited Language (Toddlers)

Intake Information	
Client name:	Date of evaluation:
Date of birth:	Age:
Examiner:	Agency or facility:
Reason for evaluation:	
Relevant history:	
Comments:	

Prepare the Work Area for Testing, Adapted for Young Children
(instructions in manual, Chapters 1 and 4)
Checklist
Place a check mark in the column to the left after completing each preparatory step in the list below.

	Inventory equipment and supplies listed in Table 1–2 and described in Appendix B.
	Check batteries that power battery-operated equipment. Replace weak or dead batteries.
	Verify that all cords and strings were removed. If not, remove and dispose of them.
	Sanitize the work area and unwrapped equipment as instructed in Chapter 1.
	Wash hands thoroughly.
	Put on examination gloves, using procedures provided in Chapter 1.
	Arrange equipment in a small plastic box.

Instruct the Examinee (and Significant Other if Appropriate)

Use your own words and developmentally appropriate language to communicate the following talking points before you begin.

- The oral-facial evaluation is a customary part of every speech-language evaluation.
- It involves inspecting all observable body parts necessary for speaking so that we may learn whether all parts are present, complete, and working properly.
- This is done to look into whether there is a physical explanation for the speech problem that brought you here or if there is any physical problem that we should address while we are helping you.
- None of the procedures are painful or harmful.
- For some people, oral-facial evaluation findings may lead to more detailed testing or possibly referral to another professional, although this is not the case for everyone.
- You may ask questions before we begin or at any time. Do you have any questions now? (If *yes*, either answer briefly or diplomatically table the question for a more appropriate time. If *no*, move on.)
- Are you ready? Let's get started!

Routine Clinical Observations

As a matter of course, complete eight specified clinical observations for all toddlers:

- Routine Clinical Observation 1: Social Interchange (A), Facial Region Inspection (B), and Breathing Observations (C) for Children With Limited Language
- Routine Clinical Observation 2: Lip and Tongue Strength and Mobility
- Routine Clinical Observation 3: Dental Alignment and Bite for Toddlers
- Routine Clinical Observation 4: Dental Occlusion
- Routine Clinical Observation 5: Oral Interior for Infants and Toddlers
- Routine Clinical Observation 6: Velar Movement
- Discretionary Clinical Observation 22: Amblyopia Screening (routine for this population)
- Discretionary Clinical Observation 23: Screening for Selected Primitive Reflexes (routine for this population)

Routine Clinical Observations 1(A): Social Interchange, Amended for Child With Limited Language (Toddler) (instructions in manual, Chapters 2 and 4)		

Rate comprehensibility for child's use of gestures, vocalizations, and other nonverbal methods. Check the one that applies.

	Consistent communication success.
	Communication success more than half the time.
	Communication success about half of the time.
	Communication success less than half of the time.
	Communication success achieved rarely if ever.

Comment on whether communication is appropriate.

Place a minus sign (−) to the left of any feature noted as atypical during vocalization.

Check all that apply.

	Articulation.		Resonance.
	Voice.		Fluency.

Describe concerns.

		Routine Clinical Observations 1(B): Facial Region Inspection (instruction in manual, Chapter 2)
		Use a minus sign (−) to mark all features noted during facial region inspection. If multiple options appear on the same line, circle those that apply.

Resting	Speaking or Vocalizing	Feature
		Facial or oral asymmetry, drooping, tremor, fasciculation, spasm.
		Poor saliva management (compared to others of similar age and development).
		Scarring.
		Thin upper lip, cleft lip.
		Micrognathia, macrognathia, retrognathic jaw, prognathic jaw.
		Hypoplastic midface, flat philtrum, epicanthal folds.
		Malformed ears, low-set ears.
		Eyelid ptosis, strabismus, wandering eye.
		Wide-set eyes.
		Forward tongue posture.
		Cranial asymmetry, prominent forehead, microcephaly, macrocephaly.
		Other dysmorphic features:

	After completing above checklist, place a minus sign (−) in the column for any applicable condition.
	Facial features suggest need for referral to genetics, neurology, or otorhinolaryngology if doctor-patient relationship has not yet been established.
	Facial features appear to possibly contribute to atypical speaking pattern. Specify.

APPENDIX A

	Routine Clinical Observation 1(C): Breathing Observations, Adapted for Young Child (instructions in manual, Chapters 2 and 4)		
Identify the type of breathing noted upon observation. For all examinees, *nasal* and *diaphragmatic* breathing are optimal; upper thoracic breathing is acceptable. Place a check mark in the far-left column if any of the features on the left apply. For the features on the right, place a minus sign (–) in the corresponding column if any are noted.			
	Type of Breathing		
	Nasal.		Oral.
	Diaphragmatic.		Upper thoracic, clavicular.
	Lower thoracic.		Noisy, evidence of respiratory distress or struggle.
Describe concerns.			

Routine Clinical Observation 2: Lip and Tongue Mobility and Strength (instruction in manual, Chapter 2)		
Place a check mark in the column to the left if the examinee performs the act smoothly, accurately, completely, and in a timely manner. Place a minus sign (−) in the column if noting any other response, and use the space below to provide additional descriptive data.			

Action			
	Pucker.		Quick repetitions of /b/ or /p/.
	Spread.		Smack the lips.
	Sustain exaggerated /u/.		

Describe atypical responses; comment on possible relationship to speech concern.

Lip Strength and Seal

Place a check mark in the box to the left if the act is judged to be within normal limits. Place a minus sign (−) in the column if noting any other response, and use the space below to provide additional descriptive data.

Action			
	Seal.		Resistance.

Describe atypical responses; comment on possible relationship to speech concern.

Tongue Mobility

Place a check mark in the column to the left of each action if the examinee performs the act smoothly, accurately, completely, and in a timely manner. Place a minus sign (−) in the column if noting any other response, and use the space below to provide additional descriptive data.

Action			
	Protrusion.		Wiggle to the left and to the right.
	Elevation.		Rotation.
	Lateralization.		

continues

APPENDIX A

Routine Clinical Observation 2: Lip and Tongue Mobility and Strength *continued*

Describe atypical responses; comment on possible relationship to speech concern.

Other Tongue Observations
Place a check mark in box to the left if feature is observed to be within normal limits. Place a minus sign (–) in the column if noting any other response, and use the space below to provide additional descriptive data.

Feature			
	Shape of tongue tip.		Lingual frenum length.

Describe atypical features; comment on possible relationship to speech concern.

Tongue Strength
Place a check mark in the column on the left if the act is judged to be within normal limits. Place a minus sign (–) in the column if noting any other response, and use the space below to provide additional descriptive data.

Action	
	Resistance.

Describe atypical responses; comment on possible relationship to speech concern.

Routine Clinical Observation 3: Dental Bite and Alignment, Amended for Toddler or Preschooler (instructions in manual, Chapters 2 and 4)

Dental Bite

For examinees with an unremarkable bite pattern, place a check mark in the column to the left corresponding to the word *normal*. If any other bite pattern is noted, place a minus sign (–) in the column that resides directly to the left of the term that best describes the person's bite. (Typically one applies; there are exceptions.)

Bite

	Normal.		Edge-to-edge bite.		Overjet.
	Open bite.		Under bite.		Flared bite.
	Closed bite.		Cross bite.		

Add descriptive information if needed; describe relationship (or potential relationship) to speech, if any.

Alignment and Condition of Teeth

Mark dental chart below to indicate dental alignment concerns noted.

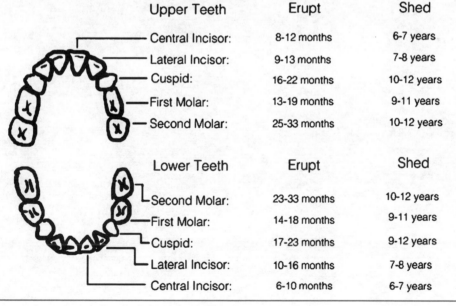

Upper Teeth	Erupt	Shed
Central Incisor:	8-12 months	6-7 years
Lateral Incisor:	9-13 months	7-8 years
Cuspid:	16-22 months	10-12 years
First Molar:	13-19 months	9-11 years
Second Molar:	25-33 months	10-12 years

Lower Teeth	Erupt	Shed
Second Molar:	23-33 months	10-12 years
First Molar:	14-18 months	9-11 years
Cuspid:	17-23 months	9-12 years
Lateral Incisor:	10-16 months	7-8 years
Central Incisor:	6-10 months	6-7 years

Describe concerns.

APPENDIX A

Routine Clinical Observation 4: Dental Occlusion (instruction in manual, Chapter 2)					
Dental Occlusion					
For examinees with neutroclusion, place a check mark in the column that resides directly to the left of that term. For examinees with distoclusion or mesioclusion, place a minus sign (–) in the column that corresponds to that classification.					
Dental Occlusion Classification					
	Neutroclusion (typical).		Distoclusion.		Mesioclusion.
Describe occlusal relationship. Comment on any possible relationship to speech production.					

Routine Clinical Observation 5: Oral Interior, Amended for Toddler or Preschooler (instructions in manual, Chapters 2 and 4)		
Tongue Surface, Size, and Shape		

Place a check mark in the box on the left if the feature is judged to be within normal limits. Place a minus sign (–) in the column if noting any atypical trait. Write *N.O.* (not observed) in the column if unable to observe. Use the space below to provide additional descriptive data.

Feature		
	Texture.		Shape.
	Size.		Other noteworthy feature:

Describe concern with the feature noted.

Hard Palate

Place a check mark in the box on the left if the feature is judged to be within normal limits. Place a minus sign (–) in the column if noting any atypical trait. Write *N.O.* (not observed) in the column if unable to observe. Use the space below to provide additional descriptive data.

Feature		
	Alveolar ridge.		Posterior nasal spine.
	Palatal arch.		Foveae palate.
	Median raphe.		Scarring.
	Mucous membrane.		Coloring.

Describe concerns.

Posterior Soft Tissue

Place a check mark in the box on the left if the feature is judged to be within normal limits. Place a minus sign (–) in the column if noting any atypical trait. Write *N.O.* (not observed) in the column if unable to observe. Use the space below to provide additional descriptive data.

Feature		
	Velum (structure only).		Palatine tonsils.
	Uvula.		Posterior pharyngeal wall.
	Faucial pillars.		

Describe concerns.

APPENDIX A

Routine Clinical Observation 6: Velar Movement (instructions in manual, Chapter 2)
Velar Movement
Place a check mark beside "velum moves up and back symmetrically on /ɑ/ phonation" if that is the case. Place a minus sign (−) in the column corresponding to any other trait noted; use the space below to provide additional descriptive data.

	Velar response to /ɑ/ phonation
	Velum moves up and back symmetrically on /ɑ/ phonation.
	Velum moves up and back asymmetrically on /ɑ/ phonation.
	Velum moves sluggishly on /ɑ/ phonation.
	Velum is not observed to move on /ɑ/ phonation.
	Misplaced velar dimple noted on /ɑ/ phonation.
Describe concerns. Comment on possible relationship to speech pattern.

Discretionary Clinical Observation 22: Amblyopia Screening (instructions in manual, Chapter 4)
Amblyopia screening is considered a discretionary procedure since it is only administered to select examinees. For children younger than 6 years, however, it is considered a routine part of the inspection.
Place a check mark in the "L" column that corresponds to "no change" for children who exhibit no negative response to covering the left eye, and place a check mark in the "R" column that corresponds to "no change" for children who exhibit no negative response to covering the right eye. Place a minus sign (−) in "L" or "R" column if the "child makes a determined attempt to see around the eye test paddle or exhibits signs of distress" when either eye was covered.

L	R	Response to Covering One Eye During Conversation or Visual Activity
		No change.
		Child makes determined effort to see around the eye test paddle or exhibited signs of distress.
		Place a minus sign (−) in the column to the left if the child tries to peer around the paddle or shows signs of distress when either eye is covered. Refer to ophthalmologist.

	Discretionary Clinical Observation 23: Screening for Selected Primitive Reflexes (instructions in manual, Chapter 4)	

Place a check mark in the column to the left for reflexes that are found to be present within the appropriate age boundaries. Place a minus sign (–) in the column to the left for reflexes that are found to be absent during the developmental period identified as appropriate for the reflex to occur. Place an arrow (→) in the column to the left for reflexes that persist beyond the age of normal suppression for that reflex.

	Reflex	Age Boundaries for Response
	Rooting.	Present at birth; inhibited between ages of 6 and 12 months.
	Sucking.	Present at birth; inhibited between ages of 2 and 3 months.
	Palmar grasp.	Present at birth; normal up to 6 months.
	Tongue-thrust reflex (not to be confused with tongue-thrust swallow).	Present at birth; normal up to 6 months.
	Babinski.	Always abnormal.

Comments.

If you believe there is a reason to omit one or more of the routine procedures, clearly mark your decision on the recording form and proceed.

Identifying and Completing Appropriate Discretionary Clinical Observations

In most cases, the inspection ends with routine clinical observations. Yet once routine procedures are complete, the next step is to determine whether the evidence indicates a need for any discretionary clinical observations. For the sake of convenience, a series of decision boxes provides structure that can facilitate identifying discretionary clinical observations that should be considered.

Bear in mind that none of the decision boxes is intended to prompt a perfunctory decision that results in a discretionary procedure. Certainly, an understanding of the examinee's overall symptom pattern combined with a rich bank of clinical experience and intuition should also contribute, albeit such intangibles are highly individualized and therefore difficult to place on a form. Even so, strategically considering tangible client-centered evidence as it appears on the form can contribute to a good decision relative to proceeding with a discretionary clinical observation, and that is the intended purpose of the decision boxes.

Once a decision box is evaluated, if it flags the corresponding discretionary clinical observation, the inspection can proceed to that discretionary observation if the examining clinician deems appropriate.

Generally, no more than three discretionary observations are flagged for a single individual. However, there are exceptions, especially when working with children who present multiple anomaly conditions.

Only six discretionary clinical observations are considered relevant for this age group:

- Discretionary Clinical Observation 9: Nasal Cavity Clearance Screening
- Discretionary Clinical Observation 10: Facial Dimension Estimates
- Discretionary Clinical Observation 13: Developmental Apraxia of Speech
- Discretionary Clinical Observation 15: Submucous Cleft Screening
- Discretionary Clinical Observation 16: Surplus Nasal Airflow Screening
- Discretionary Clinical Observation 20: Gag Reflex Stimulation

Decision Box for Nasal Cavity Clearance Screening: Discretionary Clinical Observation 9		
Place a minus sign (–) in the column to the left if noting any of the following indicators. Proceed to nasal cavity clearance screening (i.e., Discretionary Clinical Observation 9) if indicators are noted.		
	Symptom	Clinical Observation Noted
	Hyponasal resonance detected during any speech or vocalization event.	
	Nasal asymmetry.	1
	Visible or audible symptoms of congestion[a] (including mouth breathing).	

[a] May table the procedure if the person exhibits symptoms of temporary obstruction such as a cold or allergy.

Discretionary Clinical Observation 9: Nasal Cavity Clearance Screening (instructions in manual, Chapter 3)	
Screening for Nasal Cavity Clearance	
Place a minus sign (–) in column to left for all symptoms that apply.	
	Nasal asymmetry.
	Nasal obstruction due to mucosal swelling, deviated septum, hypertrophied conchae, excess mucus.
	Difficulty admitting or discharging air via the nasal passages.
	Difficulty expelling air through either nare when the other is occluded.
	Difficulty with prolonging /m/: /m→/.
Describe concerns. Comment on potential relevance to speech.	

Decision Box for Facial Dimension Estimates: Discretionary Clinical Observation 10	
Place a minus sign (–) in left column if noting any of the following indicators. Proceed to facial dimension estimates (i.e., Discretionary Clinical Observation 10) if indicators are present.	
Symptom	Clinical Observation Noted
Facial profile appears disproportionate and the person is likely to be referred for follow-up (e.g., genetics or otorhinolaryngology).	1
Malocclusion.	4
Tongue tip does not line up with alveolar ridge.	5

Discretionary Clinical Observation 10: Facial Dimension Estimates
(instructions in manual, Chapter 3)

Facial Dimension Estimates

Place a minus sign (–) to left for all that apply. If a minus sign (–) is placed in the left column in the first three rows, measure distances in millimeters and record the measurements in the divided mm column on right. Then calculate percentage for each measurement and record it in the % column on far right. Any minus sign (–) on the left should be reported to the referral recipient.

			mm	%
	Overall Facial Dimension: Distances between (1) hairline and glabella, (2) glabella and subnasale, and (3) subnasale and pogonion are not segments of approximate equal length.	1		
		2		
		3		
	Dimensions for Lower Third of Face: Distances between (1) subnasale and stomian, (2) stomian and supramentale, and (3) supramentale and pogonion are not segments of approximate equal length.	1		
		2		
		3		
	Size and Spacing of Eyes: (1) Length of palpebral fissures and (2) distance between eyes are not segments of approximate equal length.	1		
		2		
	Facial Angle: Facial angle deviates grossly from 90° or misses subnasale plane completely.			
	Frankfurt Horizontal Plane: Tragion is lower than ipsilateral lid-cheek junction.			

Describe concerns.

APPENDIX A

Decision Box for Developmental Apraxia of Speech Observations: Discretionary Clinical Observation 13	
Place a minus sign (−) in the column to the left if noting any of the following indicators in a child. Proceed to developmental apraxia of speech observations (i.e., Discretionary Clinical Observation 13) if indicators are present.	
Symptom	Clinical Observation Noted
History of speech production problems in the family or history of speech therapy in family.	Case history intake.
Delayed speech development.	
Did not engage in canonical babbling between the ages of 5 and 10 months.	
Persisting unintelligible speech, not explained by phonological disorder or organic pathology.	1
Difficulty with multisyllabic words.	
Sound transpositions (i.e., metathetic errors).	
Perseveration across word boundaries.	
Apparent disfluency or choppiness, not consistent with stuttering or cluttering.	
Difficulty with volitional tongue or lip movements in the absence of difficulty with automatic tongue or lip movements. (Symptom may be indicative or oral apraxia, which is not the same as verbal apraxia but can co-occur with it.)	2
Difficulty with sequencing movements for volitional speech.	7

Discretionary Clinical Observation 13: Developmental Apraxia of Speech Observation (instructions in manual, Chapter 3)

Observations for Preverbal or Limited Language Children

Place a minus sign (–) in the column to the left for all that apply. Parental reports are a good source for some of this information.

	Child did not engage in canonical babble between the ages of 5 and 10 months.
	Child was an unusually quiet infant.
	Child is 18 months or older and prefers to communicate using gesture.
	Child is 18 months or older and single-word utterances that are frequently holophrastic or supported by gesture dominate.
	Child frequently supplements unintelligible speech with gestures and environmental sounds.
	Child makes unusual speech sound production errors (e.g., vowel distortions, consonant insertions, voicing confusions, metathetic errors, perseveration across word boundaries, nonspeech sounds).

Describe concerns.

Observations for Verbal Children

Place a check mark in the column to the left of each word if the child makes any of the following error types when saying the words and sentences below: manner-type substitutions, additions, prolongations, repetitions, nonphonemic productions, voicing and nasality errors, vowel and diphthong errors, difficulty with sequencing phonemes in syllables, inconsistent errors, articulatory groping, silent posturing, unusual prosodic patterns, dysfluency, or choppiness.

	Alligator.		Eucalyptus.		Macaroni.
	Buttercup.		Elephant.		Vegetable.
	Cucumber.		Hippopotamus.		Washing machine.

My hippopotamus' name is Buttercup.
An alligator eats macaroni and eucalyptus every day.

Describe concerns.

APPENDIX A

Decision Box for Submucous Cleft Screening: Discretionary Clinical Observation 15		
Place a minus sign (−) in the column to the left if noting any of the following indicators. Proceed to screening for submucous cleft (i.e., Discretionary Clinical Observation 15) if indicators are noted.		
	Symptom	Clinical Observation Noted
	Hypernasal resonance.	1
	Difficulty with pressure consonants (i.e., plosives, stops, affricates, fricatives; particularly voiceless).	
	History of otitis media with effusion or nasal reflux.	
	Posterior or superior leakage of air during labial seal activity.	2
	Palatal asymmetry.	5
	Dark or bluish shading at palatal midline (i.e., median palatal raphe).	
	Palatal translucency.	
	Bifid uvula.	
	Anterior or posterior placement of velar dimple.	
	Notch in posterior hard palate, implying absence of nasal spine.	
	Hypernasality or difficulty with pressure consonants during verbal diadochokinesis.	7
	Hypernasal resonance during sustained vowel.	8

Discretionary Clinical Observation 15: Submucous Cleft Screening (instructions in manual, Chapter 3)	
Screening for Submucous Cleft	
Place a minus sign (−) in the box to the left for all that apply.	
	Notch is noted instead of nasal spine.
	Any area palpated was noted to have decreased tactile resistance. Identify the area to which this applies:
	Palatal torus noted.
Describe concerns.	

Decision Box for Surplus Nasal Airflow Screening: Discretionary Clinical Observation 16	
Place a minus sign (–) in the column to the left if noting any of the following indicators. Proceed to surplus nasal airflow screening (i.e., Discretionary Clinical Observation 16) if indicators are present.	
Symptom	Clinical Observation Noted
Perception of any of the following during speech or vocalization event.	1
Hypernasal resonance.	
Audible nasal airflow.	
Short utterance length.	
Difficulty with obstruent consonants with or without hypernasality.	
Atypical voice.	
Compensatory articulation substitutions for obstruents (i.e., plosives, stops, affricates, fricatives; particularly voiceless):	
Glottal stops.	
Pharyngeal stops, fricatives, or affricates.	
Velar fricatives.	
Posterior nasal fricative (i.e., nasal snort).	
Anterior nasal fricative (i.e., facial grimace).	
Posterior or superior air leakage during labial seal activity.	2
Velar movement on /ɑ/ phonation is asymmetrical, weak, or absent.	6
Localized velar contractions on /ɑ/ phonation.	7
Hypernasal resonance during sustained vowel.	8

Discretionary Clinical Observation 16: Surplus Nasal Airflow Screening (instructions in manual, Chapter 3)
Screening for Surplus Nasal Airflow During Speech
Place a minus sign (–) in the column to the left if the following applies.
Mirror condensation noted for oral consonants during speech.
Describe concerns.

APPENDIX A

Decision Box for Gag Reflex Stimulation: Discretionary Clinical Observation 20, Amended for Infant or Toddler	
If any of the following indicators is noted, plan to stimulate gag reflex (i.e., Discretionary Clinical Observation 20). Instructions are found in Chapter 3.	
If gag reflex is stimulated, in most cases, it should be the last activity of the evaluation since it is somewhat invasive and may negatively affect compliance in some cases, particularly for younger examinees.	
Symptom	Clinical Observation Noted
Any craniofacial symptom leading to a genetic referral.	1
Suspected inadequate velar movement.	6
Any symptom suggesting a need for neurologic referral.	1–8

Discretionary Clinical Observation 20: Gag Reflex Stimulation (instructions in manual, Chapter 3)	
Gag Reflex Stimulation	
Place a minus sign (−) in the column to the left for any that apply.	
	Absent gag reflex: no response.
	Hypoactive gag reflex: weak response.
	Hyperactive gag reflex: forceful response.
	Premature gag reflex: response prior to touching the pharyngeal wall.
	Delayed or latent gag reflex: delay between stimulating pharyngeal wall and the reflexive response.
Describe concerns.	

Summarize the Findings and Make Recommendations

Summarize the Findings: Infant or Toddler		
Review the evidence collected. Note minus signs (–) and descriptions of concerns. Record evidence of structural or performance anomaly that has potential to negatively influence speech production or result in a need for clinical follow-up. Use additional space provided at bottom if needed.		
Anomaly Was Noted When Evaluating:	**Anomaly Observed**	**Comment on Performance**
Facial region.		
Respiration.		
Lip/tongue strength/mobility.		
Emerging dentition.		
Oral interior.		
Spontaneous velar movement.		
Amblyopia screening.		
Primitive reflexes.		
Nasal cavity clearance.		
Facial dimensions.		
Developmental Apraxia of Speech.		
Submucous cleft.		
Surplus Nasal Airflow.		
Gag reflex stimulation.		

	Recommendations for Individualized Plan of Care		
	Place a check mark in the column to the left for all that apply. Supply descriptive information as suggested.		
	Clinical Implications		
	Result of oral-facial inspection is unremarkable. No impact on speech production is suspected. No follow-up is needed.		
	Oral-facial inspection yields evidence that may support a particular diagnosis or plan of care. If so, specify evidence and suspected diagnosis:		
	Oral-facial inspection yields evidence that clearly supports a particular diagnosis or plan of care. If so, specify evidence and diagnosis:		
	Plan of Care		
	Next Step	**Rationale** Circle all that apply.	**Responsible Party** Circle all that apply
	Additional testing is needed.	• Part of oral-facial inspection that was not yet completed requires more time or clinical teaching to perform. • Testing that is beyond the scope of oral-facial inspection is identified as needed. • Other (specify).	• Examiner, follow-up. • Speech-language pathologist receiving case for therapy. • Specialist speech-language pathologist referral. • Health care provider outside speech-language pathology referral. • Other (specify).
	Recommend that therapy plan include objectives/procedures designed to address concerns identified through inspection.	Specify:	Specify:

Oral-Facial Evaluation for Speech-Language Pathologists
Barbara Ann Johnson-Root, PhD, CCC-SLP

Special Recording Form: Preschoolers (Age 4 to School Age)

Intake Information	
Client name:	Date of evaluation:
Date of birth:	Age:
Examiner:	Agency or facility:
Reason for evaluation:	
Relevant history:	
Comments:	

Prepare the Work Area for Testing, Adapted for Young Children (instructions in manual, Chapters 1 and 4)	
Checklist Place a check mark in the column to the left after completing each preparatory step in the list below.	
	Inventory equipment and supplies listed in Table 1–2 and described in Appendix B.
	Check batteries that power battery-operated equipment. Replace weak or dead batteries.
	Verify that all cords and strings were removed. If not, remove and dispose of them.
	Sanitize the work area and unwrapped equipment as instructed in Chapter 1.
	Wash hands thoroughly.
	Put on examination gloves, using procedures provided in Chapter 1.
	Arrange equipment in a small plastic box.

Instruct the Examinee (and Guardian if Appropriate)

Use your own words and developmentally appropriate language to communicate the following talking points before you begin.

- The oral-facial evaluation is a customary part of every speech-language evaluation.
- It involves inspecting all observable body parts necessary for speaking so that we may learn whether all parts are present, complete, and working properly.
- This is done to look into whether there is a physical explanation for the speech problem that brought you here or if there is any physical problem that we should address while helping you.
- None of the procedures are painful or harmful.
- For some people, oral-facial evaluation findings may lead to more detailed testing or possibly referral to another professional, although this is not the case for everyone.
- You may ask questions before we begin or at any time. Do you have any questions now? (If *yes*, either answer briefly or diplomatically table the question for a more appropriate time. If *no*, move on.)
- Are you ready? Let's get started!

Routine Clinical Observations

Routinely complete nine clinical observations for all children functioning at a preschool level:

- Routine Clinical Observation 1: Conversational Speech Sample (A), Facial Region Inspection (B), Breathing Observations (C)
- Routine Clinical Observation 2: Lip and Tongue Strength and Mobility
- Routine Clinical Observation 3: Dental Alignment and Bite for Young Children
- Routine Clinical Observation 4: Dental Occlusion
- Routine Clinical Observation 5: Oral Interior for Young Children
- Routine Clinical Observation 6: Velar Movement
- Routine Clinical Observation 7: Verbal Diadochokinesis for Young Children
- Routine Clinical Observation 8: Vowel Prolongation
- Discretionary Clinical Observation 22: Amblyopia Screening (routine for this population)

Routine Clinical Observation 1(A): Conversational Speech Sample
(instructions in manual, Chapter 2)

Rate intelligibility. Check the one that applies.

Place a check mark in the corresponding column to the left if intelligibility is judged as "good." For all intelligibility ratings that are less than "good," place a minus sign (−) in the corresponding column.

	Good: Completely or nearly completely intelligible.
	Slightly Compromised: Intelligible more than half the time.
	Fair: Intelligible about half of the time.
	Poor: Intelligible less than half of the time.
	Unintelligible: Completely unintelligible (or nearly so).

Comment on age appropriateness for speech intelligibility.

Area(s) Noted as Difficult During Conversational Speech

Use a minus sign (−) to mark areas identified as possibly deficient during conversational speech.

	Articulation/phonology.		Fluency.
	Language.		Resonance.
	Voice.		Motor-speech.

Describe speech difficulty.

APPENDIX A

		Routine Clinical Observations 1(B): Facial Region Inspection (instruction in manual, Chapter 2)
		Use a minus sign (−) to mark all features noted during facial region inspection. If multiple options appear on the same line, circle those that apply.
Resting	Speaking or Vocalizing	Feature
		Facial or oral asymmetry, drooping, tremor, fasciculation, spasm.
		Poor saliva management (as compared to others of similar age and development).
		Scarring.
		Thin upper lip, cleft lip.
		Micrognathia, macrognathia, retrognathic jaw, prognathic jaw.
		Hypoplastic midface, flat philtrum, epicanthal folds.
		Malformed ears, low-set ears.
		Eyelid ptosis, strabismus, wandering eye.
		Wide-set eyes.
		Forward tongue posture.
		Cranial asymmetry, prominent forehead, microcephaly, macrocephaly.
		Other dysmorphic features:
After completing above checklist, place minus sign (−) in column for any applicable condition.		
	Facial features suggest need for referral to genetics, neurology, or otorhinolaryngology if doctor-patient relationship has not yet been established.	
	Facial features appear to possibly contribute to atypical speaking pattern. Specify.	

Routine Clinical Observation 1(C): Breathing Observations, Adapted for Young Child (instructions in manual, Chapters 2 and 4)	
Identify the type of breathing noted upon observation. For all examinees, *nasal* and *diaphragmatic* breathing are optimal; upper thoracic breathing is acceptable. Place a check mark in the far-left column if any of the features on the left apply. For the features on the right, place a minus sign (–) in the corresponding column if any are noted.	
Type of Breathing	
Nasal.	Oral.
Diaphragmatic.	Upper thoracic, clavicular.
Lower thoracic.	Noisy, evidence of respiratory distress or struggle.
Describe concerns.	

APPENDIX A

	Routine Clinical Observation 2: Lip and Tongue Mobility and Strength (instruction in manual, Chapter 2)		

Place a check mark in the column to the left if the examinee performs the act smoothly, accurately, completely, and in a timely manner. Place a minus sign (−) in the column if noting any other response, and use the space below to provide additional descriptive data.

	Action		
	Pucker.		Quick repetitions of /b/ or /p/.
	Spread.		Smack the lips.
	Sustain exaggerated /u/.		

Describe atypical responses; comment on possible relationship to speech concern.

Lip Strength and Seal

Place a check mark in the box to the left if the act is judged to be within normal limits. Place a minus sign (−) in the column if noting any other response, and use the space below to provide additional descriptive data.

	Action		
	Seal.		Resistance.

Describe atypical responses; comment on possible relationship to speech concern.

Tongue Mobility

Place a check mark in the column to the left of each action if examinee performs the act smoothly, accurately, completely, and in a timely manner. Place a minus sign (−) in the column if noting any other response, and use the space below to provide additional descriptive data.

	Action		
	Protrusion.		Wiggle to the left and to the right.
	Elevation.		Rotation.
	Lateralization.		

Describe atypical responses; comment on possible relationship to speech concern.

Other Tongue Observations
Place a check mark in box to the left if feature is observed to be within normal limits. Place a minus sign (−) in the column if noting any other response, and use the space below to provide additional descriptive data.

Feature		
Shape of tongue tip.		Lingual frenum length.

Describe atypical features; comment on possible relationship to speech concern.

Tongue Strength
Place a check mark in the column on the left if the act is judged to be within normal limits. Place a minus sign (−) in the column if noting any other response, and use the space below to provide additional descriptive data.

Action
Resistance.

Describe atypical responses; comment on possible relationship to speech concern.

APPENDIX A

Routine Clinical Observation 3: Dental Bite and Alignment, Amended for Toddler or Preschooler (instructions in manual, Chapters 2 and 4)		

Dental Bite

For examinees with an unremarkable bite pattern, place a check mark in the column to the left corresponding to the word *normal*. If any other bite pattern is noted, place a minus sign (−) in the column that resides directly to the left of the term that best describes the person's bite. (Typically one applies; there are exceptions.)

	Bite				
	Normal.		Edge-to-edge bite.		Overjet.
	Open bite.		Under bite.		Flared bite.
	Closed bite.		Cross bite.		

Add descriptive information if needed; describe relationship (or potential relationship) to speech, if any.

Alignment and Condition of Teeth

Mark dental chart below to indicate dental alignment concerns noted.

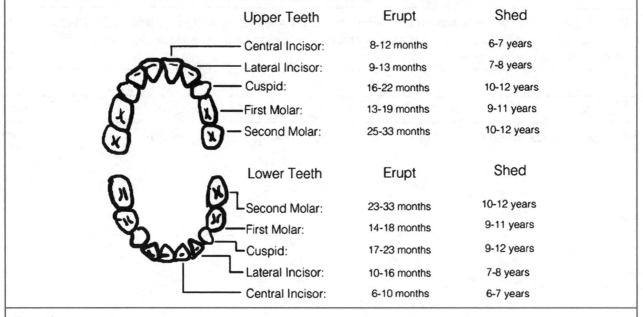

Upper Teeth	Erupt	Shed
Central Incisor:	8-12 months	6-7 years
Lateral Incisor:	9-13 months	7-8 years
Cuspid:	16-22 months	10-12 years
First Molar:	13-19 months	9-11 years
Second Molar:	25-33 months	10-12 years

Lower Teeth	Erupt	Shed
Second Molar:	23-33 months	10-12 years
First Molar:	14-18 months	9-11 years
Cuspid:	17-23 months	9-12 years
Lateral Incisor:	10-16 months	7-8 years
Central Incisor:	6-10 months	6-7 years

Describe concerns.

Routine Clinical Observation 4: Dental Occlusion (instruction in manual, Chapter 2)		
Dental Occlusion		
For examinees with neutroclusion, place a check mark in the column that resides directly to the left of that term. For examinees with distoclusion or mesioclusion, place a minus sign (–) in the column that corresponds to that classification.		
Dental Occlusion Classification		
Neutroclusion (typical).	Distoclusion.	Mesioclusion.
Describe occlusal relationship. Comment on any possible relationship to speech production.		

APPENDIX A

Routine Clinical Observation 5: Oral Interior, Amended for Toddler or Preschooler (instructions in manual, Chapters 2 and 4)			
Tongue Surface, Size, and Shape			
Place a check mark in the box on the left if the feature is judged to be within normal limits. Place a minus sign (−) in the column if noting any atypical trait. Write *N.O.* (not observed) in the column if unable to observe. Use the space below to provide additional descriptive data.			
Feature			
	Texture.		Shape.
	Size.		Other noteworthy feature:
Describe concern with the feature noted.			
Hard Palate			
Place a check mark in the box on the left if the feature is judged to be within normal limits. Place a minus sign (−) in the column if noting any atypical trait. Write *N.O.* (not observed) in the column if unable to observe. Use the space below to provide additional descriptive data.			
Feature			
	Alveolar ridge.		Posterior nasal spine.
	Palatal arch.		Foveae palate.
	Median raphe.		Scarring.
	Mucous membrane.		Coloring.
Describe concerns.			
Posterior Soft Tissue			
Place a check mark in the box on the left if the feature is judged to be within normal limits. Place a minus sign (−) in the column if noting any atypical trait. Write *N.O.* (not observed) in the column if unable to observe. Use the space below to provide additional descriptive data.			
Feature			
	Velum.		Palatine tonsils.
	Uvula.		Posterior pharyngeal wall.
	Faucial pillars.		
Describe concerns.			

Routine Clinical Observation 6: Velar Movement (instructions in manual, Chapter 2)	
Velar Movement	
Place a check mark beside "velum moves up and back symmetrically on /ɑ/ phonation" if that is the case. Place a minus sign (–) in the column corresponding to any other trait noted; use the space below to provide additional descriptive data.	
Velar response to /ɑ/ phonation	
	Velum moves up and back symmetrically on /ɑ/ phonation.
	Velum moves up and back asymmetrically on /ɑ/ phonation.
	Velum moves sluggishly on /ɑ/ phonation.
	Velum is not observed to move on /ɑ/ phonation.
	Misplaced velar dimple noted on /ɑ/ phonation.
Describe concerns. Comment on possible relationship to speech pattern.	

APPENDIX A

Routine Clinical Observation 7: Verbal Diadochokinesis, Amended for Preschooler (instructions in manual, Chapters 2 and 4)					
Speech-Alternating Motion: Rate					
Record syllables produced per second in the column that appears to the left of each syllable designation.					
Syllables/Second	Syllable	Syllables/Second	Syllable	Syllables/Second	Syllable
	/pə/		/tə/		/kə/
Speech-Alternating Motion: Perceptual Evaluation					
Place a minus sign (–) in the box on the left for all that apply.					
	Reduced range of motion for the articulators (i.e., jaw, tongue, lips).				
	Arrhythmic or unsteady performance.				
	Poor articulatory precision; specify consonant:				
	Rate, precision, or volume decreased over time; specify:				
Describe concerns. Comment on possible relevance to speech pattern.					

Speech-Sequential Motion: Rate	
Syllables/Second	Syllables
	/pə tə kə/
Speech-Sequential Motion: Subjective Evaluation	
Place a minus sign (–) in the column to the left for all that apply.	
	Difficulty rapidly sequencing the three distinctively different syllables in succession (i.e., syllable transpositions, perseveration across syllable boundaries).
	Decrease in rate, precision, or volume over time.
Describe concerns. Comment on possible relevance to speech pattern.	

Routine Clinical Observation 8: Vowel Prolongation (instructions in manual, Chapter 2)		
Vowel Prolongation: Duration		
Measure vowel duration according to instructions in the Chapter 2. Write results for each of three trials in the designated column. Circle the longest duration.		
	Trial 1	Trial 2	Trial 3
/ɑ/			
Vowel Prolongation: Subjective Evaluation		
Place a minus sign (–) in column to the left for all that apply.		
	Adult sustains /ɑ/ for fewer than 20 seconds, or child sustains /ɑ/ for fewer than 10 seconds.		
	Decrease in duration across three trials.		
	Voice quality or volume deteriorates.		
	Atypical resonance.		
	Atypical vocal quality or pitch.		
Describe concern. Comment on relevance to speech.		

APPENDIX A

Discretionary Clinical Observation 22: Amblyopia Screening (instructions in manual, Chapter 4)		
Amblyopia screening is considered a discretionary procedure since it is only administered to select examinees. For children younger than 6 years, however, it is considered a routine part of the inspection.		
Place a check mark in the "L" column that corresponds to "no change" for children who exhibit no negative response to covering the left eye, and place a check mark in the "R" column that corresponds to "no change" for children who exhibit no negative response to covering the right eye. Place a minus sign (–) in "L" or "R" column if the "child makes a determined attempt to see around the eye test paddle or exhibits signs of distress" when either eye was covered.		
L	**R**	**Response to Covering One Eye During Conversation or Visual Activity**
		No change.
		Child makes determined effort to see around the eye test paddle or exhibited signs of distress.
		Place a minus sign (–) in the column to the left if the child tries to peer around the paddle or shows signs of distress when either eye is covered. Refer to ophthalmologist.

If you believe there is a reason to omit one or more of the routine procedures, clearly mark your decision on the recording form. Then proceed with the inspection.

Identifying and Completing Appropriate Discretionary Clinical Observations

In most cases, the inspection ends with routine clinical observations. Yet once routine procedures are complete, the next step is to determine whether the evidence indicates a need for any discretionary clinical observations. For the sake of convenience, a series of decision boxes provides structure that can facilitate identifying discretionary clinical observations that should be considered.

Bear in mind that none of the decision boxes is intended to prompt a perfunctory decision that results in a discretionary procedure. Certainly, an understanding of the examinee's overall symptom pattern combined with a rich bank of clinical experience and intuition should also contribute, albeit such intangibles are highly individualized and therefore difficult to place on a form. Even so, strategically considering tangible client-centered evidence as it is arranged on the form can contribute to a good decision relative to proceeding with a discretionary clinical observation, and that is the intended purpose of the decision boxes.

Once a decision box is evaluated, if it flags the corresponding discretionary clinical observation, the inspection can proceed to that discretionary observation if the examining clinician deems it appropriate. Generally, no more than three discretionary observations are flagged for an individual. However, there are exceptions, especially when working with children who have multiple anomaly conditions.

Ten discretionary clinical observations are considered appropriate for this age group:

- Discretionary Clinical Observation 9: Nasal Cavity Clearance Screening
- Discretionary Clinical Observation 10: Facial Dimension Estimates
- Discretionary Clinical Observation 13: Developmental Apraxia of Speech Observations
- Discretionary Clinical Observation 15: Submucous Cleft Screening

- Discretionary Clinical Observation 16: Surplus Nasal Airflow Screening
- Discretionary Clinical Observation 17: Dysarthria Observations
- Discretionary Clinical Observation 18: Speech Sound Stimulability Screening
- Discretionary Clinical Observation 19: Laryngeal and Respiratory Efficiency Screening
- Discretionary Clinical Observation 20: Gag Reflex Stimulation
- Discretionary Clinical Observation 23: Screening for Selected Primitive Reflexes

Decision Box for Nasal Cavity Clearance Screening: Discretionary Clinical Observation 9	
Place a minus sign (–) in the column to the left if noting any of the following indicators. Proceed to nasal cavity clearance screening (i.e., Discretionary Clinical Observation 9) if indicators are noted.	
Symptom	Clinical Observation Noted
Hyponasal resonance detected during any speech or vocalization event.	
Nasal asymmetry.	1
Visible or audible symptoms of congestion[a] (including mouth breathing).	

[a]May table the procedure if the person exhibits symptoms of temporary obstruction such as a cold or allergy.

Discretionary Clinical Observation 9: Nasal Cavity Clearance Screening   (instructions in manual, Chapter 3)
Screening for Nasal Cavity Clearance
Place a minus sign (–) in column to left for all symptoms that apply.
Nasal asymmetry.
Nasal obstruction due to mucosal swelling, deviated septum, hypertrophied conchae, excess mucus.
Difficulty admitting or discharging air via the nasal passages.
Difficulty expelling air through either nare when the other is occluded.
Difficulty with prolonging /m/: /m→/.
Describe concerns. Comment on potential relevance to speech.

APPENDIX A

Decision Box for Facial Dimension Estimates: Discretionary Clinical Observation 10		
Place a minus sign (–) in left column if noting any of the following indicators. Proceed to facial dimension estimates (i.e., Discretionary Clinical Observation 10) if indicators are present.		
	Symptom	Clinical Observation Noted
	Facial profile appears disproportionate and the person is likely to be referred for follow-up (e.g., genetics or otorhinolaryngology).	1
	Malocclusion.	4
	Tongue tip does not line up with alveolar ridge.	5

Discretionary Clinical Observation 10: Facial Dimension Estimates
(instructions in manual, Chapter 3)

Facial Dimension Estimates

Place a minus sign (–) to left for all that apply. If a minus sign (–) is placed in the left column in the first three rows, measure distances in millimeters and record the measurements in the divided mm column on right. Then calculate percentage for each measurement and record it in the % column on far right. Any minus sign (–) on the left should be reported to the referral recipient.

			mm	%
	Overall Facial Dimension: Distances between (1) hairline and glabella, (2) glabella and subnasale, and (3) subnasale and pogonion are not segments of approximate equal length.	1		
		2		
		3		
	Dimensions for Lower Third of Face: Distances between (1) subnasale and stomian, (2) stomian and supramentale, and (3) supramentale and pogonion are not segments of approximate equal length.	1		
		2		
		3		
	Size and Spacing of Eyes: (1) Length of palpebral fissures and (2) distance between eyes are not segments of approximate equal length.	1		
		2		
	Facial Angle: Facial angle deviates grossly from 90° or misses subnasale plane completely.			
	Frankfurt Horizontal Plane: Tragion is lower than ipsilateral lid-cheek junction.			
Describe concerns.				

Decision Box for Developmental Apraxia of Speech Observations: Discretionary Clinical Observation 13	
Place a minus sign (−) in the column to the left if noting any of the following indicators in a child. Proceed to developmental apraxia of speech observations (i.e., Discretionary Clinical Observation 13) if indicators are present.	

	Symptom	Clinical Observation Noted
	History of speech production problems in the family, or history of speech therapy in family.	Case history intake
	Delayed speech development.	
	Did not engage in canonical babbling between the ages of 5 and 10 months.	
	Persisting unintelligible speech, not explained by phonological disorder or organic pathology.	1
	Difficulty with multisyllabic words.	
	Sound transpositions (i.e., metathetic errors).	
	Perseveration across word boundaries.	
	Apparent disfluency or choppiness, not consistent with stuttering or cluttering.	
	Difficulty with volitional tongue or lip movements in the absence of difficulty with automatic tongue or lip movements. (Symptom may be indicative or oral apraxia, which although is not the same as verbal apraxia, can co-occur with it.)	2
	Difficulty with sequencing movements for volitional speech.	7

APPENDIX A

Discretionary Clinical Observation 13: Developmental Apraxia of Speech Observation (instructions in manual, Chapter 3)	
Observations for Preverbal or Limited Language Children	
Place a minus sign (–) in the column to the left for all that apply. Parental reports are a good source for some of this information.	
	Child did not engage in canonical babble between the ages of 5 and 10 months.
	Child was an unusually quiet infant.
	Child is 18 months or older and prefers to communicate using gesture.
	Child is 18 months or older and single-word utterances that are frequently holophrastic or supported by gesture dominate.
	Child frequently supplements unintelligible speech with gestures and environmental sounds.
	Child makes unusual speech sound production errors (e.g., vowel distortions, consonant insertions, voicing confusions, metathetic errors, perseveration across word boundaries, nonspeech sounds).
Describe concerns.	

Observations for Verbal Children	
Place a check mark in the column to the left of each word if the child makes any of the following error types when saying the words and sentences below: manner-type substitutions, additions, prolongations, repetitions, nonphonemic productions, voicing and nasality errors, vowel and diphthong errors, difficulty with sequencing phonemes in syllables, inconsistent errors, articulatory groping, silent posturing, unusual prosodic patterns, dysfluency, or choppiness.	

	Alligator.		Eucalyptus.		Macaroni.
	Buttercup.		Elephant.		Vegetable.
	Cucumber.		Hippopotamus.		Washing machine.

	My hippopotamus' name is Buttercup.
	An alligator eats macaroni and eucalyptus every day.
Describe concerns.	

	Decision Box for Submucous Cleft Screening: Discretionary Clinical Observation 15	
	Place a minus sign (–) in the column to the left if noting any of the following indicators. Proceed to screening for submucous cleft (i.e., Discretionary Clinical Observation 15) if indicators are noted.	
	Symptom	Clinical Observation Noted
	Hypernasal resonance.	1
	Difficulty with pressure consonants (i.e., plosives, stops, affricates, fricatives; particularly voiceless).	
	History of otitis media with effusion or nasal reflux.	
	Posterior or superior leakage of air during labial seal activity.	2
	Palatal asymmetry.	5
	Dark or bluish shading at palatal midline (i.e., median palatal raphe).	
	Palatal translucency.	
	Bifid uvula.	
	Anterior or posterior placement of velar dimple.	
	Notch in posterior hard palate, implying absence of nasal spine.	
	Hypernasality or difficulty with pressure consonants during verbal diadochokinesis.	7
	Hypernasal resonance during sustained vowel.	8

Discretionary Clinical Observation 15: Submucous Cleft Screening (instructions in manual, Chapter 3)	
	Screening for Submucous Cleft
	Place a minus sign (–) in the box to the left for all that apply.
	Notch is noted instead of nasal spine.
	Any area palpated was noted to have decreased tactile resistance. Identify the area to which this applies:
	Palatal torus noted.
	Describe concerns.

APPENDIX A

Decision Box for Surplus Nasal Airflow Screening: Discretionary Clinical Observation 16	
Place a minus sign (–) in the column to the left if noting any of the following indicators. Proceed to surplus nasal airflow screening (i.e., Discretionary Clinical Observation 16) if indicators are present.	

	Symptom	Clinical Observation Noted
	Perception of any of the following during speech or vocalization event.	1
	Hypernasal resonance.	
	Audible nasal airflow.	
	Short utterance length.	
	Difficulty with obstruent consonants with or without hypernasality.	
	Atypical voice.	
	Compensatory articulation substitutions for obstruents (i.e., plosives, stops, affricates, fricatives; particularly voiceless):	
	Glottal stops.	
	Pharyngeal stops, fricatives, or affricates.	
	Velar fricatives.	
	Posterior nasal fricative (i.e., nasal snort).	
	Anterior nasal fricative (i.e., facial grimace).	
	Posterior or superior air leakage during labial seal activity.	2
	Velar movement on /ɑ/ phonation is asymmetrical, weak, or absent.	6
	Localized velar contractions on /ɑ/ phonation.	7
	Hypernasal resonance during sustained vowel.	8

Discretionary Clinical Observation 16: Surplus Nasal Airflow Screening (instructions in manual, Chapter 3)	
Screening for Surplus Nasal Airflow During Speech.	
Place a minus sign (–) in the column to the left if the following applies.	
	Mirror condensation noted for oral consonants during speech.
Describe concerns.	

Decision Box for Dysarthria Observation: Discretionary Clinical Observation 17	
Place a minus sign (–) in the column to the left if noting any of the following indicators. Proceed to dysarthria observations (i.e., Discretionary Clinical Observation 17) if indicators are noted.	
Symptom	Clinical Observation Noted
Imprecise consonants or slurred speech.	1
Hypernasality.	
Mixed resonance.	
Jaw hangs in open position when at rest, mandible deviates to the right or left at rest or in motion.	
Oral asymmetry at rest or in motion, fasciculations in perioral area.	
Atypical voice (e.g., breathy, harsh, strained-strangled).	
Labial asymmetry at rest or in motion, unilateral or bilateral labial seal weakness.	2
Tongue: Extraneous movements at rest or in motion, deviation at rest or in motion, weakness, imprecise movements, reduced range of motion, fatigue.	
Mandible: Deviates to right or left when lowered, weak resistance, extraneous movements at rest or in motion.	5
Tongue: Asymmetry, deviations, signs of atrophy, fasciculations, extraneous movements at rest or in motion.	
Velum: Asymmetry at rest or in motion, rhythmic or arrhythmic movements at rest or in motion, unilateral or bilateral weakness.	
Weak, absent, or asymmetrical velar movement on /ɑ/ phonation.	6
Motion activities: Imprecise consonants, reduced range of motion for articulators, decreasing rate or precision, slow rate, evidence of fatigue.	7
Evidence of hypernasality or fatigue on /ɑ/ phonation.	8

APPENDIX A

	Discretionary Clinical Observation 17: Dysarthria Observation, Amended for Preschooler (instructions in manual, Chapters 3 and 4)	
	Dysarthria Observation	
	Place a minus sign (–) in the column to the left for all symptoms noted during spontaneous speech.	
	Symptoms	
	Imprecise articulation.	Articulation
	Intermittent, sudden, or unpredictable articulation breakdown.	
	Difficulty initiating articulation.	
	Unpredictable vowel distortions.	
	Hypernasal resonance with nasal airflow emissions.	Resonance
	Hypernasal resonance without nasal airflow emissions.	
	Mixed resonance.	
	Low pitch.	Voice
	Irregular pitch.	
	Sudden elevation of pitch.	
	Reduced variation in pitch and loudness.	
	Sudden bursts of loudness, irregular loudness.	
	Increased loudness overall.	
	Reduced loudness or inaudible voice.	
	Harsh, hoarse, or strained-strangled quality.	
	Breathy quality.	
	Unpredictable interruptions in speech flow (e.g., variations in pitch and loudness).	Prosody
	Monotone.	
	Slow rate.	
	Short distorted phrases.	
	Dysrhythmia.	
	Sound prolongations.	
	Equal syllable stress.	
	Prolonged intervals between syllables and words.	

	Seemingly measured pace.	Prosody
	Reduced vocal emphasis.	
	Pitch peaks and valleys.	
	Loudness variability that flattens to a monotone.	
	Short rushes of speech with illogically placed pauses.	
	Variable or accelerated rate.	
	Inappropriate silences.	
	Repetitions of initial sounds.	
	Audible inspiration.	Respiration
	Breathy exhalation.	
	Sudden gusts of exhaled air.	
	Altered breathing cycle.	
	Much effort required for speech.	Overall
	Muscular weakness.	
	Extraneous movements.	
	Imprecise movements.	

Describe concerns.

APPENDIX A

Decision Box for Speech Sound Stimulability Screening: Discretionary Clinical Observation 18		
Place a minus sign (–) in the column to the left if noting any of the following indicators. Proceed to speech sound stimulability screening (i.e., Discretionary Clinical Observation 18) if indicators are present.		
	Symptom	Clinical Observation Noted
	Speech sound errors are not fully attributable to organic anomaly; stimulability testing was not completed earlier.	Any routine clinical observation.

Discretionary Clinical Observation 18: Speech Sound Stimulability Screening (instructions in manual, Chapter 3)							
Speech Sound Stimulability Screening							
List selected speech sound stimulability targets in the columns marked "target 1," "target 2," "target 3," and "target 4." In the column to the left of each target, write "HS" for highly stimulable targets, "S" for stimulable targets, and "NS" for not-stimulable targets.							
	Target 1		Target 2		Target 3		Target 4
Describe concerns.							

Decision Box for Respiratory and Laryngeal Efficiency Screening: Discretionary Clinical Observation 19	
Place a minus sign (–) in the column to the left if noting any of the following indicators. Proceed to respiratory and laryngeal efficiency screening (i.e., Discretionary Clinical Observation 19) if indicators are present.	

	Symptom	Clinical Observation Noted
	Evidence of respiratory inefficiency or distress during any speech or nonspeech activity.	1, 7, 8
	Voice quality that indicates possible inefficient use of the larynx (e.g., breathiness, harshness, hoarseness, or strained quality).	
	Failure to sustain the vowel /ɑ/ for at least 20 seconds for adults and 10 seconds for children.	8

Discretionary Clinical Observation 19: Screening for Laryngeal and Respiratory Efficiency (instructions in manual, Chapter 3)
Screening for Laryngeal and Respiratory Efficiency (i.e., S:Z ratio)
Place a minus sign (–) in column to the left for any symptom noted.

	For child examinee, measured duration was less than 10 seconds.
	Audible symptoms of vocal pathology.
	Duration decreased with consecutive trials.
	S:Z ratio was calculated as 1.2 or greater.

Describe concerns.

APPENDIX A

	Decision Box for Gag Reflex Stimulation: Discretionary Clinical Observation 20	
	Place a minus sign (−) in the column to the left if noting any of the following indicators. Proceed to gag reflex stimulation (i.e., Discretionary Clinical Observation 20) if indicators are present.	
	Note: If gag reflex is stimulated, in most cases it should be the last activity of the evaluation since it is somewhat invasive and may negatively affect compliance in some cases, particularly for younger examinees.	
	Symptom	Clinical Observation Noted
	Hypernasal resonance during speech.	1
	Difficulty with obstruent sounds.	
	Any symptoms suggesting possible neurologic involvement.	
	Any craniofacial symptom leading to a genetic referral.	
	Possible inadequate velar movement.	6
	Any symptom leading to observations for motor-speech disorder (e.g., developmental apraxia of speech, acquired apraxia of speech, dysarthria).	7
	Hypernasal resonance during sustained vowel.	8
	Any symptom suggesting a need for neurologic referral.	1–8

	Discretionary Clinical Observation 20: Gag Reflex Stimulation (instructions in manual, Chapter 3)	
	Gag Reflex Stimulation	
	Place a minus sign (−) in the column to the left for any that apply.	
	Absent gag reflex: no response.	
	Hypoactive gag reflex: weak response.	
	Hyperactive gag reflex: forceful response.	
	Premature gag reflex: response prior to touching the pharyngeal wall.	
	Delayed or latent gag reflex: delay between stimulating pharyngeal wall and the reflexive response.	
	Describe concerns.	

	Decision Box for Screening Selected Primitive Reflexes: Discretionary Clinical Observation 23

Primitive reflex stimulation may be relevant for some children older than 36 months, particularly if residual reflexes are suspected to interfere with speech production, motor-development progress, or may support a referral to evaluate for cerebral palsy. However, primitive reflex screening is not needed for most children in this age group.

Place a minus sign (–) in the column to the left if any symptom listed below applies. Proceed with screening for selected primitive reflexes (i.e., Discretionary Clinical Observation 23) if indicators are noted.

	Symptom	Clinical Observation Noted
	Any evidence of injury to the immature neurologic system (e.g., weakness, discoordination, asymmetry).	Any

Discretionary Clinical Observation 23: Screening for Selected Primitive Reflexes (instructions in manual, Chapter 4)

Place a check mark in the column to the left for reflexes that are found to be present within the appropriate age boundaries. Place a minus sign (–) in the column to the left for reflexes that are found to be absent during the developmental period identified as appropriate for the reflex to occur. Place an arrow (→) in the column to the left for reflexes that persist beyond the age of normal suppression for that reflex.

	Reflex	Age Boundaries for Response
	Rooting.	Present at birth; inhibited between ages of 6 and 12 months.
	Sucking.	Present at birth; inhibited between ages of 2 and 3 months.
	Palmar grasp.	Present at birth; normal up to 6 months.
	Tongue-thrust reflex (not to be confused with tongue-thrust swallow).	Present at birth; normal up to 6 months.
	Babinski.	Always abnormal.

Comments.

APPENDIX A

Summarize Findings and Make Recommendations

Summarize the Findings: Preschooler		
Review the evidence collected. Note minus signs (–) and descriptions of concerns. Record evidence of structural or performance anomaly that has potential to negatively influence speech production or result in a need for clinical follow-up. Use additional space provided at bottom if needed.		
Anomaly Was Noted When Evaluating:	**Anomaly Observed**	**Comment on Performance**
Facial region.		
Respiration.		
Lip/tongue strength/mobility.		
Dental alignment or bite.		
Dental occlusion.		
Oral interior.		
Velar movement.		
Verbal diadochokinesis.		
Vowel prolongation.		
Amblyopia screening.		
Nasal cavity clearance.		
Facial dimensions.		
Childhood apraxia of speech.		
Submucous cleft.		
Surplus nasal airflow.		
Dysarthria.		
Speech sound stimulability.		
Laryngeal/respiratory efficiency.		
Gag reflex stimulation.		
Screening for primitive reflexes.		

Recommendations for Individualized Plan of Care		
Place a check mark in the column to the left for all that apply. Supply descriptive information as suggested.		
Clinical Implications		
	Result of oral-facial inspection is unremarkable. No impact on speech production is suspected. No follow-up is needed.	
	Oral-facial inspection yields evidence that may support a particular diagnosis or plan of care. If so, specify evidence and suspected diagnosis:	
	Oral-facial inspection yields evidence that clearly supports a particular diagnosis or plan of care. If so, specify evidence and diagnosis:	
Plan of Care		
Next Step	**Rationale** Circle all that apply.	**Responsible Party** Circle all that apply
Additional testing is needed.	• Part of oral-facial inspection that was not yet completed requires more time or clinical teaching to perform. • Testing that is beyond the scope of oral-facial inspection is identified as needed. • Other (specify).	• Examiner, follow-up. • Speech-language pathologist receiving case for therapy. • Specialist speech-language pathologist referral. • Health care provider outside speech-language pathology referral. • Other (specify).
Recommend that therapy plan include objectives/procedures designed to address concerns identified through inspection.	Specify:	Specify:

APPENDIX A

Oral-Facial Evaluation for Speech-Language Pathologists
Barbara Ann Johnson-Root, PhD, CCC-SLP

Special Recording Form: Adults With History of Neurologic Episode

Intake Information	
Client name:	Date of evaluation:
Date of birth:	Age:
Examiner:	Agency or facility:
Reason for evaluation:	
Relevant history:	
Comments:	

Prepare the Work Area for Testing (instructions in manual, Chapter 1)
Checklist
Place a check mark in the column to the left after completing each preparatory step in the list below.
Inventory equipment and supplies listed Table 1–2 and described in Appendix B.
Check batteries that power battery-operated equipment. Replace weak or dead batteries.
Verify that all cords and strings were removed from equipment. If not, remove and dispose of them.
Sanitize the work area, and unwrap equipment as instructed in Chapter 1.
Wash hands thoroughly.
Put on examination gloves, using procedures provided in Chapter 1.
Arrange equipment as shown in Figure 1–1.

Instruct the Examinee (and Significant Other if Appropriate)

Use your own words and developmentally appropriate language to communicate the following talking points before you begin.

- The oral-facial evaluation is a customary part of every speech-language evaluation.
- It involves inspecting all observable body parts necessary for speaking so that we may ascertain whether all parts are present, complete, and working properly.
- This is done to look into whether there is a physical explanation for the speech problem that brought you here or if there is any physical problem that we should address to help you.
- None of the procedures are painful or harmful.
- A few items situated on the table may not be needed.
- For some people, oral-facial evaluation findings may lead to more detailed testing or possibly referral to another professional, although this is not the case for everyone.
- You may ask questions before we begin or at any time. Do you have any questions now?
  (If *yes*, either answer briefly or diplomatically table the question for a more appropriate time. If *no*, move on.)
- Are you ready? Let's get started!

Routine Clinical Observations

Routinely complete the 10 clinical observations listed for all examinees in this group:

- Routine Clinical Observation 1: Conversational Speech Sample (A), Facial Features (B), and Breathing Observations (C)
- Routine Clinical Observation 2: Lip and Tongue Strength and Mobility
- Routine Clinical Observation 3: Dental Alignment and Bite for Older Adults
- Routine Clinical Observation 4: Dental Occlusion
- Routine Clinical Observation 5: Oral Interior
- Routine Clinical Observation 6: Velar Movement
- Routine Clinical Observation 7: Verbal Diadochokinesis
- Routine Clinical Observation 8: Vowel Prolongation
- Discretionary Clinical Observation 20: Gag Reflex Stimulation (routine for this population)
- Discretionary Clinical Observation 21: Prompt for Dysphagia Screening (routine for this population, unless already scheduled for the screening)

Routine Clinical Observation 1(A): Conversational Speech Sample (instructions in manual, Chapter 2)	
Rate intelligibility. Check the one that applies.	
Place a check mark in the corresponding column to the left if intelligibility is judged as "good." For all intelligibility ratings that are less than "good," place a minus sign (–) in the corresponding column.	
	Good: Completely or nearly completely intelligible.
	Slightly Compromised: Intelligible more than half the time.
	Fair: Intelligible about half of the time.
	Poor: Intelligible less than half of the time.
	Unintelligible: Completely unintelligible (or nearly so).
Comment on age appropriateness for speech intelligibility.	
Area(s) Noted as Difficult During Conversational Speech	
Use a minus sign (–) to mark areas identified as possibly deficient during conversational speech.	

	Articulation/phonology.		Fluency.
	Language.		Resonance.
	Voice.		Motor-speech.

Describe speech difficulty.

		Routine Clinical Observations 1(B): Facial Region Inspection, Amended for Older Adult Examinees (instructions in manual, Chapters 2 and 4)
	Use a minus sign (−) to mark all features noted during facial region inspection. If multiple options appear on the same line, circle any that apply.
Resting	Speaking	Feature
		Facial or oral asymmetry, drooping.
		Tremor.
		Fasciculation, spasm.
		Poor saliva management.
		Scarring.
		Dysmorphic features:
	After completing checklist, place a minus sign (−) in column for any applicable condition.
		Facial features suggest neuromuscular involvement. Specify.
		Facial features appear to possibly contribute to atypical speaking pattern. Specify.

APPENDIX A

Routine Clinical Observation 1(C): Breathing Observations (instructions in manual, Chapter 2)		
Does the examinee's daily life require vocal projection? If yes, place a check mark in the box and circle the role that demands vocal projection. If the examinee has vocal projection needs not included in the list, write that information in the space provided.		
Teacher, singer, actor, attorney, clergy, public speaker.		
Identify the type of breathing noted. For all examinees, *nasal* and *diaphragmatic* breathing are optimal. *Lower thoracic* breathing is acceptable for examinees whose life does not require vocal projection. For the list on the left, place a check mark in the far-left column for all that apply. If any pattern described in the column on the right is observed, place a minus sign (−) to its left, since this is an atypical pattern. Also, where multiple options occupy the same line, circle those that apply.		
Type of Breathing		
	Nasal.		Oral.
	Diaphragmatic.		Upper thoracic, clavicular.
	Lower thoracic.		Noisy, evidence of respiratory distress or struggle.
Describe.		

Routine Clinical Observation 2: Lip and Tongue Mobility and Strength (instruction in manual, Chapter 2)			
Place a check mark in the column to the left if the examinee performs the act smoothly, accurately, completely, and in a timely manner. Place a minus sign (−) in the column if noting any other response, and use the space below to provide additional descriptive data.			
Action			
	Pucker.		Quick repetitions of /b/ or /p/.
	Spread.		Smack the lips.
	Sustain exaggerated /u/.		
Describe atypical responses; comment on possible relationship to speech concern.			

Lip Strength and Seal			
Place a check mark in the box to the left if the act is judged to be within normal limits. Place a minus sign (−) in the column if noting any other response, and use the space below to provide additional descriptive data.			
Action			
	Seal.		Resistance.
Describe atypical responses; comment on possible relationship to speech concern.			

Tongue Mobility			
Place a check mark in the column to the left of each action if examinee performs the act smoothly, accurately, completely, and in a timely manner. Place a minus sign (−) in the column if noting any other response, and use the space below to provide additional descriptive data.			
Action			
	Protrusion.		Wiggle to the left and to the right.
	Elevation.		Rotation.
	Lateralization.		

continues

APPENDIX A

Routine Clinical Observation 2: Lip and Tongue Mobility and Strength *continued*

Describe atypical responses; comment on possible relationship to speech concern.

Other Tongue Observations
Place a check mark in box to the left if feature is observed to be within normal limits. Place a minus sign (−) in the column if noting any other response, and use the space below to provide additional descriptive data.

Feature		
	Shape of tongue tip.	Lingual frenum length.

Describe atypical features; comment on possible relationship to speech concern.

Tongue Strength
Place a check mark in the column on the left if the act is judged to be within normal limits. Place a minus sign (−) in the column if noting any other response, and use the space below to provide additional descriptive data.

Action
Resistance.

Describe atypical responses; comment on possible relationship to speech concern.

Routine Clinical Observation 3: Dental Bite and Alignment, Amended for Older Adults (instructions in manual, Chapters 2 and 4)

Place a minus sign (–) in the column to the left for all that apply.

	The examinee is edentulous.
	The examinee is wearing dentures or other dental appliance.
	The dental appliance is reportedly uncomfortable.
	The examinee exhibits misarticulations that may be attributed to poorly fitted dental appliance.

Dental Bite

For examinees with unremarkable bite pattern, place a check mark in the column to the left corresponding to the word *normal*. If any other bite pattern is noted, place a minus sign (–) in the column that resides directly to the left of the term that best describes the person's bite. (Typically one applies; there are exceptions.)

Dental Bite for Examinees With Natural Teeth					
	Normal.		Edge-to-edge bite.		Overjet.
	Open bite.		Underbite.		Flared bite.
	Closed bite.		Cross bite.		

Add descriptive information if needed; describe relationship to speech, if any.

continues

APPENDIX A

Routine Clinical Observation 3: Dental Bite and Alignment, Amended for Older Adults *continued*

Alignment and Condition of Teeth for Examinees With Natural Teeth
Mark the dental chart below to indicate dental alignment concerns noted.

Upper Teeth

Central Incisor: 7-8 Years
Lateral Incisor: 8-9 Years
Cuspid: 11-12 Years
First Premolar (First Bicuspid): 10-11 Years
Second Premolar (Second Bisucpid): 11-12 Years
First Molar: 6-7 Years
Second Molar: 12-13 Years
Third Molar (Wisdom Tooth): 17-21 Years

Lower Teeth

Third Molar (Wisdom Tooth): 17-21 Years
Second Molar: 11-13 Years
First Molar: 6-7 Years
Second Premolar (Second Bicuspid): 11-12 Years
First Premolar (First Bicuspid): 10-12 Years
Cuspid: 9-10 Years
Lateral Incisor: 7-8 Years
Central Incisor: 6-7 Years

Describe dental misalignment concerns, and comment on their possible effect on speech production, if any.

Routine Clinical Observation 4: Dental Occlusion (instruction in manual, Chapter 2)					
Dental Occlusion					
For examinees with neutroclusion, place a check mark in the column that resides directly to the left of that term. For examinees with distoclusion or mesioclusion, place a minus sign (–) in the column that corresponds to that classification.					
Dental Occlusion Classification					
	Neutroclusion (typical).		Distoclusion.		Mesioclusion.
Describe occlusal relationship. Comment on any possible relationship to speech production.					

APPENDIX A

Routine Clinical Observation 5: Oral Interior (instructions in manual, Chapter 2)		
Response to Request to Open the Mouth: **Freedom of Mandibular Movement and Response to Resistance**		
Place a minus sign (–) in the column to the left, corresponding to any statements that apply.		
Activity		
	Difficulty with opening the mouth adequately for observing oral interior.	
	Pain or other sensation reported when opening the mouth for oral inspection.	
	Mandible deviates to left or right when lowered.	
	Extraneous mandibular movements at rest or in motion.	
	Not successful in resisting examiner's attempt to prevent mandibular movement.	
Place a minus sign (–) in the column to the left of any statements that describe examinee's condition.		
	Symptoms suggest *possible* temporomandibular joint disorder.	
	Symptoms suggest evidence of muscle weakness, asymmetry, discoordination, or difficulty with motor planning.	
Describe additional concerns.		
Tongue Surface, Size, and Shape		
Place a check mark in the column to the left if the feature is judged to be within normal limits. Place a minus sign (–) in the column if noting any atypical trait, and use the space below to provide additional descriptive data.		
Feature		
	Texture.	Shape.
	Size.	Other noteworthy feature:
Describe concern with the feature noted particularly as it may or may not relate to speech production.		

Hard Palate		
Place a check mark in the column to the left if the feature is judged to be within normal limits. Place a minus sign (−) in the column if noting any atypical trait, and use the space below to provide additional descriptive data.		
Feature		
	Alveolar ridge.	Posterior nasal spine.
	Palatal arch.	Foveae palate.
	Median raphe.	Scarring.
	Mucous membrane.	Coloring.
Describe concerns; comment on possible relationship to speech pattern.		

Posterior Soft Tissue		
Place a check mark in the column to the left if the feature is judged to be within normal limits. Place a minus sign (−) in the column if noting any atypical trait, and use the space below to provide additional descriptive data.		
Feature		
	Velum.	Palatine tonsils.
	Uvula.	Posterior pharyngeal wall.
	Faucial pillars.	
Describe concern. Comment on possible relationship to speech problem.		

APPENDIX A

Routine Clinical Observation 6: Velar Movement (instructions in manual, Chapter 2)
Velar Movement
Place a check mark beside "velum moves up and back symmetrically on /ɑ/ phonation" if that is the case. Place a minus sign (−) in the column corresponding to any other trait noted; use the space below to provide additional descriptive data.

	Velar response to /ɑ/ phonation
	Velum moves up and back symmetrically on /ɑ/ phonation.
	Velum moves up and back asymmetrically on /ɑ/ phonation.
	Velum moves sluggishly on /ɑ/ phonation.
	Velum is not observed to move on /ɑ/ phonation.
	Misplaced velar dimple noted on /ɑ/ phonation.

Describe concerns. Comment on possible relationship to speech pattern.

Routine Clinical Observation 7: Verbal Diadochokinesis (instructions in manual, Chapter 2)					
Speech-Alternating Motion: Rate					
Record syllables produced per second in the column that appears to the left of each syllable designation.					
Syllables/Second	Syllable	Syllables/Second	Syllable	Syllables/Second	Syllable
	/pə/		/tə/		/kə/

Speech-Alternating Motion: Perceptual Evaluation

Place a minus sign (–) in the box on the left for all that apply.

	Fewer than five syllables/second; specify consonant:
	Reduced range of motion for the articulators (i.e., jaw, tongue, lips).
	Arrhythmic or unsteady performance.
	Poor articulatory precision; specify consonant:
	Rate, precision, or volume decreased over time; specify:

Describe concerns. Comment on possible relevance to speech pattern.

Speech-Sequential Motion: Rate

Syllables/Second	Syllables
	/pə tə kə/

Speech-Sequential Motion: Subjective Evaluation

Place a minus sign (–) in the column to the left for all that apply.

	Fewer than five syllables/second.
	Difficulty rapidly sequencing the three distinctively different syllables in succession (i.e., syllable transpositions, perseveration across syllable boundaries).
	Decrease in rate, precision, or volume over time.

Describe concerns. Comment on possible relevance to speech pattern.

APPENDIX A

Routine Clinical Observation 8: Vowel Prolongation (instructions in manual, Chapter 2)		
Vowel Prolongation: Duration		
Measure vowel duration according to instructions in Chapter 2. Write results for each of three trials in the designated column. Circle the longest duration.		

	Trial 1	Trial 2	Trial 3
/ɑ/			

Vowel Prolongation: Subjective Evaluation	
Place a minus sign (–) in column to the left for all that apply.	
	Adult sustains /ɑ/ for fewer than 20 seconds, or child sustains /ɑ/ for fewer than 10 seconds.
	Decrease in duration across three trials.
	Voice quality or volume deteriorates.
	Atypical resonance.
	Atypical vocal quality or pitch.
Describe concern. Comment on relevance to speech.	

Discretionary Clinical Observation 20: Gag Reflex Stimulation (instructions in manual, Chapter 3)	
Gag Reflex Stimulation	
Place a minus sign (–) in the column to the left for any that apply.	
	Absent gag reflex: no response.
	Hypoactive gag reflex: weak response.
	Hyperactive gag reflex: forceful response.
	Premature gag reflex: response prior to touching the pharyngeal wall.
	Delayed or latent gag reflex: delay between stimulating pharyngeal wall and the reflexive response.
Describe concerns.	

Discretionary Clinical Observation 21: Dysphagia Screening Prompt
(instructions in manual, Chapter 3)

Dysphagia Screening Prompt

Place a minus sign (−) in the column to the left if any of the following apply. Proceed to dysphagia screening if two or more symptoms are noted or if the person has a history of recent neurologic incident. If in doubt, refer to screening.

	Recent history or cerebrovascular accident, neurologic incident or disease, or laryngectomy (required dysphagia screening).
	Cough after swallow.
	Voice change after swallow.
	Reduced lingual range of motion (Routine Clinical Observation 2) or incomplete facial symmetry (Routine Clinical Observation 1).
	Patient is flagged to be observed for any motor-speech disorders procedure (Discretionary Clinical Observations 15, 16, and 17).
	Abnormal volitional cough.
	Abnormal gag reflex.

Describe concerns.

If you believe there is a reason to omit one or more of the routine procedures, clearly mark your decision on the recording form. Then proceed with the inspection.

Identifying and Completing Appropriate Discretionary Clinical Observations

In most cases, the inspection ends with routine clinical observations. Yet once routine procedures are complete, the next step is to determine whether the evidence indicates a need for any discretionary clinical procedures. For the sake of convenience, a series of decision boxes provides structure that can facilitate identifying discretionary clinical observations that should be considered.

Bear in mind that none of the decision boxes is intended to prompt a perfunctory decision that results in a discretionary procedure. Certainly, an understanding of the examinee's overall symptom pattern combined with a rich bank of clinical experience and intuition should also contribute, albeit such intangibles are highly individualized and therefore difficult to place on a form. Even so, strategically considering tangible client-centered evidence as it is arranged on the form can contribute to a good decision relative to proceeding with a discretionary clinical observation, and that is the intended purpose of the decision boxes.

Once a decision box is evaluated, if it flags the corresponding discretionary clinical observation, the inspection can proceed to that discretionary observation if the examining clinician deems appropriate. Generally, no more than three discretionary observations are flagged or a single person. However, there are exceptions.

Six observations are considered discretionary for this group:

- Discretionary Clinical Observation 9: Nasal Cavity Clearance Screening
- Discretionary Clinical Observation 11: Temporomandibular Joint Disorder Screening
- Discretionary Clinical Observation 14: Acquired Apraxia of Speech
- Discretionary Clinical Observation 16: Surplus Nasal Airflow Screening
- Discretionary Clinical Observation 17: Observations for Dysarthria
- Discretionary Clinical Observation 19: Laryngeal and Respiratory Efficiency Screening

Decision Box for Nasal Cavity Clearance Screening: Discretionary Clinical Observation 9		
Place a minus sign (−) in the column to the left if noting any of the following indicators. Proceed to nasal cavity clearance screening (i.e., Discretionary Clinical Observation 9) if indicators are noted.		
	Symptom	Clinical Observation Noted
	Hyponasal resonance detected during any speech or vocalization event.	
	Nasal asymmetry.	1
	Visible or audible symptoms of congestion[a] (including mouth breathing).	

[a] May table the procedure if the person exhibits symptoms of temporary obstruction such as a cold or allergy.

Discretionary Clinical Observation 9: Nasal Cavity Clearance Screening (instructions in manual, Chapter 3)
Screening for Nasal Cavity Clearance
Place a minus sign (–) in column to left for all symptoms that apply.

	Nasal asymmetry.
	Nasal obstruction due to mucosal swelling, deviated septum, hypertrophied conchae, excess mucous.
	Difficulty admitting or discharging air via the nasal passages.
	Difficulty expelling air through either nare when the other is occluded.
	Difficulty with prolonging /m/: /m→/.

Describe concerns. Comment on potential relevance to speech.

Decision Box for Temporomandibular Joint Disorder Screening: Discretionary Clinical Observation 11	
Place a minus sign (–) in the column to the left if noting any of the following indicators. Proceed to screening for temporomandibular joint disorder (i.e., Discretionary Clinical Observation 11) if indicators are present.	

	Symptom	Clinical Observation Noted
	Limited mandibular excursion during speech activities.	1
	Limited mandibular excursion during nonspeech activities.	5
	Reported sensation of localized or referred pain when moving the jaw.	

	Discretionary Clinical Observation 11: Temporomandibular Joint Disorder Screening (instructions in manual, Chapter 3)
	Screening for Temporomandibular Joint Disorder
	Place a minus sign (–) in the box to the left for all that apply.
	Maximum opening height of oral orifice is less than 40 mm.
	Range of side-to-side jaw movement is less than 7 mm.
	Range of motion for jaw protrusion is less than 6 mm.
	Popping, clicking, grinding of temporomandibular joint is palpable during rapid opening and closing of jaw or while moving jaw from side-to-side.
	Examinee reports sensation of popping, snapping, or grinding during opening and closing of jaw or while moving jaw from side-to-side.
	Examinee reports pain in jaw, ear, or lower molar during opening and closing of the jaw or while moving jaw from side-to-side and rates pain at 2 to 5 on 5-point scale.
	Describe concerns.

Decision Box for Acquired Apraxia of Speech Observation: Discretionary Clinical Observation 14	
Place a minus sign (–) in the column to the left if noting any of the following indicators in a person who has experienced a neurologic episode postlingually or is suspected as such. Proceed to acquired apraxia of speech observation (i.e., Discretionary Clinical Observation 14) if indicators are present.	
Symptom	Clinical Observation Noted
Difficulty with multisyllabic words or words of increased length and complexity.	1
Sound transpositions (or metathetic errors).	
Perseveration across word boundaries.	
Apparent disfluency or choppiness.	
Difficulty with volitional tongue or lip movements in the absence of difficulty with automatic tongue or lip movements. (Symptom may be indicative or oral apraxia, which although is not the same as verbal apraxia, can co-occur with it.)	2
Difficulty with sequencing movements for volitional speech.	7

Discretionary Clinical Observation 14: Acquired Apraxia of Speech Observation (instructions in manual, Chapter 3)		
Observations for Acquired Apraxia of Speech		
Observations for Oral Apraxia		
Place a minus sign (−) in the column to the left for any behavior for which the examinee exhibits difficulty performing volitionally.		

	Cough.		Bite the lower lip.
	Click the tongue.		Puff the cheeks.
	Blow.		

Describe concerns.

Observations for Acquired Apraxia of Speech	
Place a check mark in the box to the left for all that apply.	

	Marked difference in the fluidity of speech for counting to five compared to naming numbers one to five on command, with counting being the more fluid of the two.
	Marked difference between fluidity of speech when counting backward from 20 to 11 compared to counting backward from 10 to 1, with the 10-to-1 countdown sequence being the more fluid.
	Marked difference between saying the word *November* in series, compared to saying the same word in response to a question, with saying the word in series being more fluid.
	Increasing difficulty with words of increased length and complexity. Place a minus sign (−) to the left of the triad(s) with increasing difficulty:
	But . . . Butter . . . Buttercup.
	Wash . . . Washing . . . Washing machine.
	Lead . . . Leader . . . Leadership.
	You . . . You call . . . Eucalyptus.
	Chalk... Chocolate . . . Chocolate cake.
	Straw . . . Strawberry . . . Strawberry shortcake.

Describe concerns.

APPENDIX A

Decision Box for Surplus Nasal Airflow Screening: Discretionary Clinical Observation 16	
Place a minus sign (–) in the column to the left if noting any of the following indicators. Proceed to surplus nasal airflow screening (i.e., Discretionary Clinical Observation 16) if indicators are present.	

	Symptom	Clinical Observation Noted
	Perception of any of the following during speech or vocalization event.	1
	Hypernasal resonance.	
	Audible nasal airflow.	
	Short utterance length.	
	Difficulty with obstruent consonants with or without hypernasality.	
	Atypical voice.	
	Compensatory articulation substitutions for obstruents (i.e., plosives, stops, affricates, fricatives; particularly voiceless):	
	Glottal stops.	
	Pharyngeal stops, fricatives, or affricates.	
	Velar fricatives.	
	Posterior nasal fricative (i.e., nasal snort).	
	Anterior nasal fricative (i.e., facial grimace).	
	Posterior or superior air leakage during labial seal activity.	2
	Velar movement on /ɑ/ phonation is asymmetrical, weak, or absent.	6
	Localized velar contractions on /ɑ/ phonation.	7
	Hypernasal resonance during sustained vowel.	8

Discretionary Clinical Observation 16: Surplus Nasal Airflow Screening (instructions in manual, Chapter 3)	
Screening for Surplus Nasal Airflow During Speech	
Place a minus sign (–) in the column to the left if the following applies.	
	Mirror condensation noted for oral consonants during speech.
Describe concerns.	

| | **Decision Box for Dysarthria Observation: Discretionary Clinical Observation 17** |

Place a minus sign (–) in the column to the left if noting any of the following indicators. Proceed to dysarthria observations (i.e., Discretionary Clinical Observation 17) if indicators are noted.

	Symptom	Clinical Observation Noted
	Imprecise consonants or slurred speech.	
	Hypernasality.	
	Mixed resonance.	
	Jaw hangs in open position when at rest, mandible deviates to the right or left at rest or in motion.	1
	Oral asymmetry at rest or in motion, fasciculations in perioral area.	
	Atypical voice (e.g., breathy, harsh, strained-strangled).	
	Labial asymmetry at rest or in motion, unilateral or bilateral labial seal weakness.	
	Tongue: Extraneous movements at rest or in motion, deviation at rest or in motion, weakness, imprecise movements, reduced range of motion, fatigue.	2
	Mandible: Deviates to right or left when lowered, weak resistance, extraneous movements at rest or in motion.	
	Tongue: Asymmetry, deviations, signs of atrophy, fasciculations, extraneous movements at rest or in motion.	5
	Velum: Asymmetry at rest or in motion, rhythmic or arrhythmic movements at rest or in motion, unilateral or bilateral weakness.	
	Weak, absent, or asymmetrical velar movement on /ɑ/ phonation.	6
	Motion activities: Imprecise consonants, reduced range of motion for articulators, decreasing rate or precision, slow rate, evidence of fatigue.	7
	Evidence of hypernasality or fatigue on /ɑ/ phonation.	8

APPENDIX A

Discretionary Clinical Observation 17: Dysarthria Observation (instructions in manual, Chapter 3)			
Dysarthria Observation			
Place a minus sign (–) in the column to the left that is marked "S" for all symptoms noted during spontaneous speech. Place a minus sign (–) in the column marked "R" for all symptoms noted during reading.			

S	R	Symptoms	
		Imprecise articulation.	Articulation
		Intermittent, sudden, or unpredictable articulation breakdown.	
		Difficulty initiating articulation.	
		Unpredictable vowel distortions.	
		Hypernasal resonance with nasal airflow emissions.	Resonance
		Hypernasal resonance without nasal airflow emissions.	
		Mixed resonance.	
		Low pitch.	Voice
		Irregular pitch.	
		Sudden elevation of pitch.	
		Reduced variation in pitch and loudness.	
		Sudden bursts of loudness, irregular loudness.	
		Increased loudness overall.	
		Reduced loudness or inaudible voice.	
		Harsh, hoarse, or strained-strangled quality.	
		Breathy quality.	
		Unpredictable interruptions in speech flow (e.g., variations in pitch and loudness).	Prosody
		Monotone.	
		Slow rate.	
		Short distorted phrases.	
		Dysrhythmia.	
		Sound prolongations.	
		Equal syllable stress.	

S	R	Symptoms	
		Prolonged intervals between syllables and words.	Prosody
		Seemingly measured pace.	
		Reduced vocal emphasis.	
		Pitch peaks and valleys.	
		Loudness variability that flattens to a monotone.	
		Short rushes of speech with illogically placed pauses.	
		Variable or accelerated rate.	
		Inappropriate silences.	
		Repetitions of initial sounds.	
		Audible inspiration.	Respiration
		Breathy exhalation.	
		Sudden gusts of exhaled air.	
		Altered breathing cycle.	
		Much effort required for speech.	Overall
		Muscular weakness.	
		Extraneous movements.	
		Imprecise movements.	

Describe concerns.

APPENDIX A

Decision Box for Respiratory and Laryngeal Efficiency Screening: Discretionary Clinical Observation 19	
Place a minus sign (–) in the column to the left if noting any of the following indicators. Proceed to respiratory and laryngeal efficiency screening (i.e., Discretionary Clinical Observation 19) if indicators are present.	
Symptom	Clinical Observation Noted
Evidence of respiratory inefficiency or distress during any speech or nonspeech activity.	1, 7, 8
Voice quality that indicates possible inefficient use of the larynx (e.g., breathiness, harshness, hoarseness, or strained quality).	1, 7, 8
Failure to sustain the vowel /ɑ/ for at least 20 seconds for adults and 10 seconds for children.	8

Discretionary Clinical Observation 19: Screening for Laryngeal and Respiratory Efficiency (instructions in manual, Chapter 3)
Screening for Laryngeal and Respiratory Efficiency (i.e., S:Z ratio)
Place a minus sign (–) in column to the left for any symptom noted.
For adult examinee, measured duration was less than 20 seconds. For child examinee, measured duration was less than 10 seconds.
Audible symptoms of vocal pathology.
Duration decreased with consecutive trials.
S:Z ratio was calculated as 1.2 or greater.
Describe concerns.

Summarize the Findings and Make Recommendations

Summarize the Findings: Adults with Recent Neurologic Episode		
Review the evidence collected. Note minus signs (–) and descriptions of concerns. Record evidence of structural or performance anomaly that has potential to negatively influence speech production or result in a need for clinical follow-up. Use additional space provided at bottom if needed.		
Anomaly Was Noted When Evaluating:	**Anomaly Observed**	**Comment on Performance**
Facial region.		
Respiration.		
Lip/tongue strength/mobility.		
Dental alignment or bite.		
Dental occlusion.		
Oral interior.		
Velar movement.		
Verbal diadochokinesis.		
Vowel prolongation.		
Gag reflex stimulation.		
Dysphagia.		
Nasal cavity clearance.		
Temporomandibular joint.		
Acquired apraxia of speech.		
Surplus nasal airflow.		
Dysarthria.		
Laryngeal/respiratory efficiency.		

Recommendations for Individualized Plan of Care			
Place a check mark in the column to the left for all that apply. Supply descriptive information as suggested.			
Clinical Implications			
	Result of oral-facial inspection is unremarkable. No impact on speech production is suspected. No follow-up is needed.		
	Oral-facial inspection yields evidence that may support a particular diagnosis or plan of care. If so, specify evidence and suspected diagnosis:		
	Oral-facial inspection yields evidence that clearly supports a particular diagnosis or plan of care. If so, specify evidence and diagnosis:		
Plan of Care			
	Next Step	**Rationale** Circle all that apply.	**Responsible Party** Circle all that apply
	Additional testing is needed.	• Part of oral-facial inspection that was not yet completed requires more time or clinical teaching to perform. • Testing that is beyond the scope of oral-facial inspection is identified as needed. • Other (specify).	• Examiner, follow-up. • Speech-language pathologist receiving case for therapy. • Specialist speech-language pathologist referral. • Health care provider outside speech-language pathology referral. • Other (specify).
	Recommend that therapy plan include objectives/procedures designed to address concerns identified through inspection.	Specify:	Specify:

Oral-Facial Evaluation for Speech-Language Pathologists
Barbara Ann Johnson-Root, PhD, CCC-SLP

Special Recording Form: Preoperative Laryngectomy

Intake Information	
Client name:	Date of evaluation:
Date of birth:	Age:
Examiner:	Agency or facility:
Reason for evaluation:	
Relevant history:	
Comments:	

Prepare the Work Area for Testing (instructions in manual, Chapter 1)
Checklist
Place a check mark in the column to the left after completing each preparatory step in the list below.
Inventory equipment and supplies listed Table 1–2 and described in Appendix B.
Check batteries that power battery-operated equipment. Replace weak or dead batteries.
Verify that all cords and strings were removed from equipment. If not, remove and dispose of them.
Sanitize the work area, and unwrap equipment as instructed in Chapter 1.
Wash hands thoroughly.
Put on examination gloves, using procedures provided in Chapter 1.
Arrange equipment as shown in Figure 1–1.

Instruct the Examinee (and Significant Other if Appropriate)

Use your own words and developmentally appropriate language to communicate the following talking points before you begin.

- The oral-facial evaluation is a customary part of every speech-language evaluation.
- It involves inspecting all observable body parts necessary for speaking so that we may ascertain whether all parts are present, complete, and working properly.
- This is done to look into whether there is a physical explanation for the speech problem that brought you here or if there is any physical problem that we should address while helping you.
- None of the procedures are painful or harmful.
- A few items situated on the table may not be needed.
- For some people, oral-facial evaluation findings may lead to more detailed testing or possibly referral to another professional, although this is the not case for everyone.
- You may ask questions before we begin or at any time. Do you have any questions now?
  (If *yes*, either answer briefly or diplomatically table the question for a more appropriate time. If *no*, move on.)
- Are you ready? Let's get started!

Routine Clinical Observations

Routinely complete the following eight clinical observations for all examinees scheduled for surgical removal of the larynx:

- Routine Clinical Observation 1: Conversational Speech Sample (A), Facial Features (B), and Breathing Observations (C) for Preoperative Laryngectomee
- Routine Clinical Observation 2: Lip and Tongue Strength and Mobility
- Routine Clinical Observation 3: Dental Alignment and Bite for Older Adults
- Routine Clinical Observation 4: Dental Occlusion
- Routine Clinical Observation 5: Oral Interior
- Routine Clinical Observation 6: Velar Movement
- Routine Clinical Observation 7: Verbal Diadochokinesis
- Routine Clinical Observation 8: Vowel Prolongation

Routine Clinical Observation 1(A): Conversational Speech Sample for Preoperative Laryngectomee (instructions in manual, Chapters 2 and 4)	
Rate intelligibility. Check the one that applies.	
Place a check mark in the corresponding column to the left if intelligibility is judged as "good." For all intelligibility ratings that are less than "good," place a minus sign (–) in the corresponding column.	
	Good: Completely or nearly completely intelligible.
	Slightly compromised: Intelligible more than half the time.
	Fair: Intelligible about half of the time.
	Poor: Intelligible less than half of the time.
	Unintelligible: Completely unintelligible (or nearly so).
Area(s) Noted as Difficult During Conversational Speech	
Use a minus sign (–) to mark areas identified as possibly deficient during conversational speech.	
Articulation/phonology.	Fluency.
Language.	Resonance.
Voice.	Motor-speech.
Describe any speaking patterns that may potentially interfere with achieving intelligible alaryngeal speech.	

APPENDIX A

		Routine Clinical Observations 1(B): Facial Region Inspection, Amended for Older Adult Examinees (instructions in manual, Chapters 2 and 4)
		Use a minus sign (−) to mark all features noted during facial region inspection. If multiple options appear on the same line, circle any that apply.

Resting	Speaking	Feature
		Facial or oral asymmetry, drooping.
		Tremor.
		Fasciculation, spasm.
		Poor saliva management.
		Scarring.
		Dysmorphic features:

After completing checklist, place a minus sign (−) in the column for any applicable condition.	
	Facial features suggest neuromuscular involvement. Specify.
	Facial features appear to possibly contribute to atypical speaking pattern. Specify.

Routine Clinical Observation 1(C): Breathing Observations, Adapted for Preoperative and Postoperative Laryngectomee (instructions in manual, Chapters 2 and 4)	

Identify the type of breathing noted upon observation. For all examinees, *diaphragmatic* breathing is optimal, and *lower thoracic* breathing is acceptable.

For the list on the left, place a check mark in the far-left column for all that apply. If any pattern described in the column on the right is observed, place a minus sign (–) to its left, since this is an atypical pattern. Also, where multiple options occupy the same line, circle those that apply.

Type of Breathing

	Diaphragmatic.		Upper thoracic, clavicular.
	Lower thoracic.		Noisy, evidence of respiratory distress or struggle.

Describe.

	Refer examinee to specialist for pulmonary testing. Place a check mark in column to the left to confirm that this is part of the plan of care.

APPENDIX A

Routine Clinical Observation 2: Lip and Tongue Mobility and Strength		
(instruction in manual, Chapter 2)		

Place a check mark in the column to the left if the examinee performs the act smoothly, accurately, completely, and in a timely manner. Place a minus sign (−) in the column if noting any other response, and use the space below to provide additional descriptive data.

Action			
	Pucker.		Quick repetitions of /b/ or /p/.
	Spread.		Smack the lips.
	Sustain exaggerated /u/.		

Describe atypical responses; comment on possible relationship to speech concern.

Lip Strength and Seal

Place a check mark in the box to the left if the act is judged to be within normal limits. Place a minus sign (−) in the column if noting any other response, and use the space below to provide additional descriptive data.

Action			
	Seal.		Resistance.

Describe atypical responses; comment on possible relationship to speech concern.

Tongue Mobility

Place a check mark in the column to the left of each action if examinee performs the act smoothly, accurately, completely, and in a timely manner. Place a minus sign (−) in the column if noting any other response, and use the space below to provide additional descriptive data.

Action			
	Protrusion.		Wiggle to the left and to the right.
	Elevation.		Rotation.
	Lateralization.		

Describe atypical responses; comment on possible relationship to speech concern.

	Other Tongue Observations

Place a check mark in box to the left if feature is observed to be within normal limits. Place a minus sign (–) in the column if noting any other response, and use the space below to provide additional descriptive data.

Feature	
Shape of tongue tip.	Lingual frenum length.

Describe atypical features; comment on possible relationship to speech concern.

	Tongue Strength

Place a check mark in the column on the left if the act is judged to be within normal limits. Place a minus sign (–) in the column if noting any other response, and use the space below to provide additional descriptive data.

Action
Resistance.

Describe atypical responses; comment on possible relationship to speech concern.

APPENDIX A

Routine Clinical Observation 3: Dental Bite and Alignment, Amended for Older Adults (instructions in manual, Chapters 2 and 4)		
Place a minus sign (–) in the column to the left for all that apply.		

	The examinee is edentulous.		
	The examinee is wearing dentures or other dental appliance.		
	The dental appliance is reportedly uncomfortable.		
	The examinee exhibits misarticulations that may be attributed to poorly fitted dental appliance.		

Dental Bite		
For examinees with unremarkable bite pattern, place a check mark in the column to the left corresponding to the word *normal*. If any other bite pattern is noted, place a minus sign (–) in the column that resides directly to the left of the term that best describes the person's bite. (Typically one applies; there are exceptions.)		

Dental Bite for Examinees With Natural Teeth					
	Normal.		Edge-to-edge bite.		Overjet.
	Open bite.		Underbite.		Flared bite.
	Closed bite.		Cross bite.		

Add descriptive information if needed; describe relationship to speech, if any

Alignment and Condition of Teeth for Examinees With Natural Teeth

Mark the dental chart below to indicate dental alignment concerns noted.

Upper Teeth

Central Incisor: 7-8 Years
Lateral Incisor: 8-9 Years
Cuspid: 11-12 Years
First Premolar (First Bicuspid): 10-11 Years
Second Premolar (Second Bisucpid): 11-12 Years
First Molar: 6-7 Years
Second Molar: 12-13 Years
Third Molar (Wisdom Tooth): 17-21 Years

Lower Teeth

Third Molar (Wisdom Tooth): 17-21 Years
Second Molar: 11-13 Years
First Molar: 6-7 Years
Second Premolar (Second Bicuspid): 11-12 Years
First Premolar (First Bicuspid): 10-12 Years
Cuspid: 9-10 Years
Lateral Incisor: 7-8 Years
Central Incisor: 6-7 Years

APPENDIX A

Describe dental misalignment concerns, and comment on their possible effect on speech production, if any.

Routine Clinical Observation 4: Dental Occlusion (instruction in manual, Chapter 2)					
Dental Occlusion					
For examinees with neutroclussion, place a check mark in the column that resides directly to the left of that term. For examinees with distoclusion or mesioclusion, place a minus sign (−) in the column that corresponds to that classification.					
Dental Occlusion Classification					
	Neutroclusion (typical).		Distoclusion.		Mesioclusion.
Describe occlusal relationship. Comment on any possible relationship to speech production.					

Routine Clinical Observation 5: Oral Interior (instructions in manual, Chapter 2)	
Response to Request to Open the Mouth: **Freedom of Mandibular Movement and Response to Resistance**	

Place a minus sign (−) in the column to the left, corresponding to any statements that apply.

	Activity
	Difficulty with opening the mouth adequately for observing oral interior.
	Pain or other sensation reported when opening the mouth for oral inspection.
	Mandible deviates to left or right when lowered.
	Extraneous mandibular movements at rest or in motion.
	Not successful in resisting examiner's attempt to prevent mandibular movement.

Place a minus sign (−) in the column to the left of any statements that describe examinee's condition.

	Symptoms suggest *possible* temporomandibular joint disorder.
	Symptoms suggest evidence of muscle weakness, asymmetry, discoordination, or difficulty with motor planning.

Describe additional concerns.

Tongue Surface, Size, and Shape	

Place a check mark in the column to the left if the feature is judged to be within normal limits. Place a minus sign (−) in the column if noting any atypical trait, and use the space below to provide additional descriptive data.

	Feature		
	Texture.		Shape.
	Size.		Other noteworthy feature:

Describe concern with the feature noted particularly as it may or may not relate to speech production.

continues

Routine Clinical Observation 5: Oral Interior *continued*

Hard Palate	
Place a check mark in the column to the left if the feature is judged to be within normal limits. Place a minus sign (−) in the column if noting any atypical trait, and use the space below to provide additional descriptive data.	

	Feature		
	Alveolar ridge.		Posterior nasal spine.
	Palatal arch.		Foveae palate.
	Median raphe.		Scarring.
	Mucous membrane.		Coloring.

Describe concerns; comment on possible relationship to speech pattern.

Posterior Soft Tissue	
Place a check mark in the column to the left if the feature is judged to be within normal limits. Place a minus sign (−) in the column if noting any atypical trait, and use the space below to provide additional descriptive data.	

	Feature		
	Velum (structure only).		Palatine tonsils.
	Uvula.		Posterior pharyngeal wall.
	Faucial pillars.		

Describe concern. Comment on possible relationship to speech problem.

Routine Clinical Observation 6: Velar Movement (instructions in manual, Chapter 2)	
Velar Movement	
Place a check mark beside "velum moves up and back symmetrically on /ɑ/ phonation" if that is the case. Place a minus sign (−) in the column corresponding to any other trait noted; use the space below to provide additional descriptive data.	
Velar response to /ɑ/ phonation	
	Velum moves up and back symmetrically on /ɑ/ phonation.
	Velum moves up and back asymmetrically on /ɑ/ phonation.
	Velum moves sluggishly on /ɑ/ phonation.
	Velum is not observed to move on /ɑ/ phonation.
	Misplaced velar dimple noted on /ɑ/ phonation.
Describe concerns. Comment on possible relationship to speech pattern.	

Routine Clinical Observation 7: Verbal Diadochokinesis (instructions in manual, Chapter 2)					
Speech-Alternating Motion: Rate					
Record syllables produced per second in the column that appears to the left of each syllable designation.					
Syllables/Second	Syllable	Syllables/Second	Syllable	Syllables/Second	Syllable
	/pə/		/tə/		/kə/

Speech-Alternating Motion: Perceptual Evaluation	
Place a minus sign (–) in the box on the left for all that apply.	
	Fewer than five syllables/second; specify consonant:
	Reduced range of motion for the articulators (i.e., jaw, tongue, lips).
	Arrhythmic or unsteady performance.
	Poor articulatory precision; specify consonant:
	Rate, precision, or volume decreased over time; specify:
Describe concerns. Comment on possible relevance to speech pattern.	

Speech-Sequential Motion: Rate	
Syllables/Second	Syllables
	/pə tə kə/

Speech-Sequential Motion: Subjective Evaluation	
Place a minus sign (–) in the column to the left for all that apply.	
	Fewer than five syllables/second.
	Difficulty rapidly sequencing the three distinctively different syllables in succession (i.e., syllable transpositions, perseveration across syllable boundaries).
	Decrease in rate, precision, or volume over time.
Describe concerns. Comment on possible relevance to speech pattern.	

Routine Clinical Observation 8: Vowel Prolongation (instructions in manual, Chapter 2)			
Vowel Prolongation: Duration			
Measure vowel duration according to instructions in Chapter 2. Write results for each of three trials in the designated column. Circle the longest duration.			
	Trial 1	Trial 2	Trial 3
/ɑ/			
Vowel Prolongation: Subjective Evaluation			
Place a minus sign (–) in column to the left for all that apply.			
	Adult sustains /ɑ/ for fewer than 20 seconds, or child sustains /ɑ/ for fewer than 10 seconds.		
	Decrease in duration across three trials.		
	Voice quality or volume deteriorates.		
	Atypical resonance.		
	Atypical vocal quality or pitch.		
Describe concern. Comment on relevance to speech.			

If you believe there is a reason to omit one or more of the routine procedures, clearly mark your decision on the recording form. Then proceed with the inspection.

Identifying and Completing Appropriate Discretionary Clinical Observations

In most cases, the inspection ends with routine clinical observations. Yet once routine procedures are complete, the next step is to determine whether the evidence indicates a need for any discretionary clinical observations. For the sake of convenience, a series of decision boxes provides structure that can facilitate identifying discretionary clinical observations that should be considered.

Bear in mind that none of the decision boxes is intended to prompt a perfunctory decision that results in a discretionary procedure. Certainly, an understanding of the examinee's overall symptom pattern combined with a rich bank of clinical experience and intuition should also contribute, albeit such intangibles are highly individualized and therefore difficult to place on a form. Even so, strategically considering tangible client-centered evidence as it is arranged on the form can contribute to a good decision relative to proceeding with a discretionary clinical observation, and that is the intended purpose of the decision boxes.

Once a decision box is evaluated, if it flags the corresponding discretionary clinical observation, the inspection can proceed to that discretionary observation if the examining clinician deems it appropriate.

Only two discretionary clinical observations are considered appropriate for this group:

- Discretionary Clinical Observation 11: Temporomandibular Joint Disorder Screening
- Discretionary Clinical Observation 21: Prompt for Dysphagia Screening

Decision Box for Temporomandibular Joint Disorder Screening: Discretionary Clinical Observation 11		
Place a minus sign (–) in the column to the left if noting any of the following indicators. Proceed to screening for temporomandibular joint disorder (i.e., Discretionary Clinical Observation 11) if indicators are present.		
	Symptom	Clinical Observation Noted
	Limited mandibular excursion during speech activities.	1
	Limited mandibular excursion during nonspeech activities.	
	Reported sensation of localized or referred pain when moving the jaw.	5

Discretionary Clinical Observation 11: Temporomandibular Joint Disorder Screening (instructions in manual, Chapter 3)	
Screening for Temporomandibular Joint Disorder	
Place a minus sign (–) in the box to the left for all that apply.	
	Maximum opening height of oral orifice is less than 40 mm.
	Range of side-to-side jaw movement is less than 7 mm.
	Range of motion for jaw protrusion is less than 6 mm.
	Popping, clicking, grinding of temporomandibular joint is palpable during rapid opening and closing of jaw or while moving jaw from side-to-side.
	Examinee reports sensation of popping, snapping, or grinding during opening and closing of jaw or while moving jaw from side-to-side.
	Examinee reports pain in jaw, ear, or lower molar during opening and closing of the jaw or while moving jaw from side-to-side and rates pain at 2 to 5 on 5-point scale.
Describe concerns.	

Decision Box for Dysphagia Screening Prompt: Discretionary Clinical Observation 21		
Regulations require that all poststroke patients should be screened for dysphagia as soon as the acute phase of the illness has passed and before returning to an oral diet. However, stroke is not the only etiology resulting in dysphagia. Recently laryngectomized patients and aging nonstroke patients should also be considered for dysphagia referral if experiencing any of the following symptoms.		
Place a minus sign (−) in the column to the left for any symptom noted.		
	Symptom	Occasion Noted
	Older adult.	Case history intake
	Patient reports difficulty with feeding or swallowing.	

Discretionary Clinical Observation 21: Dysphagia Screening Prompt (instructions in manual, Chapter 3)	
Dysphagia Screening Prompt	
Place a minus sign (−) in the column to the left if any of the following apply. Proceed to dysphagia screening if two or more symptoms are noted or if the person has a history of recent neurologic incident. If in doubt, refer for screening.	
	Recent history or cerebrovascular accident, neurologic incident or disease, or laryngectomy (required dysphagia screening).
	Cough after swallow.
	Voice change after swallow.
	Reduced lingual range of motion (Routine Clinical Observation 2) or incomplete facial symmetry (Routine Clinical Observation 1).
	Patient is flagged to be observed for any motor-speech disorders procedure (Discretionary Clinical Observations 15, 16, and 17).
	Abnormal volitional cough.
	Abnormal gag reflex.
Describe concerns.	

APPENDIX A

Summarize the Findings and Make Recommendations

Summarize the Findings: Preoperative Laryngectomee		
Review the evidence collected. Note minus signs (−) and descriptions of concerns. Record evidence of structural or performance anomaly that has potential to negatively influence speech production or result in a need for clinical follow-up. Use additional space provided at bottom if needed.		
Anomaly Was Noted When Evaluating:	**Anomaly Observed**	**Comment on Performance**
Facial region.		
Respiration.		
Lip/tongue strength/mobility.		
Dental alignment or bite.		
Dental occlusion.		
Oral interior.		
Velar movement.		
Verbal diadochokinesis.		
Vowel prolongation.		
Temporomandibular joint.		
Dysphagia.		

	Recommendations for Individualized Plan of Care		
	Place a check mark in the column to the left for all that apply. Supply descriptive information as suggested.		
	Clinical Implications		
	Result of oral-facial inspection is unremarkable. No impact on speech production is suspected. No follow-up is needed.		
	Oral-facial inspection yields evidence that may support a particular diagnosis or plan of care. If so, specify evidence and suspected diagnosis:		
	Oral-facial inspection yields evidence that clearly supports a particular diagnosis or plan of care. If so, specify evidence and diagnosis:		
	Plan of Care		
	Next Step	**Rationale** Circle all that apply.	**Responsible Party** Circle all that apply
	Additional testing is needed.	• Part of oral-facial inspection that was not yet completed requires more time or clinical teaching to perform. • Testing that is beyond the scope of oral-facial inspection is identified as needed. • Other (specify).	• Examiner, follow-up. • Speech-language pathologist receiving case for therapy. • Specialist speech-language pathologist referral. • Health care provider outside speech-language pathology referral. • Other (specify).
	Recommend that therapy plan include objectives/procedures designed to address concerns identified through inspection.	Specify:	Specify:

APPENDIX A

Oral-Facial Evaluation for Speech-Language Pathologists
Barbara Ann Johnson-Root, PhD, CCC-SLP

Special Recording Form: Postoperative Laryngectomy

Intake Information	
Client name:	Date of evaluation:
Date of birth:	Age:
Examiner:	Agency or facility:
Reason for evaluation:	
Relevant history:	
Comments:	

Prepare the Work Area for Testing (instructions in manual, Chapter 1)	
Checklist	
Place a check mark in the column to the left after completing each preparatory step in the list below.	
	Inventory equipment and supplies listed Table 1–2 and described in Appendix B.
	Check batteries that power battery-operated equipment. Replace weak or dead batteries.
	Verify that all cords and strings were removed from equipment. If not, remove and dispose of them.
	Sanitize the work area, and unwrap equipment as instructed in Chapter 1.
	Wash hands thoroughly.
	Put on examination gloves, using procedures provided in Chapter 1.
	Arrange equipment as shown in Figure 1–1.

Instruct the Examinee (and Significant Other if Appropriate)

Use your own words and developmentally appropriate language to communicate the following talking points before you begin.

- The oral-facial evaluation is a customary part of every speech-language evaluation.
- It involves inspecting all observable body parts necessary for speaking so that we may ascertain whether all parts are present, complete, and working properly.
- This is done to look into whether there is a physical explanation for the speech problem that brought you here or if there is any physical problem that we should address while helping you.
- None of the procedures are painful or harmful.
- A few items situated on the table may not be needed.
- For some people, oral-facial evaluation findings may lead to more detailed testing or possibly referral to another professional, although this is not the case for everyone.
- You may ask questions before we begin or at any time. Do you have any questions now?
  (If *yes*, either answer briefly or diplomatically table the question for a more appropriate time. If *no*, move on.)
- Are you ready? Let's get started!

Routine Clinical Observations

Only six clinical observations are routinely performed for recently laryngectomized examinees. Furthermore, some of the procedures on the list may be eliminated if they were completed prior to surgery whenever the only clinically noteworthy change since that time was surgical removal of the larynx.

The six procedures to be performed routinely for this group are as follows:

- Routine Clinical Observation 1: Facial Features (B) and Breathing Observations (C)
- Routine Clinical Observation 2: Lip and Tongue Strength and Mobility
- Routine Clinical Observation 3: Dental Alignment and Bite for Older Adults
- Routine Clinical Observation 4: Dental Occlusion
- Routine Clinical Observation 5: Oral Interior
- Discretionary Clinical Observation 21: Prompt for Dysphagia Screening (routine for this population)
- Discretionary Clinical Observation 24: Screen for Esophageal Speech Candidacy (routine for this population)

APPENDIX A

Routine Clinical Observation 1(B): Facial Region Inspection, Amended for Recent Postoperative Laryngectomee (instructions in manual, Chapters 2 and 4)	
Feature	
	Scarring.
	Facial or oral asymmetry.
	Poor saliva management.
Comments:	

Routine Clinical Observation 1(C): Breathing Observations, Adapted for Preoperative and Postoperative Laryngectomee (instructions in manual, Chapters 2 and 4)			
Identify the type of breathing noted upon observation. For all examinees, *diaphragmatic* breathing is optimal, and *lower thoracic* breathing is acceptable.			
For the list on the left, place a check mark in the far-left column for all that apply. If any pattern described in the column on the right is observed, place a minus sign (–) to its left, since this is an atypical pattern. Also, where multiple options occupy the same line, circle those that apply.			
Type of Breathing			
	Diaphragmatic.		Upper thoracic, clavicular.
	Lower thoracic.		Noisy, evidence of respiratory distress or struggle.
Describe.			
	Refer the examinee to a specialist for pulmonary testing. Place a check mark in the column to the left to confirm that this is part of the plan of care.		

Routine Clinical Observation 2: Lip and Tongue Mobility and Strength
(instruction in manual, Chapter 2)

Place a check mark in the column to the left if the examinee performs the act smoothly, accurately, completely, and in a timely manner. Place a minus sign (−) in the column if noting any other response, and use the space below to provide additional descriptive data.

Action			
	Pucker.		Quick repetitions of posture for /b/ or /p/.
	Spread.		Smack the lips.
	Sustain exaggerated /u/.		

Describe atypical responses; comment on possible relationship to speech concern.

Lip Strength and Seal

Place a check mark in the box to the left if the act is judged to be within normal limits. Place a minus sign (−) in the column if noting any other response, and use the space below to provide additional descriptive data.

Action			
	Seal.		Resistance.

Describe atypical responses; comment on possible relationship to speech concern.

Tongue Mobility

Place a check mark in the column to the left of each action if examinee performs the act smoothly, accurately, completely, and in a timely manner. Place a minus sign (−) in the column if noting any other response, and use the space below to provide additional descriptive data.

Action			
	Protrusion.		Wiggle to the left and to the right.
	Elevation.		Rotation.
	Lateralization.		

continues

APPENDIX A

Routine Clinical Observation 2: Lip and Tongue Mobility and Strength *continued*

Describe atypical responses; comment on possible relationship to speech concern.

Other Tongue Observations
Place a check mark in box to the left if feature is observed to be within normal limits. Place a minus sign (−) in the column if noting any other response, and use the space below to provide additional descriptive data.

Feature			
	Shape of tongue tip.		Lingual frenum length.

Describe atypical features; comment on possible relationship to speech concern.

Tongue Strength
Place a check mark in the column on the left if the act is judged to be within normal limits. Place a minus sign (−) in the column if noting any other response, and use the space below to provide additional descriptive data.

Action	
	Resistance.

Describe atypical responses; comment on possible relationship to speech concern.

	Routine Clinical Observation 3: Dental Bite and Alignment, Amended for Older Adults (instructions in manual, Chapters 2 and 4)				
	Place a minus sign (−) in the column to the left for all that apply.				
	The examinee is edentulous.				
	The examinee is wearing dentures or other dental appliance.				
	The dental appliance is reportedly uncomfortable.				
	The examinee exhibits misarticulations that may be attributed to poorly fitted dental appliance.				

Dental Bite					
For examinees with unremarkable bite pattern, place a check mark in the column to the left corresponding to the word *normal*. If any other bite pattern is noted, place a minus sign (−) in the column that resides directly to the left of the term that best describes the person's bite. (Typically one applies; there are exceptions.)					

Dental Bite for Examinees With Natural Teeth					
	Normal.		Edge-to-edge bite.		Overjet.
	Open bite.		Underbite.		Flared bite.
	Closed bite.		Cross bite.		

Add descriptive information if needed; describe relationship to speech, if any.

continues

APPENDIX A

Routine Clinical Observation 3: Dental Bite and Alignment, Amended for Older Adults *continued*

Alignment and Condition of Teeth for Examinees With Natural Teeth
Mark the dental chart below to indicate dental alignment concerns noted.

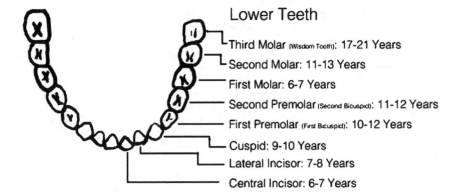

Upper Teeth

- Central Incisor: 7-8 Years
- Lateral Incisor: 8-9 Years
- Cuspid: 11-12 Years
- First Premolar (First Bicuspid): 10-11 Years
- Second Premolar (Second Bisucpid): 11-12 Years
- First Molar: 6-7 Years
- Second Molar: 12-13 Years
- Third Molar (Wisdom Tooth): 17-21 Years

Lower Teeth

- Third Molar (Wisdom Tooth): 17-21 Years
- Second Molar: 11-13 Years
- First Molar: 6-7 Years
- Second Premolar (Second Bicuspid): 11-12 Years
- First Premolar (First Bicuspid): 10-12 Years
- Cuspid: 9-10 Years
- Lateral Incisor: 7-8 Years
- Central Incisor: 6-7 Years

Describe dental misalignment concerns, and comment on their possible effect on speech production, if any.

Routine Clinical Observation 4: Dental Occlusion (instruction in manual, Chapter 2)				
Dental Occlusion				
For examinees with neutroclusion, place a check mark in the column that resides directly to the left of that term. For examinees with distoclusion or mesioclusion, place a minus sign (–) in the column that corresponds to that classification.				
Dental Occlusion Classification				
	Neutroclusion (typical).		Distoclusion.		Mesioclusion.
Describe occlusal relationship. Comment on any possible relationship to speech production.				

Routine Clinical Observation 5: Oral Interior (instructions in manual, Chapter 2)	
Response to Request to Open the Mouth: **Freedom of Mandibular Movement and Response to Resistance**	
Place a minus sign (–) in the column to the left, corresponding to any statements that apply.	
Activity	
	Difficulty with opening the mouth adequately for observing oral interior.
	Pain or other sensation reported when opening the mouth for oral inspection.
	Mandible deviates to left or right when lowered.
	Extraneous mandibular movements at rest or in motion.
	Not successful in resisting examiner's attempt to prevent mandibular movement.
Place a minus sign (–) in the column to the left of any statements that describe examinee's condition.	
	Symptoms suggest *possible* temporomandibular joint disorder.
	Symptoms suggest evidence of muscle weakness, asymmetry, discoordination, or difficulty with motor planning.
Describe additional concerns.	

Tongue Surface, Size, and Shape	
Place a check mark in the column to the left if the feature is judged to be within normal limits. Place a minus sign (–) in the column if noting any atypical trait, and use the space below to provide additional descriptive data.	
Feature	

	Texture.		Shape.
	Size.		Other noteworthy feature:

Describe concern with the feature noted particularly as it may or may not relate to speech production.

Hard Palate

Place a check mark in the column to the left if the feature is judged to be within normal limits. Place a minus sign (–) in the column if noting any atypical trait, and use the space below to provide additional descriptive data.

	Feature		
	Alveolar ridge.		Posterior nasal spine.
	Palatal arch.		Foveae palate.
	Median raphe.		Scarring.
	Mucous membrane.		Coloring.

Describe concerns; comment on possible relationship to speech pattern.

Posterior Soft Tissue

Place a check mark in the column to the left if the feature is judged to be within normal limits. Place a minus sign (–) in the column if noting any atypical trait, and use the space below to provide additional descriptive data.

	Feature		
	Velum (structure only).		Palatine tonsils.
	Uvula.		Posterior pharyngeal wall.
	Faucial pillars.		

Describe concern. Comment on possible relationship to speech problem.

	Discretionary Clinical Observation 21: Dysphagia Screening Prompt (instructions in manual, Chapter 3)
	Dysphagia Screening Prompt
	Place a minus sign (–) in the column to the left if any of the following apply. Proceed to dysphagia screening if two or more symptoms are noted or if the person has a history of recent neurologic incident. If in doubt, refer for screening.
	Recent history or cerebrovascular accident, neurologic incident or disease, or laryngectomy (required dysphagia screening.)
	Cough after swallow.
	Voice change after swallow.
	Reduced lingual range of motion (Routine Clinical Observation 2) or incomplete facial symmetry (Routine Clinical Observation 1).
	Patient is flagged to be observed for any motor-speech disorders procedure (Discretionary Clinical Observations 15, 16, and 17).
	Abnormal volitional cough.
	Abnormal gag reflex.
	Describe concerns.

Discretionary Clinical Observation 24: Esophageal Speech Pretreatment Check (instructions in manual, Chapter 4)	
The following procedures can be incorporated into the initial oral-facial inspection, and a positive response may indicate an aptitude for esophageal speech. However, poor performance on the screening does not eliminate the person from training for esophageal speech. Instead, if not achieved during the oral-facial inspection, they can be addressed in therapy in preparation for esophageal speech training. Place a check mark in the column to the left if the activity is performed successfully. If not, place a minus sign (–) in the column.	
	Use the tongue to inject air into the esophagus, while simultaneously using it to articulate with precision.
Once the speaker has achieved the above, assess the following. Scoring instructions appear on the same line as the prompt.	
	Inject air and use it to phonate /ɑ/ for as long as possible. Place a check mark in the column to the left if the phonation lasts for 0.4 seconds or more. Place a check minus (✓–) in the column to the left if phonation is achieved but does not last for 0.4 seconds. Place Ø in the column to the left if phonation is not achieved.
	Inject air and use it to phonate /ɑ/ as soon as possible after injecting the air, then repeat for 10 trials. Place a check mark in the column to the left if latency time between injection and phonation consistently does not exceed 0.6 seconds. Place a check minus (✓–) in the column if phonation is achieved, but latency exceeds 0.6 seconds some of the time. Place Ø in the column to the left if phonation is not achieved but latency consistency exceeds 0.6 seconds.
	Inject air; use it to say /ɑ/, and hold the vowel for as long as possible. Repeat for 10 trials. Place a check mark in the column if the examinee repeatedly sustains the vowel for 2.2 seconds or more. Place a check minus (✓–) in the column if the examinee fails to repeatedly sustain the vowel for 2.2 seconds or more. Place Ø in the column to the left if the examinee fails to sustain the vowel for 2.2 seconds.
	Inject air; then use it to say the syllable /dɑ/ repeatedly for eight trials. Place a check mark in the column if the examinee produces eight syllables on only one injection. Place a minus sign (–) in the column if the examinee fails to achieve eight syllables on a single injection of air.

APPENDIX A

If you believe there is a reason to omit one or more of the routine procedures, clearly mark your decision on the recording form. Then proceed with the inspection.

Identifying and Completing Appropriate Discretionary Clinical Observations

Once routine procedures are complete, the next step is to determine whether the evidence indicates a need for discretionary clinical observation. In most cases, the inspection ends with routine clinical observations.

Only one discretionary clinical observation should be considered for this particular group of older adults. That procedure is screening for temporomandibular joint disorder (i.e., Discretionary Clinical Observation 11).

<table>
<tr><td colspan="3" align="center">**Decision Box for Temporomandibular Joint Disorder Screening:**
Discretionary Clinical Observation 11</td></tr>
<tr><td colspan="3">Place a minus sign (–) in the column to the left if noting any of the following indicators. Proceed to screening for temporomandibular joint disorder (i.e., Discretionary Clinical Observation 11) if indicators are present.</td></tr>
<tr><td></td><td align="center">Symptom</td><td align="center">Clinical Observation Noted</td></tr>
<tr><td></td><td>Limited mandibular excursion during speech activities.</td><td align="center">1</td></tr>
<tr><td></td><td>Limited mandibular excursion during nonspeech activities.</td><td rowspan="2" align="center">5</td></tr>
<tr><td></td><td>Reported sensation of localized or referred pain when moving the jaw.</td></tr>
</table>

<table>
<tr><td colspan="2" align="center">**Discretionary Clinical Observation 11: Temporomandibular Joint Disorder Screening**
(instructions in manual, Chapter 3)</td></tr>
<tr><td colspan="2" align="center">Screening for Temporomandibular Joint Disorder</td></tr>
<tr><td colspan="2">Place a minus sign (–) in the box to the left for all that apply.</td></tr>
<tr><td></td><td>Maximum opening height of oral orifice is less than 40 mm.</td></tr>
<tr><td></td><td>Range of side-to-side jaw movement is less than 7 mm.</td></tr>
<tr><td></td><td>Range of motion for jaw protrusion is less than 6 mm.</td></tr>
<tr><td></td><td>Popping, clicking, grinding of temporomandibular joint is palpable during rapid opening and closing of jaw or while moving jaw from side-to-side.</td></tr>
<tr><td></td><td>Examinee reports sensation of popping, snapping, or grinding during opening and closing of jaw or while moving jaw from side-to-side.</td></tr>
<tr><td></td><td>Examinee reports pain in jaw, ear, or lower molar during opening and closing of the jaw or while moving jaw from side-to-side and rates pain at 2 to 5 on 5-point scale.</td></tr>
<tr><td colspan="2">Describe concerns.</td></tr>
</table>

Summarize the Findings and Make Recommendations

Summarize the Findings: Recent Laryngectomee		
Review the evidence collected. Note minus signs (−) and descriptions of concerns. Record evidence of structural or performance anomaly that has potential to negatively influence speech production or result in a need for clinical follow-up. Use additional space provided at bottom if needed.		
Anomaly Was Noted in:	Structure	Performance
Facial region.		
Respiration.		
Lip/tongue strength/mobility.		
Dental alignment or bite.		
Dental occlusion.		
Oral interior.		
Dysphagia.		
Esophageal speech candidacy.		
Temporomandibular joint.		
Comments:		

APPENDIX A

Recommendations for Individualized Plan of Care		
Place a check mark in the column to the left for all that apply. Supply descriptive information as suggested.		
Clinical Implications		
Result of oral-facial inspection is unremarkable. No impact on speech production is suspected. No follow-up is needed.		
Oral-facial inspection yields evidence that may support a particular diagnosis or plan of care. If so, specify evidence and suspected diagnosis:		
Oral-facial inspection yields evidence that clearly supports a particular diagnosis or plan of care. If so, specify evidence and diagnosis:		
Plan of Care		
Next Step	**Rationale** Circle all that apply.	**Responsible Party** Circle all that apply
Additional testing is needed.	• Part of oral-facial inspection that was not yet completed requires more time or clinical teaching to perform. • Testing that is beyond the scope of oral-facial inspection is identified as needed. • Other (specify).	• Examiner, follow-up. • Speech-language pathologist receiving case for therapy. • Specialist speech-language pathologist referral. • Health care provider outside speech-language pathology referral. • Other (specify).
Recommend that therapy plan include objectives/procedures designed to address concerns identified through inspection.	Specify:	Specify:

APPENDIX B

Equipment and Supplies

In preparation for an oral-facial inspection, arrange for convenient access to essential equipment and supplies that are listed in Table 1–2. For the sake of specificity, an annotated version appears in this appendix.

Largely, the disposable items on the list can be a part of the clinical inventory that is accessible to a number of examiners; in some clinics, all equipment and supplies may be provided. However, many clinicians prefer to own their own nondisposable items.

For the most part, keep all materials in a single location so as to streamline preparation. Refer to Chapter 1 for instructions on how to prepare the work area as well as the equipment, and refer to Figure 1–1, which illustrates organization and setup for nondistractible clients.

Some materials on the annotated list are needed only for discretionary procedures, and they are identified as such. Unless absolutely certain that the discretionary procedure is not needed, prepare discretionary materials for use and lay them out as shown in the figure so that they will be available.

Equipment and Supplies Needed to Prepare the Work Area

Spare Batteries

Carry spare batteries for all battery-operated equipment, and keep them in a handy location that is isolated from other equipment and supplies so as to avoid chemical contamination. House batteries in a container that is made of something other than metal (e.g., plastic, wood, composite).

Always check batteries for power *before* the examinee arrives; replace as needed. If in doubt, replace batteries prior to testing so as to avoid losing power during the exam.

Disinfectant Soap

Use disinfectant soap for hand washing as described in Chapter 1. Repeat hand washing as needed.

Disinfectant Wipes

Use disinfectant wipes to sanitize the work area as explained in Chapter 1. Repeat if necessary.

Alcohol or Alcohol Wipes

Use alcohol wipes or rubbing alcohol applied to a disposable cloth to sanitize unwrapped equipment. Follow Chapter 1 instructions; repeat if needed.

Tissues

Place a reasonably stocked tissue box nearby. Many clients present with nasal discharge or poor saliva management, and some who sustained neurologic injury may experience sudden episodes of tearing or crying. Having the tissue box within the client's reach for older children and adults facilitates meeting this physical need discretely and efficiently. For younger children and potentially distractible individuals, however, manage the location of the tissue box so that it does not compete for your attention.

Small Plastic Box (for Birth-to-5 and Distractible People)

If working with small children or other potentially distractible individuals, instead of arranging the sterilized items on a table as shown in Figure 1–1, a small plastic box can be used both to store the items and to keep them out of the examinee's reach while still ensuring that they are close by for the examiner. The box should be adequate in size to house all items needed (e.g., about the size of a small shoebox). Plastic is recommended so that the inside of the box can be sanitized when preparing the work area before each use.

A plastic zipper bag is also an option. However, the plastic bag is considered disposable and should be changed between examinees, since it does not lend itself easily to sanitation.

Equipment and Supplies Needed During Inspection

Pen and Recording Form

The recording form and pen are needed for all steps, including special testing; therefore, they are not listed in the short equipment lists associated with each step.

Examination Gloves

Select properly sized examinations gloves that are latex free and powder free. Store the gloves in original packaging to avoid potential contamination. Latex-free gloves are recommended because some examinees may have latex allergy, and both types of gloves are similar in cost at the time of this writing. Powder-free gloves are also recommended because powdered gloves can leave an unpleasant residue.

Chapter 1 describes a technique for putting on the gloves and removing them while minimizing potential for contamination in the process. Other methods exist for putting on and removing gloves hygienically. If having learned another sanitary method for gloving and degloving, keep in mind that the only requirement is to minimize risk of contamination.

Gloves may need to be replaced during oral-facial inspection if they become contaminated. For that reason, keep the box of examination gloves nearby until completing the inspection.

Penlight

Select a small flashlight (i.e., approximately the size of the pen) with adequate power to illuminate the oral cavity, front to back and top to bottom. The light should have *no strings, cords, or lanyards* attached to prevent unintended contamination of sanitized equipment resulting from proximity to a nonsterilized cord. Strings or cords should be removed prior to the equipment sanitation described in Chapter 1.

Individually Wrapped Tongue Depressor

Use disposable tongue depressors that are individually wrapped. Flavored tongue depressors may be used with children but are not necessary. Pediatric tongue depressors are available through some distributors but similarly are not required.

Partially unwrap the tongue depressor when arranging materials for use. Refer to Figure 1–1 if needed.

Stopwatch (Not Needed for Infants and Toddlers)

Select a stopwatch that allows the basic function of accurately counting seconds, with a start and stop feature. Similar to the penlight, the stopwatch should have *no strings, cords, or lanyards attached*.

Some phones and other electronic devices have stopwatch features, and these may be used. However, due to the likelihood of exposure to contaminants throughout the day, a phone that is used for oral-facial inspections should be properly sanitized before clinical use. If the phone does not safely tolerate exposure to decontaminants, a dedicated stopwatch device is preferred.

Recording Device

Choose a recording device for preserving short speech samples and for readily accessing the samples at a later time. Use a recording device that has *no strings, cords, or lanyards attached* for the same reason given in the earlier section on the penlight and stopwatch. Some commonly owned electronic devices have a recording feature that may be used if it meets stated criteria and is able to be sanitized.

Millimeter Ruler

The ruler should be rigid (i.e., not a tape measure), with no sharp edges, and approximately 120 millimeters in length. The millimeter ruler is needed for two discretionary procedures only: facial dimension estimates (i.e., Discretionary Clinical Observation 10) and screening for temporomandibular joint disorder (i.e., Discretionary Clinical Observation 11).

Small Cup of Water (Not Needed for Birth-to-5 and Adults)

The cup should be small in size and disposable. A sleeve of disposable cups can be kept clean by opening the end that exposes the bottom of the first cup and removing them one at a time, for individual use.

Before placing the cup in the work area, fill it with approximately 1 ounce of water. The cup of water is needed only if checking for tongue-thrust swallow (i.e., Discretionary Clinical Observation 12).

Small Compact Mirror or Reflective Surface (Not Needed for Infants)

Select a mirror that has *no sharp edges* and is *capable of gathering condensation*. The mirror is needed if completing screening for surplus nasal airflow during speech (i.e., Discretionary Clinical Observation 16).

The most effective reflective surface that we were able to find for this purpose is a *floxite detail reflector*, which is used for laryngectomy and tracheostomy management. These can be purchased online, and a sample appears during the child evaluation on the demonstration video.

Extra-Long Cotton Swab

Use disposable extra-long cotton swabs that are individually wrapped. The cotton swab is needed if it becomes necessary to stimulate the gag reflex (i.e., Discretionary Clinical Observation 20).

Although the wrapped swab should be arranged with other equipment when preparing the work area, it may not be needed. Therefore, leave it wrapped until ready to perform gag reflex stimulation.

Eye Test Paddle (Birth-to-5 Only)

A small plastic paddle that is useful for covering one eye can be purchased. If one is not available, a small paddle can be made by cutting a 3 × 5–inch card in half and stapling it to one end of a tongue depressor. If a homemade paddle is used, it should be considered disposable. The eye test paddle is needed for amblyopia screening (i.e., Discretionary Clinical Observation 22).

Large In-Room Mirror

Assuming that a large mirror resides in each diagnostic room is reasonable. However, if one does not, make arrangements to have access to a mirror that is large enough for viewing the full face. This may be needed for speech sound stimulability screening.

Materials Needed for Interpreting Evidence Gathered

Calculator

Many electronic devices (i.e., cell phones) have a calculator function that is useful for this purpose. Calculations are important for both routine and discretionary procedures, but they can be completed after the face-to-face inspection.

APPENDIX C

Optional Rapid Review of Relevant Anatomy and Physiology

What to Expect From the Review

A Convenient and Optional Refresher

The procedures and clinical implications conveyed in the preceding chapters assume that examiners possess an operational grasp of pertinent anatomy and physiology sufficient to support a complete meaningful oral-facial inspection that leads to clinically relevant conclusions and recommendations. Yet this handbook is intended as a clinical tool for examiners at every level from student to expert, including some experienced clinicians whose recollection of anatomy and physiology details may be somewhat rusty. For that reason, in an effort to promote a reasonable degree of consistency across examiners regardless of background or years in practice, Appendix C outlines basic information intended to ensure *convenient and optional* access to a quick, worthwhile review of applicable anatomy and physiology.

Limitations of the Optional Review

The review is limited in scope, intentionally focusing on anatomic parts of interest that lend themselves to direct or indirect inspection in the absence of instrumentation. Some salient facts relative to less visible features are included as well, but only to the extent that integrity is somewhat discernible through the external observations that an oral-facial evaluation yields.

Always keep in mind that the optional review's primary objective is to expediently refresh recall of information learned previously, if in fact you deem that you need a reminder. Therefore, when reading this section, you will note that many assumptions are made as to your basic knowledge.

It is not appropriate to use these few pages as an initial introduction to the topic; neither is it appropriate to consider the rapid review as all inclusive. If you feel that you require additional information to proceed with a worthwhile oral inspection, you are encouraged to seek out resources that cover the subject matter more thoroughly (Duffy, 2013; Dworkin, Marunick, & Krouse, 2004; Fuller, Pimentel, & Peregoy, 2012; Hanson & Mason, 2003; Kummer, 2008; Lass, 2013; Peng et al., 2004; Perri & Halford, 2004; Ruda, Krakovitz, & Rose, 2012; Seikel, King, & Drumright, 2010).

Four Interdependent Subsystems

The speech production system essentially comprises four *interdependent* and *overlapping* subsystems. They are respiration, phonation, resonance, and articulation.

As we proceed, bear in mind that exactly how the parts of any organism work can only be fully appreciated when they are considered in the context of a greater whole, yet for the purpose of gaining understanding about the discrete parts, virtual dissection is needed (Box C–1).

| Box C–1. Dissection: Analogy From Biology |

When considering dissection from a biology perspective, although examining the parts of an organism (e.g., a frog or plant) postmortem provides insight, by nature it renders the organism and its parts lifeless. Similarly, discussing any part of the speech production system in isolation fails to portray an accurate picture of how the speech production system functions viably as a whole.

In recognition of this phenomenon, the ensuing pages virtually dissect the speech production system into four interdependent biologic subsystems considered necessary for speech, particularly as they can be observed either directly or indirectly through basic oral-facial inspection. Since the four subsystems perform in concert, and since they share a number of common elements, although the subsystems are discussed in discrete sections, expect frequent cross-references and commentary on overlap.

The Respiratory and Vocal Tracts

Before delving into a practical review of the four subsystems, let us first take a quick look at the respiratory and vocal tracts. These two overlapping pathways serve all four subsystems in distinct ways.

The Respiratory Tract

The respiratory tract (Figure C–1A) is the open channel that provides passage for inspiratory and expiratory breathing cycles whose primary purpose is to sustain life. Normally, the respiratory tract includes the trachea, larynx with vocal folds in the abducted position, laryngopharynx, oropharynx, nasopharynx, nasal cavities, and nares, with air usually entering and exiting the body via the nares. In a lesser way, the respiratory tract also occasionally features the oral cavity and oral orifice for some types of breathing activities.

The Vocal Tract

Although the vocal tract essentially uses the respiratory tract structures, the vocal tract's role is to accommodate expiring air that the speaker uses as the vehicle for spoken communication (Figure C–1B). The vocal tract comprises the trachea, larynx, laryngopharynx, oropharynx, oral cavity, oral orifice, nasopharynx, nasal cavities, nares, and sinuses. The airstream is modified at various levels along the tract in ways that are discussed throughout the appendix.

Characteristically, the vocal tract divides into two pathways, enabling two egress possibilities for the modified airstream. For most speech sounds, air exits through the oral orifice; however, for the purpose of producing certain phonemes, air can be redirected to exit through the nasal orifice. Exactly how the airflow is regulated for selective nasal and oral egress is covered in the subsequent sections that speak to resonance and articulation.

Structures That, When Juxtaposed, Work Together to Modify the Airstream for Speech

Decades ago, some of our professional forebears described eight structural locations that are used to modify airflow for speech as it travels upward through the vocal tract. Because of physiologic events that occur at these structural locations, they referred to them as *valves* (Darley, Aronson, & Brown, 1975). Through the years, others have referred to certain structural parts of the vocal tract as having valve-like qualities as well (Dworkin, 1991; Dworkin, Marunick, & Krouse, 2004; Edmonson & Esling, 2006; Emerick & Hatten, 1979; Forner & Hixon, 1977; Gelfer & Pazera, 2006; Itoh, Horii, Daniloff, & Binnie, 1982; Wolfe, Garnier, & Smith, 2009).

To proceed, it is important to understand the concept of valving in general so that we may later apply it to the biomechanical valves that make intelligible speech possible. Refer to Box C–2 for a general explanation of valving.

The use of the term *valve*, when describing specific anatomic locations along the vocal tract, recognizes that airflow changes occur at designated sites, reshaping the airstream and giving each place of narrowing or constriction a complex and dynamic

purpose (Edmonson & Esling, 2006). Therefore, the term *valve* is intentionally recaptured for the purpose of this manual and applied interchangeably with terms commonly used to describe the same locations along the vocal tract. The eight structural locations that virtually function as biomechanical valves are vocal folds (i.e., laryngeal valve), velopharyngeal port (i.e., velopharyngeal valve), posterior tongue blade and velum (i.e., lingua-velar valve), tongue blade and hard palate (i.e., lingua-palatal valve), tongue tip and alveolar ridge (i.e., lingua-alveolar valve), interdental (i.e., lingua-dental valve), maxillary central incisors and lower lip (i.e., labial-dental valve), and bilabial valve (see Figure C–1B).

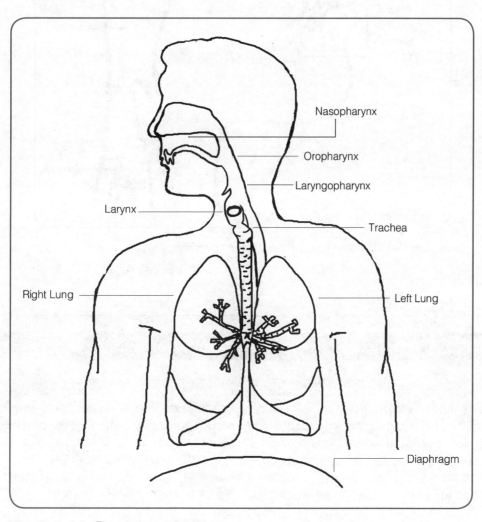

Figure C–1A. Respiratory tract.

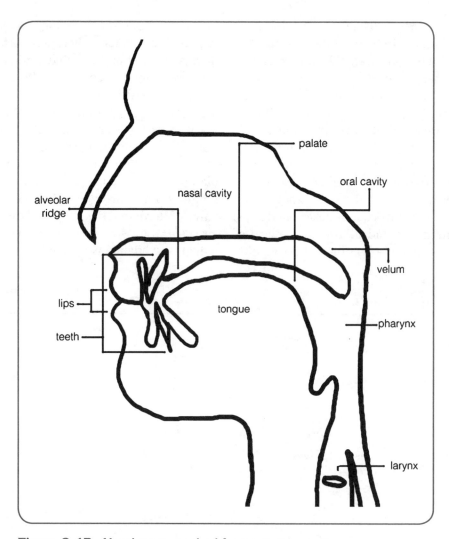

Figure C–1B. Vocal tract, marked for anatomic parts.

Box C–2. General Description of Valving

Generally speaking, valves, whether inside or outside of the body, comprise two or more parts that are capable of engaging for the purpose of controlling the flow of a fluid (i.e., liquid or gas). In some cases, valves open and close to permit or prevent flow, as is true for a simple faucet. In other cases, a valve may engage in more complex ways to accomplish a particular pattern or direction of flow, as with some multifunction shower heads and hose nozzles. Some musical instruments, particularly those of the brass family, offer an excellent example of valves being used to manage airflow traveling through a tract or tube to intentionally modify sound in distinct ways and thereby create a desired effect.

Table C–1 lists each anatomic part involved in constricting the flow of air, a designation as to whether the part is movable or stationary, and each part's contribution to speech production. The same parts are illustrated in Figure C–1B.

Table C–2 then lists the virtual valves, anatomic parts that comprise each, and the speech function potentially associated with that location. Similarly, Figure C–1C displays the location of each valve along the vocal tract.

Understanding content in Tables C–1 and C–2 as well as corresponding figures can be helpful when preparing to perform an oral-facial evalua-

tion. When viewed together, they shed light on each of the anatomic parts, providing insight into their importance to speech from two perspectives. These tables and figures are intended to augment information that addresses each part's collaboration with other parts as it contributes to the function of a virtual valve.

Before any valving takes place, however, first a speaker must generate an upward-flowing airstream that passes through the vocal tract. The moving airstream begins with the exhalation phase of respiration, originating in the lungs (i.e., below the vocal tract).

Table C–1. Movable and Stationary Structures Along the Vocal Tract That Are Involved in Modifying the Airstream for Speech

Part	Movable or Stationary	Functional Highlights
Vocal folds	Movable	The two folds work together to produce voice (i.e., phonation)
		Sound source for most phonemes
		Always abducted during quiet respiration; alternately adducted and abducted during speech to accomplish a sound source for voiced phonemes (and not assuming role of sound source for voiceless phonemes)
		In a partially abducted position, they approximate to create friction for the /h/ phoneme
		May be used to produce the glottal stop /ʔ/, which is standard in some dialects, and compensatory under the circumstance of velopharyngeal insufficiency or compromised palatal integrity
		Space between them is called the glottis
Posterior-pharyngeal wall[a]	Movable	When coupled with the velum, participates in accomplishing velopharyngeal closure, which is necessary for all vowels, as well as all but the three nasal consonants of American English
		Does not approximate the velum during quiet respiration
Velum[a]	Moveable	When coupled with the posterior-pharyngeal wall, participates in accomplishing velopharyngeal closure
		Does not approximate the pharyngeal wall during quiet respiration
		When coupled with the posterior tongue blade, participates in producing lingua-velar phonemes /k/, /g/, /ŋ/, /w/, and /r/. Both /w/ and /r/ have a more anterior point of articulation as well.

continues

Table C–1. *continued*

Part	Movable or Stationary	Functional Highlights
Tongue[a]	Movable	When posterior tongue blade is coupled with velum, it participates in producing lingua-velar phonemes /k/, /g/, /ŋ/, /w/, and /r/
		When the tongue blade is coupled with the hard palate, it participates in producing lingua-palatal phonemes /ʃ/, /ʒ/, /tʃ/, /dʒ/, /r/, and /j/
		When tongue tip is coupled with the alveolar ridge, it participates in producing lingua-alveolar phonemes /t/, /d/, /s/, /z/, /l/, and /n/
		When tongue tip is occupying the interdental space between the maxillary and mandibular incisors, it participates in producing interdental consonants /θ/ and /ð/
Hard palate[a] (including alveolar ridge)	Stationary	The bony barrier that separates the oral and nasal cavities; when structurally intact, prevents unwanted nasal resonance or nasal airflow emissions; needed for intraoral pressure
		Portion that is posterior to the alveolar ridge can be coupled with the tongue blade to participate in producing lingua-palatal phonemes /ʃ/, /ʒ/, /tʃ/, /dʒ/, /r/, and /j/
		When the alveolar ridge of the hard palate is coupled with the tongue tip, it participates in producing lingua-alveolar phonemes /t/, /d/, /s/, /z/, /l/, and /n/
Maxillary incisors[a]	Stationary	Working together with the tongue tip and mandibular incisors, participates in producing interdental sounds /θ/ and /ð/
		When coupled with the lower lip, participates in producing labial-dental consonants /f/ and /v/
Mandibular incisors[a]	Movable	Working together with the tongue tip and maxillary incisors, participates in producing interdental sounds /θ/ and /ð/
Lower lip[a]	Movable	When coupled with the maxillary incisors, participates in producing labial-dental consonants /f/ and /v/
		When coupled with the upper lip, participates in producing the bilabial consonants /p/, /b/, /m/, and /w/
Upper lip[a]	Movable	When coupled with the lower lip, participates in producing the bilabial consonants /p/, /b/, /m/, and /w/
Mandible (jaw)	Movable	Raises and lowers to change the size and shape of the oral cavity for articulation and resonance
Maxilla	Stationary	Articulates with palatine bone; partial barrier between the nasal and oral cavities; foundation for maxillary dentition

[a]Can be viewed (or partially viewed) via the oral orifice.

Table C–2. The Eight Valves That Modify the Moving Airstream for Speech

Valve	Parts	What Can Be Accomplished at that Valve Location
Laryngeal (direct visual inspection requires instrumentation)	Two vocal folds	Phonation
		Place of articulation for voiceless laryngeal fricative /h/
		Place of articulation for glottal stop /ʔ/, which is part of some dialect or may be used due to compromised palatal or velar integrity
		Place of articulation for compensatory stops and fricatives when palatal or velar integrity is compromised
Velopharyngeal	Velum and posterior-pharyngeal wall	Closed for most speech sounds of American English, permitting airflow to exit orally
		Open for nasal consonants, allowing airflow to exit nasally
		Important for balancing nasal and oral resonance
Lingua-velar	Posterior tongue blade and velum	Place of articulation for nasal consonant /ŋ/
		One of two valves operating for the glide /w/ and retroflex /r/
		Place of articulation for stop consonant /g/
		Place of articulation and sound source for stop-plosive consonant /k/
Lingua-palatal	Tongue blade and hard palate (posterior to alveolar ridge)	Place of articulation for glide /j/
		One of two places of narrowing for liquid retroflex /r/
		Place of articulation for fricatives /ʃ/ and /ʒ/
		Place of articulation for affricates /tʃ/ and /dʒ/
		Sound source for /ʃ/ and /tʃ/
Lingua-alveolar	Tongue tip and the alveolar ridge of the hard palate	Place of articulation for nasal consonant /n/
		Place of articulation for lateral /l/
		Place of articulation for fricatives /s/ and /z/
		Place of articulation for stop consonant /d/
		Place of articulation for stop-plosive consonant /t/
		Sound source for /s/ and /t/
Lingua-dental	Tongue tip, maxillary incisors, mandibular incisors	Place of articulation for fricatives /θ/ and /ð/
		Sound source for /θ/

continues

Table C–2. *continued*

Valve	Parts	What Can Be Accomplished at that Valve Location
Labial-dental	Lower lip and maxillary incisors	Place of articulation for fricatives /f/ and /v/
		Sound source for /f/
Bilabial	Upper and lower lips	Place of articulation for nasal consonant /m/
		One of two valves operating for the glide /w/
		Place of articulation for stop consonant /b/
		Place of articulation for stop-plosive consonant /p/
		Sound source for /p/

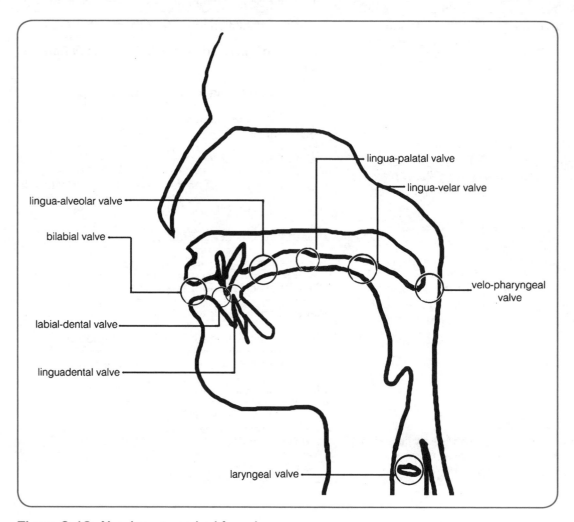

Figure C–1C. Vocal tract, marked for valves.

Respiration

Simply stated, respiration is the exchange of gases between an organism and its atmosphere (Zemlin, 1998). This process brings oxygen to the organism through inspiration, thereby supporting life, while also expelling carbon dioxide and pollutants through expiration (Merrill, 2008; Seikel et al., 2010).

Humans recycle the exhaled air very efficiently for spoken communication. Therefore, the anatomic parts that enable respiration are germane to oral-facial evaluation, even though speech is clearly not their primary function, and most of the parts are not available for direct visual inspection without instrumentation.

Basic Anatomy of the Respiratory Subsystem

The parts of the respiratory subsystem that can be viewed without instrumentation are listed and described in Table C–3. Note that no respiratory part above or below the oropharynx can be seen directly during oral-facial inspection. Therefore, clinicians

Table C–3. Parts of the Respiratory System That May Be Directly Observed Without Instrumentation

Part	Brief Description	Significant Observations Relative to Respiration
Nasal orifices	Nares	There should be no obstructions
Nasal cavities (partially available for viewing)	Nasal passages, divided into two parts by the nasal septum, posterior to nares and superior to hard palate	There should be no obstructions
Oropharynx	Pharyngeal channel directly posterior to the faucial pillars and anterior to the posterior-pharyngeal wall	There should be no obstructions
	Visible through the mouth when open	
Torso	Trunk of the human body, from shoulders to abdomen	Optimally, the lower torso expands and contracts during breathing cycles (diaphragmatic breathing)
		Rhythmic lower thoracic movement may be acceptable if the person does not have a public speaking role but is not ideal and may lead to pathology
		Rhythmic raising and lowering of the shoulders or upper thoracic expansion and contraction during respiration indicates clavicular breathing or upper thoracic breathing, respectively, neither of which adequately supports speech
		At rest, inspiration and expiration phases of the respiratory cycle are equal in duration. During speech, the inspiratory phase is short, and the expiratory phase is much longer.

APPENDIX C

inspect the components indirectly through listening and by watching the person's breathing patterns.

The remaining parts of the respiratory system are either completely or partially hidden from direct viewing. Some can be viewed directly by instrumentation, others through surgery or autopsy, both of which are beyond the scope of a routine oral-facial inspection. Since these occult parts are significant to the breath supply required for speech and their function can be judged to some extent indirectly, they are listed and briefly described in Tables C–4 and C–5.

Muscles of respiration, including those used for both inhalation and exhalation, are briefly listed and described in Tables C–6 through C–8. Note some muscles of respiration also assist with posture and serve to stabilize the body's core.

Basic Physiology of Inhalation

Since the lungs are freely suspended within the framework of the thoracic cavity and not attached to any muscles (Figure C–2), inhalation is accomplished by using muscles to expand the size of the thorax, forcing air to rush into the lungs via the respiratory tract. Air from outside the body rushes in because pressure within any chamber (e.g., thoracic cavity) seeks equilibrium with the pressure outside the chamber (e.g., atmosphere) when an opening allows passage between the two (e.g., respiratory tract). This natural physical principle is the same notion used in the design of manometers and barometers (Knight, 2013; Seikel et al., 2010).

The diaphragm is the principal muscle used to expand the thorax for inspiration (see Table C–6).

Table C–4. Soft Tissues of the Respiratory Tract and Esophagus

Part	Brief Description	Functional Highlights
Respiratory tract	Nasal passages	• Provides airway passage between external environment and the lungs • Primarily used for inspiration and expiration
	Nasopharynx	
	Oropharynx[a]	
	Laryngopharynx	
	Larynx	
	Trachea	
Lungs	A pair of free-floating organs suspended within the thorax	The structures through which the body continually refreshes the blood's oxygen supply, while at the same time ridding itself of carbon dioxide and other pollutants
	Composed of rich blood supply, connective tissue, bronchial tubes, and tissue specialized for gas exchange	
Esophagus	Not part of the respiratory tract but may become part of the vocal system in voice restoration after laryngectomy	
	Runs parallel to the trachea and immediately behind it	

[a]Only the oropharynx is available for viewing without instrumentation.

Table C–5. Internal-Bony Framework of the Respiratory System

Part	Brief Description	Functional Highlights
Pectoral girdle	Includes scapula and clavicle bones that support upper extremities	
	Provides attachment for muscles that are useful for raising the rib cage during inspiration	
	Attaches to the sternum	
Rib cage	Twelve pairs of ribs that are attached posteriorly to 12 thoracic vertebrae. Seven are attached anteriorly to the sternum, three are attached indirectly to the sternum via cartilage, and two are not attached (i.e., floating ribs).	
	Provides attachment for many muscles that provide strength, rigidity, continuity, and mobility to the rib cage for respiration	
Sternum	Articulates with the clavicle and first seven ribs	Provides the thoracic cavity with stability and protection
	Cartilaginous attachment to ribs 8 through 10 allows rib cage to rotate slightly during respiration	
Spinal column	Comprises 32 to 33 contiguous and joined vertebral segments	
	Houses spinal cord with spinal nerves	
	Spinal nerves that innervate muscles of respiration arise from cervical vertebrae 1 through 7 and thoracic vertebrae 1 through 12	
	Processes serve as attachment for several muscles	
	Articulates with rib cage, providing stability and mobility for respiration and posture	
Pelvic girdle	At the base of the spinal column	
	Coxal (i.e., hip) bones	

Table C–6. The Diaphragm: Primary Muscle of Inspiration

Brief Description of Diaphragm	Innervation	Functional Highlights of the Diaphragm
The primary muscle of inspiration	Spinal nerves arising from vertebrae C3 through C5	When contracted, increases the vertical dimension of the thorax for inspiration (shortens the central tendon)
Separates the thorax from the abdomen		Compresses the abdominal viscera on contraction
Foramen allows structures to pass through (e.g., spinal column)		When relaxed, decreases the vertical dimension of the thorax for expiration

Table C–7. Accessory Muscles of Inspiration: Muscles of Thorax, Neck, and Back

Thorax, Neck, or Back Muscle	Muscle	Innervation	Functional Highlights
Thorax	External intercostal muscles	Intercostal nerves (spinal nerves arising from T1 through T6)	Increase the transverse dimension of the thorax for inspiration
		Thoroabdominal intercostal nerves (spinal nerves arising from T7 through T11)	
	Pectoralis major and pectoralis minor	Spinal nerves arising from C5 through C8	May be useful for deep inhalation
Neck	Scalene muscles (anterior, medius, posterior)	Spinal nerves arising from C2 through C8	Assist with elevating the rib cage, allowing air to rush in. At least low-level involvement with every inhalation, increased activity with increased respiratory effort
	Sternocleidomastoid muscle	Cranial nerve XI. Spinal nerves arising from C1 through C5	Assist with elevating the rib cage, allowing air to rush in
Back	Quadratus lumborum muscle		Provide stability
	Latissimus dorsal muscle		
	Serratus posterior superior muscle	Spinal nerves arising from T2 and T3	
	Serratus posterior inferior muscle	Spinal nerves arising from T9 through T12	
	Serratus anterior muscle	Spinal nerves arising from C5 through C7, T2 and T3	
	Levator costalis muscle (brevis and longus)	Spinal nerves arising from C8 through T11	
	Subclavius	Spinal nerves arising from C5 and C6	

It is the large muscle that serves as the thoracic floor, forming a dividing wall between the thorax and abdomen. When contracted, the diaphragm descends, increasing the thorax's vertical dimension. Although quiet inspiration can be accomplished using diaphragmatic contraction alone, the accessory muscles of inhalation can assist by expanding the rib cage, thereby increasing the transverse thoracic dimension as well. Greater respiratory needs associated with forced inspiration or physical exer-

Table C–8. Muscles of Forced Expiration: Not Very Active During Passive Breathing

	Muscle or Muscle Group	Innervation	Primary Purpose/Basic Description
Abdominal muscles	Transverse abdominis	Spinal nerve arising from T7 through L1	Compresses anterior and lateral walls of the abdomen
	External oblique	Spinal nerves arising from T7 through T12	Pulls ribs downward, compresses the lateral and anterior walls of the abdomen
	Rectus abdominis	Spinal nerves arising from T7 through T12	Pulls down on the sternum, lowers the rib cage, compresses anterior abdominal wall
	Internal oblique	Spinal nerves arising from T7 through L1	Pulls rib cage downward, compresses anterior and lateral abdominal walls
Thoracic muscles	Internal intercostals	T2 to T11	Pull down on the rib cage; decrease transverse dimension of the thorax
	Lateral iliocostalis lumborum		Depresses the rib cage
	Lateral iliocostalis thoracis		Works with lateral iliocostalis lumborum to stabilize back of the rib cage wall
	Subcostal muscles	Spinal nerves arising from T1 through T11	Pulls down on the rib cage
	Transverse thoracic	Spinal nerves arising from T2 through T6	Pulls down on ribs 2 through 6
Back	Latissimus dorsi	Spinal nerves arising from C6 through C8	Contraction lowers the rib cage wall
	Quadrarus lumborum	Spinal nerves arising from T12 through L3	Pulls down on rib 12
	Serratus posterior-inferior	Spinal nerves arising from T9 through T12	Depresses ribs 8 through 12, pulling the rib cage down

tion increase the number of muscles employed for inhalation (Perri & Halford, 2004; Seikel et al., 2010). See Table C–7.

When the thoracic cavity increases its vertical and transverse dimensions, the air molecules in the lungs spread out to accommodate the larger space, resulting in lower air pressure within the cavity compared to the atmospheric pressure outside. As a result, air automatically flows into the respiratory tract, usually via the nasal orifice, finding its way to the lungs where the vital gas exchange occurs.

Basic Physiology of Exhalation

Once the gas exchange has taken place in the lungs, the air that contains waste gases must be expelled, making room for the next inspiratory phase where more oxygen-bearing air is carried into the lungs for

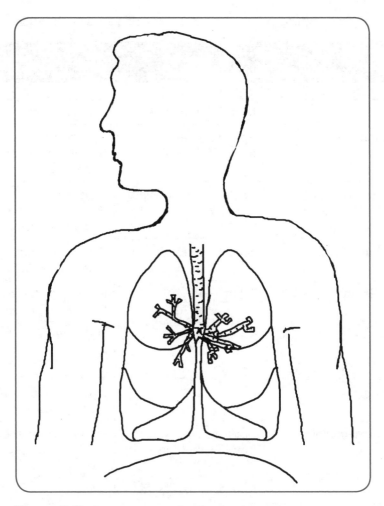

Figure C–2. Lungs suspended in the thorax.

processing. The act of exhaling is generally accomplished by relaxing the diaphragm, which causes it to ascend naturally. As a result, the thorax shrinks, resuming its previous vertical dimension. This causes air molecules inside the lungs to huddle more closely together, increasing the likelihood of collision due to crowding. The increased thoracic pressure instantly forces air molecules to exit the body as the internal chamber (i.e., lungs) and external atmosphere seek equilibrium. Consequently, exhalation is accomplished naturally and effortlessly (Knight, 2013; Seikel et al., 2010).

Forced Expiration

The act of forcing expiration, however, may require additional muscle involvement since reducing the transverse thoracic dimension is needed for the act of forcing air out of the body. The muscles of forced expiration are comparable to a cummerbund, wrapping the abdomen neatly on all sides. Contracting this muscle group essentially squeezes the abdomen, similarly forcing the air out of the lungs via the respiratory tract (Seikel et al., 2010). See Table C–8 for muscles of forced expiration.

Concluding Remarks on Respiration

Normally, resting inhalation and exhalation are accomplished via the nasal orifices and require no conscious effort. The only discernible manifestation, if any, should be a slight inaudible and rhythmic expansion and contraction of the abdomen.

The unmodified moving airstream that exits the body through the respiratory tract is the raw medium for speech production. To produce intelligible speech, however, the flow of air must be captured and then modified in three ways; the first modification is known as phonation.

Phonation

The first virtual valve that airflow encounters after it exits the lungs while traveling upward through the vocal tract is housed within the larynx and comprises the two vocal folds (see Table C–2). During nonspeech respiration, the vocal folds (i.e., laryn-geal valve) are normally in the abducted position (Figure C–3A), creating a space between the folds known as the glottis. When intending to speak, normally the person adducts the folds (Figure C–3B) at the time of exhalation, then forces air between the adducted folds, thus using airflow as a medium for voice production (Figure C–3C), as explained below.

Since none of the laryngeal parts are available for viewing in the absence of instrumentation, and since the simple oral-facial inspection does not involve instruments, our comments in this section are limited to information needed for screening vocal fold function and laryngeal integrity through listening alone. Therefore, discussion of laryngeal anatomy may seem brief.

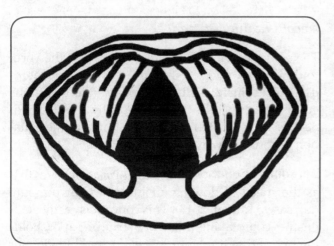

A

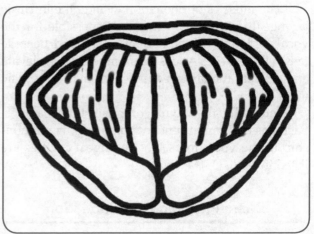

B

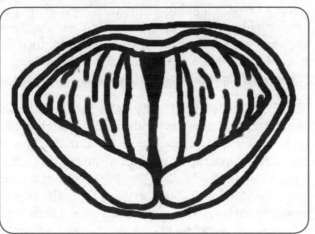

C

Figure C–3. **A.** Vocal folds, abducted position. **B.** Vocal folds, adducted position. **C.** Vocal folds, adducted, air forcing through.

Basic Laryngeal Anatomy

The larynx is a musculocartilaginous structure located at the superior end of the trachea and inferior to the pharynx. Its framework from bottom to top is essentially outlined in Table C–9. There are only two pairs of movable joints within the laryngeal structure, and these serve key functions relative to voice production. The cricoarytenoid joint permits the arytenoids to rock, glide, and minimally rotate, enabling the vocal folds to adduct, which is essential to phonation. The cricothyroid joint permits the thyroid movement that is essential to pitch control.

Extrinsic membranes connect the musculocartilaginous larynx to the hyoid bone above and the trachea below (Table C–10). Likewise, intrinsic membranes connect the laryngeal cartilages to one another (Table C–11).

The muscles of phonation include the intrinsic laryngeal muscles, which make it possible for the vocal folds to adduct, abduct, relax, and become tense (Table C–12). Additionally, muscles that elevate and depress the laryngeal mechanism are extrinsic to it (Table C–13).

Internally, the larynx comprises three cavities. Each has a different function, based on its relationship to the vocal folds. The laryngeal cavities are listed in Table C–14.

Basic Physiology of Phonation

Voice production is possible because the moving airstream is capable of setting adducted vocal folds into vibration, creating audible turbulence while the air passes through the constricted glottis (see Figure C–3C). Although the muscles of phonation mentioned earlier are responsible for positioning the folds and even adjusting their length, they do not contribute to the vibrations that are fundamental to voice production. As a matter of fact, vocal fold vibration is a passive aeromechanical event (Wolfe et al., 2009).

Although an undisputed explanation for vocal fold vibration has not yet been universally accepted or proven and many theories have been offered, the myoelastic-aerodynamic theory of phonation is most widely received. The *myoelastic-aerodynamic theory of phonation* is useful in explaining the probable relationship between air passing between the adducted folds and passive vocal fold vibrations (Behrman, 2013; Fuller et al., 2012; Seikel et al., 2010).

The theory comprises myoelastic and aerodynamic elements as its name suggests. Before delving into a full description of the theory, let us consider its three elements separately.

Myoelastic Element

The myoelastic element recognizes that vocal fold tissues are elastic. From a physical science perspective, the term *elasticity* applies to solid masses (e.g., vocal folds) that, if stretched or repositioned in response to an applied force (e.g., moving airstream), are inclined to return to their original position or dimension after the force is removed (Knight, 2013).

Aerodynamic Element

The aerodynamic element recognizes that the vocal folds and moving airstream are subject to aerodynamic principles. Two aerodynamic equations govern the principles that theoretically apply to phonation. They are Bernoulli's equation and the equation of continuity, explained as follows.

Bernoulli's Equation. *Bernoulli's equation* states that as the speed of flowing air increases, air pressure decreases (Knight, 2013). This concept is easily demonstrated by taking a narrow strip of paper, holding one end of it to your lower lip, and blowing air straight out over the top of the paper strip, thus creating a rapidly flowing airstream above the paper. One might presuppose that blowing the air above the strip would force the strip downward. Instead, in conformity to Bernoulli's equation, the strip rises toward the rapidly flowing airstream. Try it!

The Equation of Continuity. The equation of continuity states that when fluid travels through a tube (e.g., air traveling through the vocal tract), flow is faster in the narrower parts of a tube (e.g., glottis) than in wider parts (Knight, 2013). Therefore, you may assume that the air traveling through the narrower space between the folds travels at a faster rate than the air traveling above and below the glottal opening (see Figure C–1B).

Table C–9. The Cartilaginous Laryngeal Framework

Part	Brief Description and Location
Cricoid cartilage (a single cartilage)	Occupies most of the inferior part of the larynx
	A complete signet-shaped ring, narrow anterior, and broader posterior lamina
	Rests atop the superior-most tracheal ring; articulates with trachea by way of the cricotracheal ligament
	The posterior surface is larger, and posterior-superior surface articulates with the arytenoid cartilages at the cricoarytenoid joint
	Exterior lateral surfaces articulate with the paired inferior horns (i.e., cornua) of the thyroid cartilage (i.e., cricothyroid joint)
	Hosts the only movable joints of the larynx (i.e., paired cricothyroid joints and paired cricoarytenoid joints)
Thyroid cartilage (a single cartilage)	Largest cartilage, comprises most of the anterior larynx
	Protects the vocal folds
	Resides directly above the cricoid cartilage; articulates with it at the cricothyroid joint
	Thyroid notch, at the superior juncture of the two lamina (anterior thyroid)
	Angular protuberance (Adam's apple)—anterior
	Two sets of horns (superior and interior cornua)
	Paired inferior horns articulate with the external lateral surfaces of the cricoid cartilage, forming the cricothyroid joint
Epiglottis (a single cartilage)	A leaf-like structure behind the hyoid bone
	Function—cover laryngeal opening during deglutination (swallowing); a safety valve
Arytenoid cartilages (paired)	Pyramid shape
	Reside on the upper posterior surface of the cricoid cartilages
	The posterior point of attachment for the paired vocal folds
	Can approximate at midline via muscle contraction, adducting the folds
Corniculate cartilages (paired)	Rest on the superior apices of the arytenoids
	Notable landmarks on the aryepiglottic folds
Cuneiform cartilages (paired)	Embedded within the aryepiglottic folds (when present)
	Not always present
Hyoid bone	Not part of the musculocartilaginous structure but of critical importance to the laryngeal framework and provides stability to it
	Superior to musculocartilaginous laryngeal structure
	Articulates with superior paired horns of the thyroid cartilage via lateral hypothyroid ligaments

Table C–10. Extrinsic Laryngeal Membranes: Connect Laryngeal Cartilages to Hyoid Bone Above and Trachea Below

Membrane	Function
Thyrohyoid membrane	Connect thyroid cartilage to hyoid bone
Lateral thyrohyoid ligaments	Connect superior cornua of thyroid to major cornua of hyoid bone
Hyoepiglottal ligament	Connects epiglottis to hyoid bone
Thyroepiglottal ligament	Connects epiglottis to thyroid cartilage
Cricotracheal ligament	Connects cricoid cartilages to first tracheal ring

Table C–11. Intrinsic Laryngeal Membranes: Connect Laryngeal Cartilages to Each Other

Membrane	Brief Description
Conus elasticus	Comprised of medial cricothyroid ligament and lateral cricothyroid membranes
	Connects thyroid, cricoid, and arytenoid cartilages
Quadrangular membrane	Connect the epiglottis, thyroid, corniculate cartilages, and arytenoid cartilages
Aryepiglottic folds	Extends from the epiglottis to the arytenoids
Anterior lateral and posterior ceratocricoid ligaments	Reinforce cricothyroid articulation on both sides
Thyroepiglottic ligament	Attaches thyroid cartilage to epiglottis
Posterior cricoarytenoid ligament	Attaches cricoid and arytenoid cartilages

The Myoelastic-Aerodynamic Theory of Phonation

Let us combine these three ideas (i.e., elasticity relative to vocal fold composition, Bernoulli's equation, and the equation of continuity). By so doing, we can briefly explain how the myoelastic-aerodynamic theory is believed to influence vocal fold behavior during phonation.

First, although the folds normally rest in an abducted position for respiration (see Figure C–3A), a speaker adducts the folds to produce voice (see Figure C–3B). Adducting the folds places them in position of being an elastic obstruction that stands in the way of the moving airstream. Upon encountering the adducted folds, because they are elastic in nature, the force of the moving airstream in effect blows them apart (see Figure C–3C). Due to

Table C–12. Intrinsic Muscles of Phonation: Connect Laryngeal Cartilages to Each Other and Enable Vocal Folds' Abduction, Adduction, and Relaxation

Muscle or Muscle Group (With Brief Description)	Innervation	Primary Purpose
Lateral cricoarytenoid muscle	Cranial Nerve X	Vocal fold adduction and relaxation
Transverse arytenoids muscle	Cranial Nerve X	Vocal fold adduction
Oblique arytenoids muscle	Cranial Nerve X	Vocal fold adduction
Posterior cricoarytenoid muscle	Cranial Nerve X	Vocal fold abduction, by pulling arytenoids backward and outward
Cricothyroid muscle	Cranial Nerve X	Increase vocal fold tension by increasing the distance between the thyroid and arytenoid cartilages
		Depress the thyroid cartilage when cricoid cartilage is anchored
		Elevates the cricoid cartilage when thyroid cartilage is anchored
Thyrovocalis muscle (a part of thyroarytenoid muscle)	Cranial Nerve X	Increase vocal fold tension; may assist with adduction
Thyromuscularis (a part of thyroarytenoid muscle)	Cranial Nerve X	Adducts, lengthens, relaxes vocal folds
Superior thyroarytenoid muscle	Cranial Nerve X	Tilts the thyroid back to relax vocal folds; pulls muscular processes forward for medial compression
Thyroepiglottic muscle	Cranial Nerve X	Dilates the airway
Aryepiglottic muscle	Cranial Nerve X	Constricts the laryngeal opening

the equation of continuity, however, the air pressure between the folds is less than air pressure throughout the wider portions of the channel; therefore, the airflow between the folds moves faster than the airflow above and below them. Moreover according to Bernoulli's equation, the air pressure at the site of the folds is less, due to its increased velocity. This sets the stage to draw the elastic vocal folds back together, much like the strip of paper that is drawn upward in the exercise described earlier.

When the airstream is moving upward while the vocal folds are in an adducted position, the cycle of opening and closing according to these physical principles is repeated rapidly, roughly 100 to 400 cycles per second, with the range of cycles per second varying according to age and gender.

Applying the Myoelastic-Aerodynamic Theory to Vocal Physiology. During speech, vocal fold vibration is the sound source for all vowels and more than half of the consonants (i.e., voiced consonants). Yet some consonants require that the vibration not happen (i.e., voiceless consonants), relying on various other valves to serve as an alternate sound source,

Table C–13. Laryngeal Levators and Depressors

	Muscle	Innervation	Primary Purpose
Laryngeal elevators	Digastricus (anterior belly)	Cranial Nerve V	Elevates the hyoid bone (and, with it, the larynx) or depresses the mandible
	Digastricus (posterior belly)	Cranial Nerve VII	
	Stylohyoid	Cranial Nerve VII	Moves hyoid bone up and back
	Mylohyoid	Cranial Nerve V	Elevates the hyoid
			Depresses the mandible
	Geniohyoid	Cranial Nerve XII Spinal nerve arising from C1	With mandible anchored, pulls hyoid bone up and forward
	Thyropharyngeus	Cranial Nerve X	Constricts pharynx
			Elevates larynx
Laryngeal depressors	Sternohyoid	Cranial Nerve XII Spinal nerves arising from C1 through C3	Depresses hyoid
	Omohyoid		
	Sternothyroid		
	Thyrohyoid	Cranial Nerve XII Spinal nerves arising from C1 and C2	Depresses hyoid
			Elevates larynx
Tongue muscles that serve as discretionary elevators	Genioglossus	Cranial Nerve XII	Elevates hyoid to position the larynx; also serves an extrinsic muscle of the tongue
	Hyoglossus muscle	Cranial Nerve XII	Elevates hyoid, may help position larynx
			Depresses tongue (an extrinsic tongue muscle)

Table C–14. Laryngeal Cavities

Cavity	Brief Description
Vestibule	Additus larynges to ventricular vocal folds (just above true vocal folds), a part of the laryngeal resonating cavity
Ventricle	Ventricular vocal folds to true vocal folds; portion of the laryngeal resonating cavity, closest to the sound source
Subglottal region	Includes true folds, to the inferior border of the cricoid cartilage; the sound source as well as the space directly below it where pressure builds to allow for phonation

a topic whose detail is deferred to the section that addresses articulation.

Hence, normally under circumstances of connected speech, the laryngeal valve engages for phonation as needed, alternately refraining from phonation appropriately as well. As a demonstration, say the phrase "respiration and phonation" aloud (i.e., /ˈrɛs pə e ʃən ænd foʊ ˈne ʃən/). Note that the vocal folds begin and end in the adducted position, but abduct four times during the short phrase to stop the vibrations while saying voiceless /sp/, /ʃ/, /f/, and again /ʃ/.

Rapid vocal fold vibration results in an audible buzz that, although not recognizable as human voice without further modification, becomes the sound source for most speech sounds. The following sections shed light on the other two modifications that the airstream undergoes as it becomes intelligible speech: resonance and articulation.

Preliminary Comments Relevant to Discussing Resonance and Articulation

Many scholars handle resonance and articulation together (Fuller et al., 2012; Lass, 2013; Seikel et al., 2010); similarly, the two topics are frequently deliberated separately (Bauman-Waengler, 2012; Boone, McFarlane, Von Berg, & Zraick, 2010; Gordon-Brannan & Weiss, 2007; Shipley & McAfee, 2008; Wolfe, Garnier, & Smith, 2009). Clearly, there is tremendous overlap between the two subjects, and it is possible to discuss them together or separately depending on the angle of approach.

Generally, though, the lists of anatomic parts involved in both resonance and articulation are quite similar. Furthermore, the acts of resonance and articulation transpire concurrently, creating a large degree of interdependence between the two aspects of speech production. Yet, for the purpose of discussion, it can be helpful to separate them artificially, while recognizing that neither occurs independently of the other. Therefore, we present the topic of resonance first, followed by the topic of articulation and referring back to the section on resonance frequently as needed.

Resonance

Generally speaking, resonance of any kind results from vibrations within one or more chambers that are located in the vicinity of a sound source (Stedman, 2005). The chamber selectively amplifies the aspects of the sound source that are most compatible with its natural resonating frequency. Resonance, therefore, enhances the character of a raw sound produced by vibration. Box C–3 expands on this idea.

It follows, then, that in order for vocal fold vibration (i.e., phonation) to convert from a nondescript buzz into a recognizable human voice, the sound that the vocal folds emit sets a series of nearby air-filled resonating chambers into a vibrating pattern, conferring on the voice traits such as fullness, richness, and depth, giving each person's voice a distinct character based on the size and shape of the resonating chambers (Lass, 2013; Wolfe et al., 2009), which are listed in Table C–15 and illustrated in Figure C–4.

Box C–3. Resonating Chambers

The vocal tract and sinuses serve as a series of multiresonant chambers that reside within the vicinity of the vocal sound source. Each compartment amplifies the vocal sound at its own resonant frequency, creating a voice that is not only uniquely human but also distinct to the individual speaker.

The same principle applies to musical instruments. For example, a violin's resonating chamber is different in size and shape compared with that of the cello's, and this difference clearly affects the type of sound that either stringed instrument is capable of producing. Also, even within instruments, certain violins are more desirable than others because of the quality of their tone, largely attributable to the quality of the resonating chamber's size, shape, and even composition (Parker, 2009).

APPENDIX C

Table C–15. Resonating Chambers

	Part	Brief Description
Vocal tract resonating chambers	Laryngopharynx	Portion of vocal tract that is directly inferior to the oropharynx and directly superior to the vocal folds; includes the laryngeal vestibule and ventricle
	Oropharynx[a]	Space directly posterior to the oral cavity
		Anterior border: faucial pillars
		Superior border: velum
		Posterior border: pharyngeal wall
		Inferior border: hyoid bone (not visible)
	Oral cavity[b]	The interior of the mouth
		Anterior border: the lips
		Superior border: hard and soft palates
		Posterior border: faucial pillars
		Inferior border: the tongue
		Lateral borders: cheeks (including the small buccal cavities)
	Nasopharynx	The space directly above the velum
		Contains the adenoids
	Nasal passages[a]	The paired nasal passages, separated by the nasal septum
		Anterior border: nares (also called nostrils)
		Inferior border: hard palate (comprised of maxillae and palatine bone)
Noteworthy resonating sinuses	Maxillary sinus	Chambers within the skeletal structure of the cranium or face that normally contain air and contribute to resonance, have canals to equalize pneumonic pressure and drain mucus
	Frontal sinus	
	Ethmoid sinus	
	Sphenoid sinus	

[a]Partially observable without instrumentation.
[b]Directly observable without instrumentation.

Essentially, the vocal tract and sinuses function as a multicomponent resonator. Each vocal tract segment and sinus chamber selectively increases the amplitude of vocal fold vibrations that are similar to its own natural resonating frequency, producing a complex sound that is highly recognizable as human voice and unique to each person's individual vocal tract (Dworkin et al., 2004; Lass, 2013).

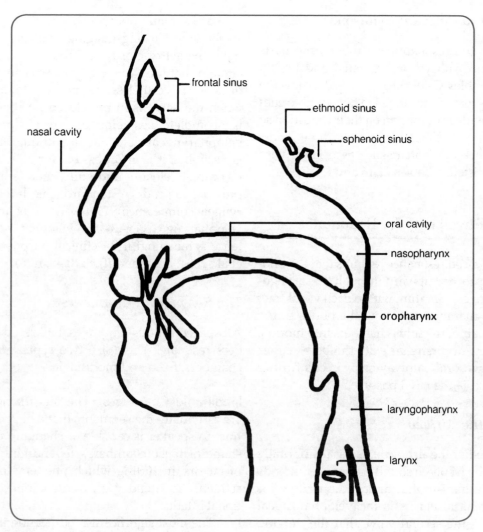

Figure C–4. Resonating chambers.

Resonance Balance and Imbalance

Normally, the entire tract functions in unison as a multiresonant tube. Properly balanced resonance results and is easily recognized perceptually. The resonating chambers involved in human speech are listed in Table C–15.

When resonance is imbalanced, the tube's equilibrium is off, and this may manifest in various ways depending on the part or parts of the tube involved in the disturbance. For example, *pharyngeal*, *hypernasal*, and *hyponasal* resonance are characterized by disproportionate focus relative to one or more of the vocal tract segments. On the other hand, the term *mixed* resonance implies disproportionate focus that shifts between or involves imbalance relative to two or more segments (Kummer, 2008).

Lastly, cul-de-sac resonance occurs when the vibrating air within the chamber or chambers is not part of a moving airstream but instead comprises stationary air vibrating within a resonating chamber. The cul-de-sac voice is perceived as muffled and has differing characteristics depending on the chamber that holds the vibrating but stationary air: oral cul-de-sac resonance, nasal cul-de-sac resonance, and pharyngeal cul-de-sac resonance (Kummer, 2008).

Basic Anatomy Relevant to Resonance

In addition to the resonating chambers, the parts of the resonance subsystem are listed and briefly described in Tables C–16 through C–20. Although some parts are visible and some are not, audible cues frequently provide information on their condition so that follow-up and clinical decisions can be made. Bony framework and soft tissues associated with resonance are listed in Tables C–16 and C–17.

Basic Physiology for Resonance

In essence, balanced resonance requires that the phonated airflow proceed upward through the laryngo- and oropharynges, vibrating within each vocal tract segment (i.e., chamber), affecting the bones of the skull to set the air of the sinus chambers into motion. Then the resonant airstream exits the body either through an open oral pathway or proceeds further upward to exit via the nasal passages.

Redirecting the Airflow

Normally, whether the airflow exits nasally or orally depends on which speech sound the speaker intends to say. The mechanism that directs the airflow for either oral or nasal egress is the velopharyngeal valve, which is the second valve that the moving airstream encounters during speech (Tables C–2 and C–19; see Figure 2–32 and Figure C–2).

The velopharyngeal valve is capable of closing with a sphincter-like action that cannot be observed via the oral orifice since the velopharyngeal act takes place beyond the palate and above the level of the oropharynx. Aspects of velopharyngeal closure that can be observed through the oral orifice are movement, symmetry, physical condition of the observable parts, and possibly some indicators of obstruction (Kummer, 2008).

However, it is important to note that when closed, the normally functioning velopharyngeal valve alternately prevents and allows the airflow from proceeding upward toward the nasal egress. Velopharyngeal closure is necessary for all vowels and nearly all consonants of American English, as well as for many nonspeech activities (e.g., kissing, swallowing, sucking, gagging, and vomiting). Essentially the act of closure is an all-or-none phenomenon in that the valve either closes completely or it does not; nevertheless, it is possible for air to escape when the valve is in the closed position if closure is incomplete (i.e., velopharyngeal incompetence or velopharyngeal deficiency). Although a tight seal is desirable, it is also possible for a person to have incomplete closure and still generate enough oral pressure to produce standard speech (i.e., velopharyngeal competence). Thus, distinguishing between velopharyngeal closure and velopharyngeal competence is meaningful for clinical purposes (Dworkin et al., 2004; Kummer, 2008; Riski, n.d.).

The Resonating Chambers

All speech sounds require that all resonating chambers resonate. There are two types of resonating chambers: fixed and modifiable.

Modifiable Chambers. The modifiable chambers are essentially the segments that comprise the vocal tract. A speaker is capable of changing the size and shape of these chambers, depending on a variety of factors, including which phoneme or phoneme sequence is intended, prosodic variations, or emotional intent.

The most significant modification that resonating chambers accomplish is the coupling and uncoupling of the nasal and oral cavities as controlled by the velopharyngeal mechanism. Changing the size and shape of the oral cavity by mandibular and lingual movements is also highly significant to resonance. More subtle changes in the upper larynx and pharynges also contribute to normal changes in resonant speech.

In addition to being subject to speaker-controlled adjustments, it is the balance between these modifiable resonating chambers that can be interrupted in the event of physical limitation or obstruction, neurologic episode, an interrupted feedback loop (e.g., deafness), or even surging emotions. Typically, symptoms of imbalance are easily recognized through listening, and some may be explored further through oral-facial inspection as described in this manual.

Table C–16. Bony Framework Required for Resonance

Part	Brief Description	Function for Resonance
Mandible	The lower jaw, including the lower dental ridge	Opens and closes to shape oral resonance
Maxillae	A paired set of bones that make up the upper jaw, including most of the hard palate, base of the nose, and upper dental ridge	Comprises most of the boundary between the oral and nasal cavities; if incomplete can interfere with balanced resonance
Palatine bones	A small complex pair of bones that make up the posterior quarter of the hard palate and extend upward to form portions of the nasal spine, nasal crest, and orbital process	Contributes to the boundary between oral and nasal cavities
		If incomplete can interfere with balanced resonance
Nasal septum	Comprises the vomer, perpendicular plate of ethmoid bone, and septal cartilage	If enlarged or significantly deviated, can interfere with nasal airflow and balanced resonance
	A dividing plate between the two nasal cavities	
Nasal conchae (nasal turbinates)	Small bones on the lateral surface of the nasal cavity; they articulate with the maxilla, palatine bone, and ethmoid bone	If overdeveloped, can interfere with nasal airflow and balanced resonance
Nasal bone	A small pair of bones that comprise the superior surface of the nose	If incomplete, may interfere with balanced resonance
	Articulate with the frontal bones, maxillae, ethmoid bone, and nasal septal cartilage	
Zygomatic bone	Also called cheekbones	
	Articulates with the maxillae, frontal bone, temporal bone, and sphenoid bone	
Lacrimal bone	Articulate with maxillae, frontal bone, nasal bone, and interior conchae	
	Comprise a small portion of the nasal wall and medial orbit	
Ethmoid bone	A complex structure at the core of the facial skeleton	
	Makes up the superior nasal septum and articulates with the middle and superior nasal conchae	
	Also articulates with the frontal bone, lacrimal bone, and maxilla	
Sphenoid bone	More complex than ethmoid bone	
	Significant in its contribution to the bony structure of the cranium	

Table C–17. Soft Tissues Associated With Resonance

Part	Brief Description	Relevance to Resonance
Velopharyngeal port[a]	The lower boundary of the nasopharynx and upper boundary of the oropharynx	• When closed, prevents expired air from exiting via the nasal cavities, forcing an oral egress; closure is important to most of the phonemes of American English
	Point of constriction for velopharyngeal closure	• When open, allows expired air to exit via the nasal passages for nasal resonance
Palatine tonsils[a]	Paired masses located on the lateral walls of the oropharynx	• If enlarged, can impede nasal resonance
	Typically pink, wrinkled, and barely peeking from behind the anterior faucial pillars	• In extreme cases, enlarged tonsils can impede velar movement • Palatine tonsils may assist with velopharyngeal closure in some cases
Pharyngeal tonsil (i.e., adenoid)	A single mass located on the posterior wall of the nasopharynx	If enlarged, can interfere with nasal resonance

[a]Directly observable without instrumentation.

Table C–18. Muscles Primarily Responsible for Velopharyngeal Closure

	Muscle	Innervation	General Function
Velar muscles	Levator veli palatine	Cranial Nerve X, also IX, XI, and XII	Elevates and retracts the posterior velum (primary elevator), in sling-like fashion; may assist in swallow reflex
	Palatopharyngus muscles (a.k.a. pharyngopalatinus)	Cranial Nerve X, possibly XI	Greater force in lowering the velum (for nasal consonants); pulls velum back; narrows the pharynx by pulling lateral walls upward and medially when velum is stable; guides bolus to lower pharynx in swallowing
	Musculus uvulae	Cranial Nerve X, possibly XI	Shortens and elevates the velum for a stronger seal, assisting levator veli palatine in velopharyngeal closure; absence can result in velopharyngeal insufficiency

Table C–18. *continued*

	Muscle	Innervation	General Function
Velar muscles *continued*	Glossopalatinus (a.k.a. palatoglossus)	Cranial Nerve X, possibly	With tongue anchored, depresses the velum, but not with as much force as palatopharyngus; elevates the tongue; may assist with pharyngeal swallow reflex
	Tensor velipalatini	Cranial Nerve V	Contraction tenses and stabilizes the velum; opens and closes eustachian tube with pumping action during swallow; unilateral action pulls velum to one side and slightly downward; bilateral contraction flattens the velum and pulls it down slightly and increases velar tension; opens lumen of the eustachian tube; may assist with pharyngeal swallow
Pharyngeal muscles	Superior pharyngeal constrictors • Buccopharyngeus • Glossopharyngeus • Mylopharyngeus • Pterygopharyngeus	Cranial Nerve X, possibly XI	Pulls the pharyngeal wall forward; constricts the diameter of the pharynx in the nasal region only; assists levatorveli palatine in creating a greater seal for velopharyngeal closure by pulling posterior-pharyngeal wall forward and lateral pharyngeal walls inward
	Middle pharyngeal constrictors • Ceratopharyngeus • Chondopharyngeus	Cranial Nerve X, possible XI	Narrows the diameter of the pharynx in the oral region only
	Inferior pharyngeal constrictors • Cricopharyngeus • Thyropharyngeus	Cranial Nerve X, possible XI	Assists in swallowing and vocal resonance by reducing the cross-sectional area of the pharyngeal lumen in the laryngeal region by forward movement of the posterior pharyngeal wall and medial movement of the lateral pharyngeal walls in sphincter-like fashion
	Salpingopharyngus	Cranial Nerve X, possible XI	Pulls lateral pharyngeal walls upward and inward, decreasing the width of the pharynx
	Stylopharyngus muscle	Cranial Nerve IX	Pulls upward on the pharynx and draws the lateral pharyngeal walls even more laterally, increasing the width of the pharynx; pulls upward on the pharynx and larynx

APPENDIX C

Table C–19. Muscles Responsible for Raising and Lowering the Mandible

	Muscle	Brief Description	Innervations
Mandibular elevators	Masseters (external and internal)	Elevates the mandible	Cranial Nerve V (trigeminal)
	Temporalis	Elevates the mandible	Cranial Nerve V (trigeminal)
		Assists with drawing back the mandible and moving it laterally	
	Internal pterygoid	Elevates the mandible	Cranial Nerve V
	Medial pterygoid (a.k.a. internal pterygoid)	Elevates the mandible; assists with protrusion	Cranial Nerve V (trigeminal)
Mandibular depressors	Digastricus anterior	Participates in depressing the mandible	Cranial Nerve V
	Digastricus posterior	Participates in depressing the mandible	Cranial Nerves VII and V
	Platysma	Depresses the mandible	Cranial Nerve VII (facial)
	Mylohyoid	With hyoid bone anchored, plays a minor role in depressing the mandible; assists with retracting the mandible	Cranial Nerve V (trigeminal)
	Geniohyoid	With hyoid bone anchored, plays minor role in depressing the mandible; assisting with retracting the mandible	Cranial Nerve XII (hypoglossal)
	Lateral (external) pterygoid	Depresses the mandible; bilateral contraction assists with protrusion; unilateral contraction assists in lateral mandibular movement	Cranial Nerve V (trigeminal)

Table C–20. Mandibular Ligaments

Ligament	Function	Connections
Temporal mandibular ligament	Vertical support	Connects mandible to zygomatic arch
Sphenomandibular ligament	Medial support	Connects mandible to sphenoid bone
Stylomandibular ligament	Posterior support	Connects mandible to styloid process

Fixed Chambers. On the other hand, fixed chambers generally retain the same size and shape regardless of speaking condition. That is, the sinuses are essentially stationary air-filled cavities within the bones of the skull for which the speaker has no effectual control over size and shape. However, speakers have within their control the ability to use the muscles of respiration to project the voice in such a way that the fixed chambers can be used more or less efficiently. For the most part, professionally trained speakers and singers skillfully exploit the benefits of the fixed chambers, while untrained speakers benefit less from the contribution that the sinus cavities may have on voice quality.

Furthermore, with regard to the fixed resonating chambers, it was mentioned that they are ideally filled with air. In cases of congestion due to infection or allergy, mucus or swollen tissue may fill or partially fill the sinus chambers temporarily. This situation impedes normal sinus resonance and influences voice quality, usually temporarily.

Auditory Feedback's Contribution to Resonance

Also, resonance balance relative to fixed and modifiable chambers is something that speakers adjust as a result of perceiving their own speech through auditory feedback. Since speakers essentially do not provide visible clues as they achieve or adjust resonance, deaf and hard-of-hearing speakers find it difficult to balance resonance in the absence of accurate and precise auditory feedback. Hence, many deaf speakers, especially those who have not had the benefit of strategically applied listening practice, use the pharyngeal chamber excessively in a cul-de-sac fashion, resulting in what may be perceived as pharyngeal cul-de-sac resonance. Atypical resonance associated with compromised hearing is not due to a problem with the resonating system but is due to the limitations in feedback system that normally enables a person to modify airflow relative to fixed and modifiable resonating chambers.

Concluding Remarks on Resonance

Balanced resonance requires that the resonating chambers and the anatomic boundaries between them are complete and intact, the velopharyngeal port opens and closes freely and symmetrically, the jaw opens and closes freely and accurately, the nasal egress is free of obstruction, the integrity of the neuromuscular system is adequate for precise and accurately timed control of the modifiable multiresonant vocal tract, the sinus chambers are filled with air and not mucous, and the speaker has adequate hearing to monitor and adjust balance accordingly. When atypical resonance is perceived, irregularities with any of these may be the source of the difficulty.

Principally, the most prominent movements that are needed to control the sizes and general shapes of the resonating chambers are the opening and closing of the velopharyngeal port, as well as the raising and lowering of the mandible, and these must be intact and properly functional. Therefore, although we recognize that finer adjustments to the multiresonant tract require ancillary muscular involvement as well, information on the muscles and ligaments required for controlling resonance is limited to those used to accomplish these two acts (see Tables C–18 through C–20).

Additionally, some adjustments to the resonating chambers result in specific speech sound productions. These are discussed in a later section.

By way of review, exhaled respiration creates the moving airstream, which becomes audible through phonation, and acquires distinct character traits by resonating in a multiresonant series of chambers.

The next and final step toward producing comprehensible speech is to alter the airflow in specific ways to create distinct speech sounds, or phonemes. Again, the eight valves (see Figure C–1C, Table C–2) are helpful in describing the exact locations and types of airflow modifications that are needed for intelligible speech.

Articulation

Basic Anatomy Relative to Articulation

The bony structures required for articulation include the hard palate, mandible, maxilla, temporomandibular joint, and dentition (Table C–21). The soft structures of articulation include the lips, tongue, and velum (Table C–22). Muscles of articulation are summarized with brief descriptions in Tables C–23 through C–25.

Table C–21. Bony Framework Associated With Articulation

	Brief Description	Function Relative to Articulation
Maxilla	An irregularly shaped bone that comprises part of the skull. It accommodates the upper teeth and participates in forming the orbits, hard palate, and nasal cavity.	Contributes to the bony barrier between the nasal and oral resonating chambers that is necessary for articulation and resonance
		Accommodates the upper teeth
Hard palate	The bony roof of the mouth and floor of the nasal cavity	Contributes to the bony barrier between the nasal and oral resonating chambers that is necessary for articulation and resonance
		Place of lingual contact for linga-alveolar and lingua-palatal consonants
Dentition	Teeth	Anterior teeth can contribute to articulation for sounds that require fricative or affricate airstream
Mandible	A U-shaped bone that forms the jaw. Posteriorly, it articulates with the temporal bone on both sides, at the location of the temporomandibular joint.	Location determines occlusion, which can influence relationship between the tongue and the palate for articulation
		Raising and lowering changes the size of the oral resonating chamber
		Raises and lowers frequently during speech
		Provides superior stability to the hyoid bone and laryngeal structure
Temporo-mandibular joint	A compound joint between the mandible and temporal bone	The primary function is to raise and lower the jaw for articulation, resonance, and eating

Table C–22. Soft Structures Associated With Articulation

	Brief Description	Function Relative to Articulation
Lips	Two muscular folds that define the anterior boundary for the oral cavity	The lips participate in articulation for the consonants /p/, /b/, /w/, and /m/, as well as for most vowels
Tongue	A moveable muscular mass that occupies the oral cavity, forms part of the floor of the oral cavity	The tongue is the principal body part used for speech articulation
Velum	Soft palate; a moveable muscular mass that extends posteriorly from the hard palate	Participates in coupling and uncoupling the oral and nasal cavities for changes in resonance
		The point of lingual contact for lingua-velar consonants
Pharyngeal wall	The visible wall located at the back of the throat	Participates in coupling and uncoupling the oral and nasal cavities for changes in resonance

Table C–23. Perioral Muscles Directly Relevant to Articulation

Muscle	Brief Description	Innervations
Obicularis oris (inferior and superior)	Constricts the oral opening; closes the mouth; puckers the lips; involved in tongue-thrust swallow	Cranial Nerve VII (facial)
Depressor angulioris (triangularis)	Helps compress upper lip against the lower lip; depresses angle of the lip and assists in compressing upper lip against lower lip	
Platysma	Helps depress the mandible; depresses and wrinkles skin of lower face and mouth	
Buccinator	Compresses the lips and cheeks against the teeth; draws corners of mouth outward	
Levatoranguli	Pulls corners of mouth upward and assists with closing the mouth by pulling lower lip upward	
Levator labii superior	Elevates and everts upper lip	
Levator labii superioris alaeque nasi	Elevates upper lip	
Mentalis	Elevates, protrudes, and everts the lower lip; wrinkles chin skin	
Risorius	Pulls mouth angle outward	
Zygomatic major	Pulls mouth angle upward and outward	
Zygomatic minor	Elevates upper lip	

APPENDIX C

As is true for all structures considered so far, many parts contributing to articulation are not directly visible in the absence of instrumentation, most notably muscles and bones. Nonetheless, some information about structure and function of these parts can be learned by inspecting the observable parts of the face and oral cavity, as instructed in Chapters 2 through 4.

Aspects of articulation that are of particular interest when inspecting the oral-facial region for speech adequacy include capacity for efficiently voicing and devoicing, adjusting resonance balance, arriving at a desired place of articulation precisely and with timeliness, and making changes to the airflow so as to adjust the manner of articulation. These aspects are discussed under the headings of sound source, resonance, place, and manner of articulation.

Sound Sources for Articulation

As mentioned previously, the first valve that the air stream encounters on its journey upward is the laryngeal valve (see Figure C–1C). It comprises two vocal folds that are capable of constricting in such a way as to produce the buzzing sound that becomes

Table C–24. Muscles of the Tongue Directly Relevant to Articulation

	Muscle	Brief Description	Innervations
Intrinsic	Superior longitudinal	Elevates, assists in protrusion, retraction, lateralization; relaxes lateral margins; deviates the tongue tip	Cranial Nerve XII (hypoglossal)
	Inferior longitudinal	Pulls tip of tongue downward, assists in retraction, shortening, protruding; deviates the tongue	
	Transverse muscles of the tongue	Provides a way for the tongue to narrow and elongate; assists in relaxing lateral margins and elevating posterior tongue	
	Vertical muscles of the tongue	Pulls the tongue down into the floor of the mouth (flattens); assists with protrusion and creating longitudinal groove	
Extrinsic	Genioglossus	Posterior fibers participate in protrusion, depression, and relaxing lateral margins of tongue; anterior fibers retract; contracting the full muscle depresses medial portion and assists with creating longitudinal groove	
	Hyoglossus	Pulls sides of tongue down; assists with retraction	
	Styloglossus	Draws tongue up and back; assists with retraction by pulling tongue toward pharynx for swallowing	
	Chondroglossus	Depresses the tongue	
	Palatoglossus	Elevates the tongue or depresses soft palate	Cranial Nerve X, possibly XI

Table C–25. Muscles That Move the Mandible Directly Relevant to Articulation

Muscle	Brief Description	Innervations
Masseter	Elevates the mandible	Cranial Nerve V (trigeminal)
Temporalis	Elevates mandible, draws it back from protrusion	
Medial pterygoid	Elevates the mandible	
Digastricus, anterior and posterior	Participate in depressing the mandible	Cranial Nerves V (trigeminal) and VII (facial)
Mylohyoid	Depresses the mandible	Cranial Nerve V (trigeminal)
Geniohyoid	Depresses the mandible	Cranial Nerve XII (hypoglossal)

the sound source for most speech sounds. Each phoneme of American English is classified according to whether it is voiced or not voiced. For all voiced phonemes, the sound source is the laryngeal buzz that was previously described as phonation. Sound sources for all standard American English consonants are displayed in Table C–26.

Table C–26. Standard Consonants of American English and Their Sound Source

Consonant	Sound Source
/h/	Laryngeal valve
/ŋ/	
/g/	
/w/	
/r/	
/dʒ/	
/ʒ/	
/j/	
/n/	
/d/	
/l/	
/z/	
/ð/	
/v/	
/m/	
/b/	
/k/	Lingua-velar valve
/tʃ/	Lingua-palatal valve
/ʃ/	
/t/	Lingua-alveolar valve
/s/	
/θ/	Lingua-dental valve
/f/	Labial-dental valve
/p/	Bilabial valve

Resonance for Articulation: Velopharyngeal Role

The second structural location that the airflow meets along its path was initially discussed under the topic of resonance (see Figure C–1C). The observable velopharyngeal valve comprises the velum and posterior-pharyngeal wall. In an open position, it redirects the airflow so that it exits through the nasal passages (see Figure 2–32B), as opposed to the oral egress that is used for most speech sounds when it is closed (see Figure 2–32A). The opening and closing of the velopharyngeal port cannot be viewed through the oral orifice during routine inspection, although velar movement can be judged superficially with regard to symmetry, condition, height, and excursion.

When the Velopharyngeal Port Is Open. A shift in airflow direction occurs when the port is open. Simultaneous to the opening of the port, the tongue rises or the lips approximate to occlude a portion of the oral orifice, allowing for partial oral resonance and full nasal resonance, while forcing the airflow to exit through the nose instead of the mouth.

This occurs for the three nasal phonemes only (i.e., /m/, /n/, /ŋ/). The amount of oral resonance for these three sounds depends on the location of constriction that prevents oral egress while the nasal and oral cavities are coupled. Specifically, the /ŋ/ phoneme's oral resonance is limited to the minuscule portion of the oral chamber that is posterior to the lingua-velar articulatory valve site (Figure C–5A). Similarly, the phoneme /n/ involves approximately two thirds of the oral chamber that lies posterior to the lingua-alveolar point of constriction (Figure C–5B), and /m/ involves nearly the full oral chamber because the bilabial barrier prevents air from exiting via the oral chamber at its anterior-most boundary (Figure C–5C).

When the Velopharyngeal Port Is Closed. The vowels and all other consonants require that the velopharyngeal valve close completely (see Figure 2–32A), preventing nasal egress of air and permitting the full impact of constriction for valves that reside within the oral chamber. Different classes of speech sounds require different levels of strength for the velopharyngeal valve, depending on manner

APPENDIX C

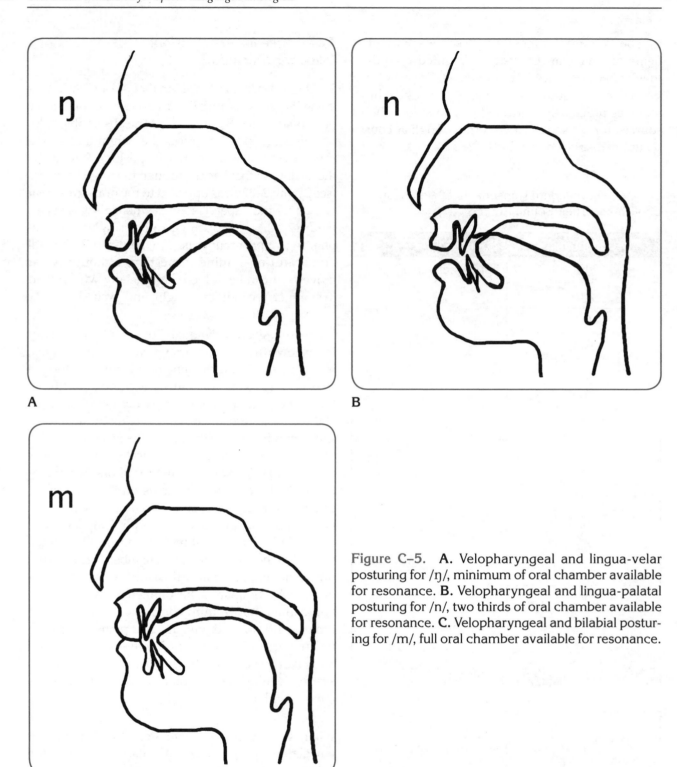

A

B

C

Figure C–5. **A.** Velopharyngeal and lingua-velar posturing for /ŋ/, minimum of oral chamber available for resonance. **B.** Velopharyngeal and lingua-palatal posturing for /n/, two thirds of oral chamber available for resonance. **C.** Velopharyngeal and bilabial posturing for /m/, full oral chamber available for resonance.

of valve constriction. For example, nasal consonants described earlier (i.e., /ŋ/, /n/, /m/) require no velopharyngeal strength since the port remains open while the nasal and oral chambers couple. Yet some phonemes are accomplished through narrowing or reshaping the oral cavity without constricting it in any way: all vowels, glides (i.e., /j/, /w/), and liquids (i.e., /r/, /l/). Due to their open-oral posture, these sounds also require very little velopharyngeal strength. Conversely, stop-plosives (i.e., /k/, /t/, /p/), stops (i.e., /g/, /d/, /b/), affricates (i.e., /tʃ/, /dʒ/), and oral fricatives (i.e., /ʃ/, /ʒ/, /s/, /z/, /θ/, /ð/, /f/, /v/) require more velopharyngeal strength, with stop-plosives requiring the most (Kent, 1994; Kummer, 2008).

Managing Velopharyngeal Action for Connected Speech. Relative to conversational speech, the three nasal consonants are peppered throughout the predominantly oral sound system. Therefore, the velopharyngeal valve must not only open and close adequately for specific speech sounds but also open and close rapidly and precisely at appropriate times during connected speech. To demonstrate, say the phrase "articulation and resonance" (i.e., /ɑɚ 'tɪk jə le ʃən ænd 'rɛ zən ɛns/) aloud. Note that your velopharyngeal valve began and ended in the closed position, while it opened and closed four times in less than 2 seconds.

Place of Articulation

Seven of the eight biomechanical valves serve as places for articulatory constriction: laryngeal, lingua-velar, lingua-palatal, lingua-alveolar, lingua-dental, labial-dental, and bilabial. Only the laryngeal valve has been discussed in detail thus far. The remaining six are fully dedicated to articulation, can be viewed for structure and function through the oral orifice, and are capable of functioning as a sound source for voiceless phonemes. Let us explore the seven valves of articulation as we continue to follow the airstream upward and outward through the vocal tract.

Laryngeal Valve as a Place of Articulation

In addition to being the sound source for all voiced phonemes, the laryngeal valve also is the place of articulation and sound source for one standard speech sound: the voiceless fricative /h/. To produce it, the vocal folds approximate while maintaining a partially abducted position, creating friction but not phonation. The vocal folds are also the articulatory

site for a phoneme that is present in many, but not all dialects of the language: the glottal stop /ʔ/. Furthermore, vocal folds can become a place of articulation for compensatory sounds when a person's oral structure does not allow for adequate intraoral pressure.

Lingua-Velar Valve as a Place of Articulation

Of the observable biomechanical valves, the posterior-most valve comprises the posterior tongue blade and velum. It is the sole place of articulation for three standard phonemes (i.e., stop-plosive /k/, stop /g/, nasal /ŋ/) and one of two points of partial constriction for the semivowels (i.e., retroflex /r/ and glide /w/).

This is the valve that closes off the oral egress entirely when the velopharyngeal port is in the open position for the nasal /ŋ/ (see Figure C–5A). All other phonemes that require constriction or partial constriction of this valve call for an open velopharyngeal port (Figure C–6A). The lingua-velar valve also serves as sound source for the voiceless consonant /k/.

Lingua-Palatal Valve as a Place of Articulation

The lingua-palatal valve comprises the tongue blade and hard palate (Figure C–6B). It is the location of articulation for two affricates (i.e., /tʃ/, /dʒ/), two fricatives (i.e., /ʃ/, /ʒ/), and one glide (i.e., /j/). The lingua-palatal valve is also one of the two points of partial approximation for the liquid retroflex (i.e., /r/). The lingua-palatal valve also serves as the sound source for voiceless phonemes /ʃ/ and /tʃ/ (see Table C–26).

Lingua-Alveolar Valve as a Place of Articulation

The lingua-alveolar valve involves the tongue tip and alveolar ridge. It is the place of articulation for one stop-plosive (i.e., /t/), one stop (i.e., /d/), two fricatives (i.e., /s/, /z/), and the lateral liquid (i.e., /l/) (Figure C–6C). It is also the site of oral egress obstruction for the nasal /n/ (see Figure C–5B). The lingua-alveolar valve is also the sound source for the voiceless phonemes /s/ and /t/ (see Table C–26).

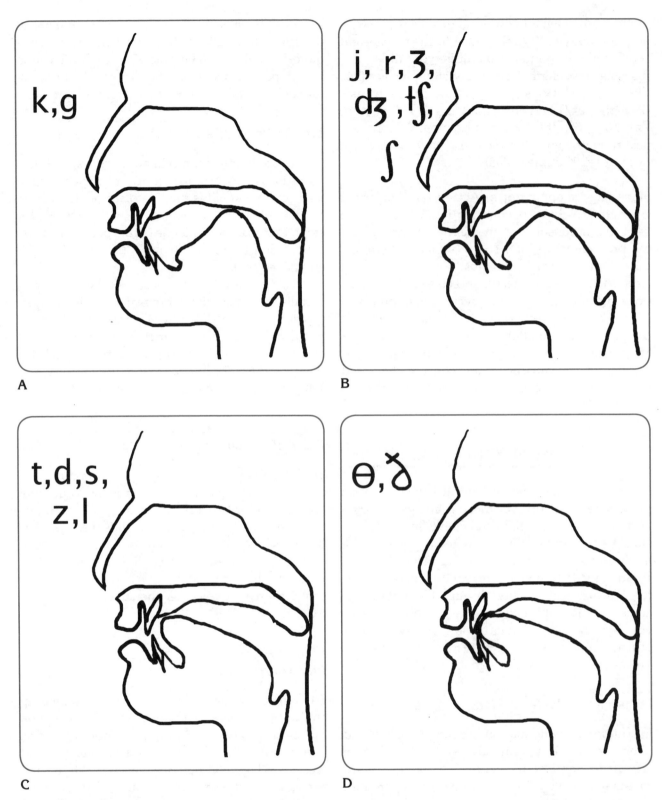

Figure C–6. **A.** Velopharyngeal and lingua-velar posturing for /k/, /g/, and /w/. **B.** Velopharyngeal and lingua-palatal posturing for /ʃ/, /ʒ/, /tʃ/, /dʒ/, /j/, and /r/. **C.** Velopharyngeal and lingua-alveolar posturing for /t/, /d/, /s/, /z/, and /l/. **D.** Velopharyngeal and lingua-dental posturing for /θ/ and /ð/. *continues*

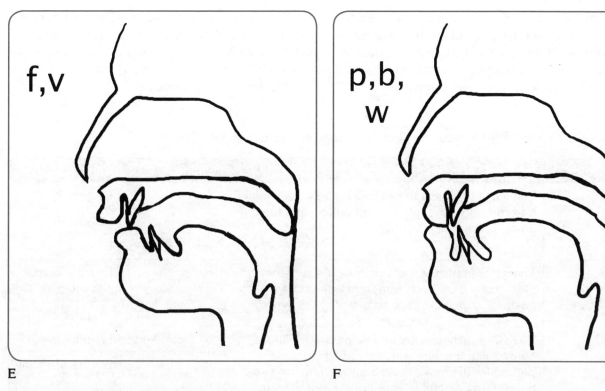

E   F

Figure C–6. *continued* **E.** Velopharyngeal and labial-dental posturing for /f/ and /v/. **F.** Velopharyngeal and bilabial posturing for /p/, /b/, and /w/.

Lingua-Dental Valve as a Place of Articulation

The lingua-dental valve, sometimes called the interdental tongue position, has three parts: maxillary incisors, mandibular incisors, and tongue tip. This valve is employed for two fricatives (i.e., /θ/, /ð/) (Figure C–6D). The lingua-dental valve is the sound source for the voiceless phoneme /θ/ (see Table C–26).

Labial-Dental Valve as a Place of Articulation

The labial-dental valve comprises the maxillary incisors and lower lip. When the two parts meet, they modify the airstream for two fricatives (i.e., /f/, /v/) (Figure C–6E). The labial-dental valve is the sound source for the voiceless phoneme /f/ (see Table C–26).

Bilabial Valve as a Place of Articulation

The bilabial valve comprises the upper and lower lips. This is the sole articulatory valve employed for one stop-plosive (i.e., /p/), one stop (i.e., /b/), and one nasal (i.e., /m/) (see Figure C–5C and Figure C–6F). It is also one of two valves that approximates when producing one glide (i.e., /w/). The bilabial valve is the sound source for the voiceless phoneme /p/ (see Table C–26).

Manner of Articulation

All eight of the valves along the vocal tract (see Table C–2 and Figure C–1C) are involved in reshaping the airstream in specific ways to form standard speech sounds used for communication. These ways of modifying the airstream are commonly called *manner of articulation.*

For most dialects of American English, the virtual valving system is capable of modifying the airflow in seven basic ways, referred to as manner of articulation. This manual uses the following labels: stop-plosive, stop, affricate, fricative, liquid, glide, and nasal. Some classification systems include additional categories for manner, but one may argue that the seven labels listed herein consume the other categories as well. For example, sibilants fit well under the category of fricative, as a subcategory.

Each biomechanical valve is capable of accomplishing at least one manner of articulation, and no one valve is used to accomplish all seven. More detailed information on the seven manners of articulation is displayed in Table C–27.

Table C–27. Manner of Articulation for American English Phonemes

Manner	How the Valve Accomplishes This Manner	Phonemes	Constricted
Nasal[a]	The valve obstructs the airflow entirely, preventing it from exiting through the oral orifice, and forcing a nasal egress of air	/ŋ/	Lingua-velar
		/n/	Lingua-alveolar
		/m/	Bilabial
Glide	The valve approximates but does not constrict, then gently transitions from that articulatory position to the next phoneme, which is a vowel	/w/	Lingua-velar and bilabial
		/j/	Lingua-palatal
Liquid	The valve reshapes the airway passage without constricting it in any way, providing a unique pattern for the moving airstream. There are two types: retroflex and lateral. For the retroflex, the tongue rises in two places, creating an airflow pattern that has a curve in it. For the lateral, the unique pathway for the airstream is divided into two parts, left and right.	/r/ (retroflex)	Lingua-palatal
		/l/ (lateral)	Lingua-alveolar
Fricative	The valve creates a narrow opening that causes noisy turbulence when the air is forced through it	/h/	Laryngeal
		/ʃ/, /ʒ/	Lingua-palatal
		/s/, /z/	Lingua-alveolar
		/θ/, /ð/	Lingua-dental
		/f/ /v/	Labial-dental
Affricate	The valve stops the airflow, then gently releases it, forcing the air through a narrow passage as with a fricative	/tʃ/, /dʒ/	Lingua-palatal
Stop	The valve stops the airflow, then releases abruptly	/g/	Lingua-velar
		/d/	Lingua-alveolar
		/b/	Bilabial
Stop-plosive	The valve stops the airflow and releases it abruptly. A stronger velar seal is required than for stops.	/k/	Lingua-velar
		/t/	Lingua-alveolar
		/p/	Bilabial

[a]Velopharyngeal valve is open; for all others, it is closed.

Tying It All Together

Speech production has been described repeatedly as one of the most, if not *the* most, complex sequential motor activity performed by humans. Clearly, the muscles of the face, mouth, tongue, mandible, and pharynx collaborate in remarkable ways to orchestrate the movements necessary to accomplish spoken language. A rapid review can hardly do justice to the full range of complexities. Be reminded, therefore, that the overview provided herein should serve only to refresh recollection of information needed when inspecting the oral-facial mechanism for structure and function.

APPENDIX D
Summary of Relevant Cranial Nerves

Although cranial nerves are sited throughout the rapid review of relevant anatomy and physiology (see Appendix C), the information is embedded in text and tables that are devoted to other content issues. To call more careful attention to symptoms that may highlight cranial nerve involvement, Appendix D is added. Since not all cranial nerves participate in speech production, only those that do are highlighted in this section (Table D–1). Resources that were consulted in creating this appendix include Culbertson, Christensen, and Tanner (2013); Gertz (2007); Purves et al. (2004); and Seikel et al. (2010).

Table D–1. Summary of Relevant Cranial Nerves

Cranial Nerve	Structure or Region	Examples of Evidence of Damage
V Trigeminal	Skin of the face Muscles of the jaw	Unilateral upper motor neuron damage results in minimal motor deficit due to bilateral innervation. Some symptoms may include the following: • Jaw-jerk reflex that can be elicited by pulling down on the open mandible • Atrophy • Jaw that deviates toward affected side when open Bilateral lower motor neuron damage may result in the following: • Jaw that hangs open, seriously affecting speech production • Hypernasal resonance if tensor veli palatine is involved Damage to the sensory component of the nerve can result in the following: • Loss of tactile sensation for anterior two thirds of the tongue • Loss of ability to feel skin of the forehead, upper face, and nose (ophthalmic branch) • Loss of ability to feel skin of the lower face (mandibular branch) Trigeminal neuralgia may occur. It is characterized by a sharp sensation of pain that traverses the course of the nerve or affected branch.
VII Facial	Muscles of facial expression Taste receptors Anterior 2/3 of tongue as well as hard palate and velum.	Unilateral upper motor neuron damage has minimal impact due to bilateral innervation. However, it may result in the following: • Paralysis of all facial muscles below the eyes • Involuntary contraction of muscles of facial expression, particularly in response to emotional stimuli Unilateral lower motor neuron damage will result in the following: • Upper and lower facial paralysis that affects the side of the lesion. This may include inability to close the eyelid on the affected side; muscle sagging; poor muscle tone; reduced wrinkling around the lips, nose, and forehead; asymmetrical smile with lips drawn toward the unaffected side; poor saliva management; or cheeks that puff out during exhalation (flaccid buccinator). History of damage to the facial nerve resulting from penetrating wound or neurologic episode, damage to the middle ear, skull fracture involving the temporal bone

Table D–1. *continued*

Cranial Nerve	Structure or Region	Examples of Evidence of Damage
IX Glossopharyngeal	Oropharynx, posterior nasopharynx, eustachian tube Taste, pain, temperature sensation for posterior one third of tongue	Loss of sensation for the posterior one third of the tongue and pharynx Reduced auricle sensation Reduced or absent gag reflex may be associated with damage to cranial nerve IX, but absent gag reflex is not useful for identifying a lesion
X Vagus	Laryngeal, pharyngeal and velar muscles Pain and touch sensation for skin or mucosal lining that covers posterior auricle, lower pharynx, larynx, and esophagus Muscles of respiration A complex muscle whose influence extends well beyond sensory and motor information derived from oral-facial inspection	Damage to pharyngeal branch may result in the following: • Swallowing deficiency • Loss of gag reflex • Unilateral damage to pharyngeal branch may result in hypernasal resonance that is secondary to failure to elevate the velum on affected side • Bilateral damage results in poor velar movement that results in hypernasal resonance, nasal regurgitation, dysphagia, and pharyngeal paralysis Damage to the superior laryngeal nerve may result in the following: • Loss of sensation in the upper larynx • Paralysis of the cricothyroid muscle Damage to the recurrent laryngeal nerve may result in the following: • Altered laryngeal sensation below the vocal folds • Unilateral damage may result in vocal fold weakness on the affected side as indicated by hoarse or breathy vocal quality • Bilateral damage may result in vocal fold paralysis, usually in the paramedian position, resulting in limited phonation with a breathy or hoarse quality, as well as limited vocal range for both pitch and inflection • Bilateral damage may also result in vocal fold paralysis in the adducted position, which can be life-threatening and characterized by laryngeal stridor that is noticeable upon both inhalation and exhalation
XI Accessory	Muscles of the neck	Unilateral lesion that affects sternocleidomastoid results in an inability to turn the head away from the affected side. Damage that affects the trapezius muscle results in restricted arm and shoulder movement, as well as drooping of the shoulder on the affected side.

continues

Table D–1. *continued*

Cranial Nerve	Structure or Region	Examples of Evidence of Damage
XII Hypoglossal	Motor and sensory muscles of the tongue	Unilateral lower motor neuron damage results in the following: • Profound impact on speech production • Loss of lingual movement on the affected side • Muscular weakness and atrophy on the affected side • Lingual deviation toward the affected side • Lingual fasciculations • At rest, tongue may deviate toward unaffected side Upper motor neuron lesion may result in the following: • Lingual weakness • Impaired volitional tongue movements, with spasticity

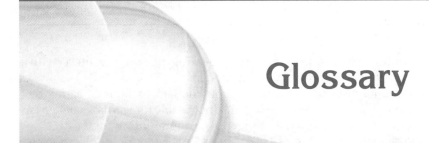

Glossary

Accommodation (special education). Slight change in testing or teaching protocol that can facilitate evaluation or learning, without making changes to content or expectations.

Accreditation. The process by which programs and institutions become authorized to provide specific services, such as offering degrees, treating patients, or teaching students. Meeting standards of practice and external review are fundamental to the accreditation process.

Acute. May refer to a disease with rapid onset and short course; may also refer to the phase of an illness that immediately follows the onset of injury.

Adenoid. See *pharyngeal tonsil.*

Adenoid facies (adenoid face). Changes in the face of a young child who has enlarged adenoids; caused by chronic mouth breathing, which results in structural changes to the face; features include elongated face, open mouth, high palatal arch, shortened upper lip, narrowing of the nostrils, and vacant expression; also associated with crowded teeth and malocclusion.

Alaryngeal speech. Speech that relies on a sound source other than the larynx for phonation; alaryngeal sound sources may be the mouth of the esophagus, tracheoesophageal puncture with valve, electronic larynx, or mechanical larynx.

Alveolar ridge. Palatal ridge that is directly posterior to the anterior maxillary dentition.

Amblyopia. Loss of vision in one eye with no apparent structural explanation; occurs in early childhood and may be the brain's way of resolving conflicting signals received from the two eyes; leading cause of monocular vision; early detection is important to successful treatment outcome.

American English. A set of dialects of the English language that are commonly used in the United States.

Ankyloglossia. A common congenital anomaly of the lingual frenum that restricts tongue movement; also called *tongue tie.*

Anomaly. A structural or functional defect that is characterized by marked deviation from the standard.

Anterior. Toward the front.

Anterior nasal fricative. Nonstandard speech sound that may be used when compensating for surplus nasal airflow; also called *facial grimace.*

Apraxia of speech. A motor-speech disorder that is characterized by difficulty with planning and programming the movements for speech; not associated with muscle weakness.

Articulation. Use of lips, teeth, mandible, tongue, alveolar ridge, palate, velum, posterior pharyngeal wall, and vocal folds to produce speech sounds.

Asymmetry. Dissimilarity in equivalent parts or organs on opposite sides of the body.

Asynchronous. Not occurring at the same time or occurring with dissimilar timing.

Atrophy. Wasting away of a body part due to lack of use or secondary to disease.

Atypical. Not corresponding to normal expectations.

Auricle. See *pinna.*

Bifid uvula. The complete or incomplete separation of the uvula into two tags; often associated with submucous cleft.

Bilabial. Pertaining to upper and lower lips.

Bilateral. Affecting both sides.

Blind. Vision that is either absent or compromised and not correctable to a functional level as diagnosed by a vision specialist.

Bruxism. Teeth grinding, clenching of the teeth; usually occurs during sleep.

Canonical babbling. Babbling that is characterized by repetitive sequences of CV syllables; occurs between 5 and 10 months of age; important to later speech development.

Catarrh. Inflammation, with increased flow of mucus.

Cerebrovascular accident. Interruption in blood supply that causes damage to a part of the brain; also called a *stroke.*

GLOSSARY

Certificate of Clinical Competence. The certificate that the American Speech-Language-Hearing Association confers on individuals who have met minimum criteria for independent clinical practice in the field of speech-language pathology or audiology.

Certification. Confirmation that a person possesses specific skills, qualifying that person to perform specific acts; clinical certification requires education, supervised clinical practice, and evaluation by an external reviewing body.

Chronic. Describes a condition that is persistent or long lasting.

Clavicular breathing. Shallow breathing, characterized by rhythmic upward and downward shoulder movement.

Cliché. Popular, overused expression.

Clinical art. The aspect of clinical practice that capitalizes on skills resulting from experience, such as clinical intuition, clinical problem solving, critical thinking, and integrating ideas.

Clinical practicum. The supervised experience that student clinicians complete as part of their education in preparation for earning a degree, certification, and licensure.

Clinical question. A question asked when seeking relevant and useful evidence that becomes fundamental to clinical decision making.

Clinical science. The aspect of clinical practice that capitalizes on gathering and reporting quantitative and qualitative evidence.

Clinical supervision. Professional oversight of students in clinical practicum; includes observation, conferencing, written and verbal feedback, and collaborative clinical problem solving.

Clinically relevant. Pertains to data that explain or partially explain the communication disorder.

Colloquial language. Form of language that is commonly used in informal conversation but is not acceptable for formal written or spoken language.

Compensatory. Serving to counterbalance a deficit or loss.

Conversational speech sample. A brief conversation between a client and clinician that is used to informally judge intelligibility, articulation, language, voice, fluency, and pragmatics.

Cranial. Pertaining to the head.

Craniofacial anomaly. A structural or functional deviation of the head or face.

Crepitus. The sound of bone rubbing on bone.

Cul-de-sac resonance. Resonance that sounds muffled or hollow; often associated with the speech of deaf people, hard-of-hearing persons, or those with a cranial-facial anomaly.

Deaf. Severe to profound lack of natural hearing that, when unaided, is not usable for learning spoken language or for spoken communication; if capitalized (i.e., Deaf), can also refer to a cultural group that embraces deafness as a way of life.

Deciduous teeth. The first set of teeth; also called primary teeth.

Dental arch. The curved framework of the maxilla and mandible that houses the teeth.

Dental bite. Relationship between maxillary and mandibular incisors.

Dental misalignment. Any relationship between the teeth that deviates from the dental arch.

Dental occlusion. Relationship between the first maxillary molar and the first mandibular molar.

Dentition. Teeth.

Diadochokinesis (verbal and nonspeech). Rapid alternating or sequential movements.

Diagnosis. A description that classifies a disorder or condition according to name of condition, individual characteristics, severity, and etiology.

Diastema. Space or spaces between adjacent teeth.

Documentation. Formal written evidence that records any event.

Dysarthria. A family of motor-speech disorders that results from damage to the central or peripheral nervous system.

Dysmorphia. Malformation or abnormality in the shape or size of a feature or body part.

Dysphagia. Neurogenic disorder that negatively affects a person's ability to swallow safely.

Dysrhythmia. Abnormal rhythm.

Edema. Accumulation of fluid in cells or tissue.

Electronic larynx. A handheld, battery-operated device that, when placed under the mandible, produces vibrations that can serve as sound source when laryngeal phonation is not an option.

Epicanthal fold. A skin fold in the upper eyelid that covers the inner corner of the eye.

Esophageal speech. A method of alaryngeal speech that relies on the speaker producing vibrations at the mouth of the esophagus in order to produce speech sounds.

Etiology. The cause or origin of a condition.

Euphemism. Using pleasant-sounding words to hide a negative meaning (e.g., *independent* may be a euphemistic way to describe a child who *resists adult-directed activities*).

Fasciculations. Involuntary contractions; twitching.

Fissure. A narrow opening or separation in the bony or mucosal framework.

Fistulus. A small hole in the bony framework that connects two spaces.

Frankfurt horizontal plane. Imaginary line between the tragion and lid-cheek junction; can be used to identify low-set ears.

Functional communication disorder. A communication disorder with no identifiable physical cause.

Glabella. Most prominent point that lies at midline directly between the eyebrows.

Glottal. Pertaining to the space between the vocal folds.

Glottal stop. A type of speech sound that is produced by stopping the airflow at the level of the vocal folds, then suddenly releasing it; sometimes is used to compensate for surplus nasal airflow; is a standard speech sound in certain dialects of American English.

Glottis. The space between the vocal folds.

Hard of hearing. Compromised hearing in the mild to moderate range.

Hemianopia/hemianopsia. Loss of left or right visual field, affecting one or both eyes.

Hemi-spatial neglect. A condition that occurs most often in brain-injured patients whose cerebral infarct involves right cerebral hemisphere areas that interpret visual information; patients with the condition experience reduced response to stimuli presented to one side of the visual field and may even behave as if that side does not exist.

Holophrase. A single-word sentence with embedded grammar; a single-word sentence that is not simply a label (e.g., Child holds up a cookie and says, "Mine," not labeling the cookie but declaring a relationship between himself and the cookie).

Hypernasal resonance. Imbalanced resonance that favors resonating cavities in the nasal region.

Hypertelorism. Abnormally increased distance between two organs; can refer to wide-set eyes.

Hypertrophied. Having increased bulk; enlarged.

Hyponasal resonance. Imbalanced resonance that lacks full participation from the resonating cavities in the nasal region.

Hypoplastic. Underdevelopment of a tissue or organ (e.g., hypoplastic midface).

Hypotelorism. Abnormally decreased distance between two organs; can refer to narrow-set eyes.

Hypothesis. Proposed explanation; educated guess.

Infant. A child in the first year of life.

Inferior. Lower or below.

Inflammation. A physiological response to injury or infection resulting in redness, pain, swelling, tenderness, perception of heat, or even low-grade function.

Intelligibility. The degree to which speech is understandable or comprehensible to others.

Interdental. Pertaining to the space between maxillary and mandibular anterior dentition.

Intraoral. Within the mouth.

Ipsilateral. Same side.

Labial. Pertaining to the lips.

Labial dental. Pertaining to contact between the maxillary incisors and the lower lip.

Laryngectomee. A person who has had the larynx surgically removed for medical reasons.

Laryngectomy. The surgical procedure that results in the removal of the larynx.

Laryngopharynx. Lower portion of the pharynx that is directly above the larynx.

Larynx. Organ of voice production; also serves to protect the airway.

Lateral. On the side.

Lid-cheek junction. The location where the inferior-most point of the orbit meets the zygomatic arch.

Lingua-alveolar. Pertaining to contact between the tongue tip and the alveolar ridge.

Lingua-palatal. Pertaining to contact between the anterior tongue blade and the palatal arch immediately posterior to the alveolar ridge.

Lingua-velar. Pertaining to contact between the posterior tongue blade and the velum.

Lingual. Pertaining to the tongue.

Lip pits. Bilateral pits on the surface of the lower lip; often associated with cleft lip.

Lungs. The organs of respiration.

Luxation. Dislocation.

Macrocephaly. The condition of having an excessively large head.

Macroglossia. The condition of having an excessively large tongue.

Macrognathia. The condition of having an excessively large mandible.

Malocclusion. Misaligned relationship between maxillary and mandibular first molars.

Mandible. The lower jaw.

Marcus Gunn jaw wink. A condition that results in winking one eye when using muscles that accomplish oral sucking.

Maxilla. An irregularly shaped bone that supports the upper teeth and contributes to the orbit, the hard palate, and the bony structure of the nasal cavity.

Medial. Toward the middle.

Median palatal raphe. Slight indentation or seam that separates left and right sides of the hard palate.

Menton. The inferior-most point on the inferior surface of the chin.

Metathetic error. Speech production error that is characterized by speech sounds trading places within a word, or even across word boundaries (e.g., pony tail →/'te nɪ 'poʊl/, caterpillar →/'kæ lə pɪ tɚ/)

Microcephaly. The condition of having an excessively small head.

Microglossia. The condition of having an excessively small tongue.

Micrognathia. The condition of having an excessively small mandible.

Modification (special education). A change in either content or minimal expectation, allowing for a lesser response due to disability or age.

Monocular vision. Having the use of one eye only.

Monoloudness. Characteristic of a voice that does not normally inflect with changes in loudness.

Monopitch. Characteristic of a voice that does not normally inflect with changes in pitch.

Myringotomy tubes. Ventilation tubes that surgically puncture the tympanic membrane for the purpose of treating chronic otitis media.

Naris (plural nares). Nostril.

Nasal regurgitation. Loss of food or liquid through the nasal egress.

Nasal snort. See *posterior nasal fricative.*

Nasopharynx. The portion of the pharynx that is directly posterior to the velum.

Neurogenic. Originating in the nervous system.

Obstruent. Consonant requiring intraoral pressure.

Occult. Hidden; not overt; not observable.

Oral breathing. Mouth breathing.

Organic etiology. Physical cause.

Orifice. An opening.

Oropharynx. Portion of the pharynx that is directly posterior to the oral cavity.

Otitis media. Middle ear infection.

Palatine tonsils. Lymphatic tissue residing directly behind the faucial pillars, bilaterally; also called *tonsils.*

Palpebral fissures. Eye slits.

Papillae (lingual). Taste buds; sensory end organs on the tongue.

Perioral. In the vicinity of the mouth.

Perseveration. Persistent repetition of a once meaningful response that is no longer meaningful.

Pharyngeal. Of the throat.

Pharyngeal fricative. A consonant speech sound characterized by pharyngeal constriction, resulting in audible friction; not a standard sound of American English.

Pharyngeal tonsil. A mass of lymphatic tissue that occupies a portion of the nasopharynx immediately posterior to the velum; also called *adenoid.*

Pharynx. The throat.

Philtrum. The vertical depression or groove at the midline directly above the upper lip.

Phonation. Production of voice using the vocal folds.

Phoneme. A single speech sound.

Phonology. The study of the sound system of a language, including the speech sounds and the rules for combining them.

Pica. Pattern of eating nonnutritive materials, such as dirt, sand, plastic, paper, hair, feces, or paint. Pattern of behavior must occur for 1 month or more in order for a diagnosis to be considered.

Pinna. The outer ear; also called the *auricle.*

Pogonion. The anterior-most point of the chin.

Posterior. Behind; near the back.

Posterior nasal fricative. A speech-like sound that may substitute for other fricatives in cases of surplus nasal airflow; also called *nasal snort.*

Preauricular. In front of the ear.

Preschool-age child. A child who is older than 36 months but not yet old enough to enter school.

Primary care physician. A physician who serves as a patient's first point of contact for health care.

Primary teeth. See *deciduous teeth.*

Primitive reflex. Any one of a group of reflexes that normally occurs during gestation and infancy; normally suppressed at an early age; may recur in some adults who have sustained an injury to the central nervous system.

Prognathia. The condition of having an excessively prominent mandible.

Prognosis. A statement of professional opinion that addresses whether a client is likely to improve, with or without treatment.

Ptosis. Drooping.

Quadrantanopia. Loss of a visual field quadrant, affecting one or both eyes.

Quasi-resonant nuclei. Vowel approximation.

Range of motion. Refers to distance and direction that a body part can move.

Rationale. A reasoned exposition, especially one defining the fundamental reasons for a course of action.

Recommendation. Advice that is not considered optional; must be completed, or a reason should be given for not completing it.

Reduplicated babbling. See *canonical babbling.*

Reflex. Involuntary action in response to a stimulus.

Remarkable. Noteworthy.

Repetitive-motion disorder. Painful condition affecting soft tissues, specifically nerves, tendons, ligaments, muscles; usually results from overuse; also called *cumulative trauma disorder, repetitive stress injury,* or *overuse syndrome.*

Resonance. Sympathetic or forced vibrations of air in cavities that are in the vicinity of a sound source.

Respiration. Breathing.

Retrognathia. The condition of having a receded mandible.

Sagittal plane. A vertical plane that passes from front to back and divides the body or body part into left and right halves.

Scientific method. A way to ask and answer questions by making observations, doing experiments, gathering evidence, and drawing conclusions.

Scope of practice. The range of responsibility and oversight for a particular profession.

Scotoma. Blind spot.

Screening. A way to identify individuals who need in-depth testing in a particular area.

Stoma. A hole or opening that is either natural or surgically created and links a body cavity with the external environment.

Stomian. The horizontal line denoting where the upper and lower lips meet.

Stress-timed language. Any spoken language whose cadence calls for equal temporal spacing between stressed syllables (e.g., American English).

Subclinical. Describing a feature that is noted but also judged as having no relevance to the communication disorder.

Subluxation. Partial dislocation.

Submucous cleft palate. Incomplete integrity of the bony palatal structure that is covered by mucous membrane.

Subnasale plane. The horizontal line that marks the junction between the nose and philtrum.

Suggestion. Advice that is optional.

Superior. Above or upward.

Supramentale. Indentation in the chin that resides below the lower lip and above pogonion.

Syllable-timed language. Any spoken language whose cadence calls for equal temporal spacing between syllables (e.g., Spanish).

Syndrome. A combination of symptoms that, when co-occurring, characterize a disease or inherited anomaly.

Toddler. An ambulatory child younger than age 3 years.

Tongue tie. See *ankyloglossia.*

Tracheoesophageal puncture. A surgical procedure that creates a small fistulus connecting the trachea and esophagus.

Tragion. Superior surface of the tragus.

Tragus. Tongue-like cartilaginous projection in the auricle that is directly anterior to the external auditory meatus.

Tunnel vision. Vision that excludes access to the peripheral visual field.

Unilateral. Affecting one side.

Unremarkable. Not worthy of comment; not clinically significant or relevant.

Uvula. A small mass of tissue that hangs at midline directly posterior to the velum and attaches to it.

Valve. Any mechanism with moveable parts that controls the flow of liquid or gas.

Velar. Pertaining to the soft palate.

Velopharyngeal. Pertaining to the velum and posterior pharyngeal wall.

Velum. Soft palate.

Viseme. A category of speech sounds that all have the same appearance on a person's face when spoken; applies to speech reading (e.g., /b/, /m/, /p/, and /w/ are all in the bilabial viseme group).

Zygoma. Cheekbone.

Zygomatic arch. The superior boundary of the cheekbone; also called *lid-cheek junction.*

References

American Speech-Language-Hearing Association. (2005). *Evidence-based practice in communication disorders* [Position statement]. Retrieved from http://www.asha.org/policy

American Speech-Language-Hearing Association. (2007a). *Childhood apraxia of speech: Ad hoc committee on apraxia of speech in children* [Position statement]. Retrieved from http://www.asha.org/policy

American Speech-Language-Hearing Association. (2007b). *Childhood apraxia of speech: Ad hoc committee on apraxia of speech in children* [Technical report]. Retrieved from http://www.asha.org/policy

Andrianopoulos, M. V. (n.d.) *Oral peripheral + neuromotor speech examinations* [PDF document]. Retrieved from http://people.umass.edu/mva/pdf/oral%20periph%20neuromotor%20exam_09.pdf

Andrianopoulos, M. V., & Hanson, M. L. (1987). Tongue-thrust and the stability of overjet correction. *The Angle Orthodontist, 57,* 121–135.

Astle, A. T., Webb, B. S., & McGraw, P. V. (2011). Can perceptual learning be used to treat amblyopia beyond the critical period of visual development? *Journal of the College of Optometrists, 31,* 564–573.

Bankaitis, A. U., Kemp, R. J., Krival, K., & Bandaranayake, D. (2006). *Infection control for speech-language pathology.* St. Louis, MO: Auban.

Bankson, N. W., Bernthal, J. E., & Flipsen, P. (2009). Phonological assessment procedures. In J. E. Bernthal, N. W. Bankson, & P. Flipsen, P. (Eds.), *Articulation and phonological disorders: Speech sound disorders in children* (pp. 187–250). Boston, MA: Allyn & Bacon.

Bauman-Waengler, J. (2011). *Articulatory and phonological impairments: A clinical focus.* Boston, MA: Allyn & Bacon.

Behrman, A. (2013). *Speech and voice science.* San Diego, CA: Plural.

Belmonte, M. K., Saxena-Chandhok, T., Cherian, R., Muneer, R., George, L., & Karanth, P. (2013). Oral-motor deficits in speech-impaired children with autism. *Frontiers in Integrative Neuroscience, 7,* 1–8.

Bergman, R. T. (1999). Cephalometric of soft tissue facial analysis. *American Journal of Orthodontics and Dentofacial Orthopedics, 116,* 373–389.

Berlin, C. I. (1963). Clinical measurement of esophageal speech: Methodology and curves of skill acquisition. *Journal of Speech and Hearing Disorders, 28,* 42–51.

Boone, D. R., McFarlane, S. C., Von Berg, S. L., & Zraick, R. I. (2010). *The voice and voice therapy.* Boston, MA: Allyn & Bacon.

Boshart, C. A. (2009). *How to do a comprehensive and worthwhile oral-facial examination.* Montgomery, TX: Speech Dynamics.

Brescovici, S., & Roithmann, R. (2008). Modified glatzel mirror test reproducibility in the evaluation of nasal patency. *Brazilian Journal of Otorhinolaryngology, 74,* 215–222.

Bresolin, D., Shapiro, G. G., Shapiro, P. A., Dassel, S. W., Furukawa, C. T., Pierson, W. E., . . . Bierman, C. W. (1984). Facial characteristics of children who breathe through the mouth. *Pediatrics, 73,* 622–625.

Buckendorf, G. R., Gordon, C. J., Goodwyn-Craine, A. (2007). Assessment of the speech mechanism. In R. Paul & W. Cascella (Eds.), *Introduction to clinical methods in communication disorders* (pp. 85–110). Baltimore, MD: Paul H. Brookes.

Buder, E. H., Chorna, L. B., Oller, D. K., & Robinson, R. B. (2006). Vibratory regime classification of infant phonation. *Journal of Voice, 22,* 553–564.

Bunton, K., Kent, R. D., Duffy, J. R., Rosenbek, J. C., & Kent, J. F. (2007). Listener agreement for auditory perceptual ratings of dysarthria. *Journal of Speech, Language, and Hearing Research, 50,* 1481–1495.

Bunton, K., Kent, R. D., Kent, J. F., & Rosenbek, J. C. (2000). Perceptuo-acoustic assessment of prosodic impairment in dysarthria. *Clinical Linguistics and Phonetics, 14,* 13–24.

Burrus, A. E., & Willis, L. B. (2013). *Professional communication in speech-language pathology: How to write, talk and act like a clinician.* San Diego, CA: Plural.

Buxbaum, L. J. (2006). On the right (and left) track: Twenty years of progress in studying hemispatial neglect. *Cognitive Neuropsychology, 23,* 184–201.

Bzoch, K. R. (2004). *Communicative disorders related to cleft lip and palate.* Austin, TX: Pro-Ed.

Canning, B. A., & Rose, M. F. (1974). Clinical measurements of the speed of tongue and lip movements in British children with normal speech. *British Journal of Disorders of Communication, 9,* 45–50.

Capute, A. J. (1979). Identifying cerebral palsy in infancy through study of primitive-reflex profiles. *Pediatric Annals, 8,* 34–42.

Chen, Y. C. (2012). A simple method for isolating filament as 'algae seed stock' from monostrumalatissimum (chlorophyta) germlings, and applications for mass cultivation. *Journal of Phycology, 48,* 246–247.

Chone, C. T., Gripp, F. M., Spina, A. L., & Crespo, A. N. (2005). Primary versus secondary tracheoesophageal puncture for speech rehabilitation in total laryngectomy: Long-term results with indwelling voice prosthesis. *Otolaryngology Head and Neck Surgery, 133,* 89–93.

Cohen, W., Waters, D., & Hewlett, N. (1998). DDK rates in the paediatric clinic: A methodological minefield. *International Journal of Language and Communication Disorders, 33,* 428–433.

Cole, E. B., & Flexer, C. (2011). *Children with hearing loss: Developing listening and talking.* San Diego, CA: Plural.

Courtney, R. (2013). The importance of correct breathing for raising healthy good looking children. *Journal of Australian Traditional-Medicine Society, 29,* 20–27.

Culbertson, W. R., Christensen, S. C., & Tanner, D. C. (2013). *Anatomy and physiology study guide for speech and hearing.* San Diego, CA: Plural.

Darley, F. L., Aronson, A. E., & Brown, J. E. (1975). *Motor speech disorders.* Philadelphia, PA: W. B. Saunders.

de Felicio, C. M., & Ferreira, C. L. P. (2008). Protocol for orofacial myofunctional evaluation with scores. *International Journal of Pediatric Otorhinolaryngology, 72,* 367–375.

de Felicio, C. M., Folha, G. A. C., Ferreira, C. L. P., & Medeiros, A. P. M. (2010). Expanded protocol of orofacial myofunctional evaluation with scores: Validity and reliability. *International Journal of Pediatric Otorhinolaryngology, 74,* 1230–1239.

Donovan, N., Daniels, S. K., Edmiaston, J., Weinhardt, J., Summers, D., & Mitchell, P. H. (2013). Dysphagia screening: State of the art. *Stroke, 44,* 24–31.

Duffy, J. R. (2000). Motor speech disorders: Clues to neurologic diagnosis. In C. H. Adler & J. E. Ahlskog (Eds.), *Parkinson's disease and movement disorders:* *Diagnosis and treatment guidelines for practicing physicians* (pp. 35–56). Rochester, MN: Mayo Foundation for Medical Education and Research.

Duffy, J. R. (2006). Apraxia of speech in degenerative neurological disease. *Aphasiology, 20,* 511–527.

Duffy, J. R. (2011, April). *Differential diagnosis among the dysarthrias: The rules of the game.* Paper presented at the annual convention of the Texas Speech-Language-Hearing Association, Houston, TX.

Duffy, J. R. (2013). *Motor-speech disorders: Substrates, strategies, differential diagnosis.* St. Louis, MO: Elsevier.

Duffy, J. R., & Josephs, K. A. (2012). The diagnosis and understanding of apraxia of speech: Why including neurodegenerative etiologies may be important. *Journal of Speech, Language, and Hearing Research, 55,* 1518–1522.

Duffy, J. R., & Kent, R. D. (2001). Darley's contribution to the understanding, differential diagnosis and scientific study of the dysarthrias. *Aphasiology, 15,* 275–289.

Duffy, J. R., Waumbaugh, J., Fredrickson, J., & Haley, K. (2013, November). *Current issues in apraxia of speech and progressive apraxia of speech.* Paper presented at the annual convention of the American Speech-Language-Hearing Association, Chicago, IL.

Dworkin, J. P. (1991). *Motor speech disorders: A treatment guide.* St. Louis, MO: Mosby Yearbook.

Dworkin, J., & Culatta, R. (1996). *Dworkin-Culatta oral mechanism exam and treatment system (D-COME-T).* Nicholasville, KY: Edgewood.

Dworkin, J. P., Marunick, M. T., & Krouse, J. H. (2004). Velopharyngeal dysfunction: Speech characteristics, variable etiologies, evaluation techniques, and differential treatments. *Language Speech and Hearing Services in Schools, 35,* 333–352.

Eadie, T. L. (2007). Application of the ICF in communication after total laryngectomy. *Seminars in Speech and Language, 28,* 291–300.

Eckels, F. C., & Boone, D. R. (1981). The s/z ratio as an indicator of laryngeal pathology. *Journal of Speech and Hearing Disorders, 46,* 147–149.

Edmiaston, J., Connor, L. T., Loehr, L., & Nassief, A. (2010). Validation of a dysphagia screening tool in acute stroke patients. *American Journal of Critical Care, 19,* 357–364.

Edmonson, J. A., & Esling, J. H. (2006). The valves of the throat and their functioning in tone, vocal register and stress: Laryngoscopic case studies. *Phonology, 23,* 157–191.

Emerick, L. L., & Hatten, J. T. (1979). *Diagnosis and evaluation in speech pathology.* Englewood Cliffs, NJ: Prentice-Hall.

Engel-Yeger, B. (2008). Evaluation of gross motor abilities and self-perception in children with amblyopia. *Disability and Rehabilitation, 30,* 243–248.

Farina, D., Bodin, C., Gandolfi, S., DeGasperi, W., Borghesi, A., & Maroldi, R. (2009). TMJ disorders and pain: Assessment by contrast-enhanced MRI. *European Journal of Radiology, 70,* 25–30.

Fletcher, S. G. (1972). Time-by-count measurement of diadochokinetic syllable rate. *Journal of Speech and Hearing Research, 15,* 763–770.

Flipsen, P., Bankson, N. W., & Bernthal, J. E. (2009). Classification and factors related to speech sound disorders. In J. E. Bernthal, N. W. Bankson, & P. Flipsen (Eds.), *Articulation and phonological disorders: Speech sound disorder in children* (pp. 121–186). Boston, MA: Allyn & Bacon.

Fluharty, N. B. (1997). *Fluharty Preschool Speech and Language Screening Test* (2nd ed.). Austin, TX: Pro-Ed.

Forner, L. L., & Hixon, T. J. (1977). Respiratory kinematics in profoundly hearing-impaired speakers. *Journal of Speech and Hearing Research, 20,* 373–407.

Frankenburg, W. K. (2002). Developmental surveillance and screening of infants and young children. *Pediatrics, 89,* 1221–1225.

Frankenburg, W. K., Dodds, J., & Archer, O. (1990). *Technical manual.* Denver, CO: Denver Developmental Materials.

Frankenburg, W. K., Dodds, J., Archer, O., Shapiro, H., & Bresnik, B. (1992). *The Denver II*: A major revision and restandardization of the *Denver Developmental Screening Test. Pediatrics, 89,* 91–97.

Fraser, C. (2006). Tongue thrust and its influence in orthodontics. *International Journal of Orthodontics, 17,* 9–18.

Fucile, S., Wright, P. M., Chan, I., Yee, S., Langlais, M., & Gisel, E. G. (1998). Functional oral-motor skills: Do they change with age? *Dysphagia, 13,* 195–201.

Fuller, D. R., Pimentel, J. T., & Peregoy, B. M. (2012). *Applied anatomy and physiology for speech-language pathology and audiology.* Philadelphia, PA: Lippincott Williams & Wilkins.

Gelfer, M. P., & Pazera, J. F. (2006). Maximum duration of sustained /s/ and /z/ and the s/z ratio with controlled intensity. *Journal of Voice, 20,* 369–379.

Gertz, S. D. (2007). *Liebman's neuroanatomy made easy and understandable.* Austin, TX: Pro-Ed.

Godnig, E. C. (2003). Tunnel vision: Its causes and treatment strategies. *Journal of Behavioral Optometry, 14,* 95–99.

Goldfarb, R., & Serpanos, Y. C. (2009). *Professional writing in speech-language pathology and audiology.* San Diego, CA: Plural.

Goldman, R., & Fristoe, M. (2000) *Goldman-Fristoe Test of Articulation-2.* Circle Pines, MN: American Guidance Service.

Gordon-Brannan, M. E., & Weiss, C. E. (2007). *Clinical management of articulatory and phonological disorders.* Philadelphia, PA: Lippincott Williams & Wilkins.

Green, J. R., Moore, C. A., Higashikawa, M., & Steeve, R. W. (2000). The physiological development of speech-motor control: Lip and jaw coordination. *Journal of Speech, Language, and Hearing Research, 43,* 239–255.

Green, J. R., Moore, C. A., & Riley, K. J. (2002). The sequential development of jaw and lip control for speech. *Journal of Speech, Language, and Hearing Research, 45,* 66–79.

Guddemi, M., & Case, B. J. (2004). *Assessment report: Assessing young children.* Boston, MA: Pearson Education.

Gupta, V. B. (1999). *Manual of developmental and behavioral problems in children.* New York, NY: Marcel Dekker.

Haley, K. L., Jacks, A., de Riesthal, M., Abou-Khalil, R., & Roth, H. L. (2012). Toward a quantitative basis for assessment and diagnosis of apraxia of speech. *Journal of Speech, Language, and Hearing Research, 55,* 1502–1517.

Hall, P. K. (2007a). Introduction and philosophy. In P. K. Hall, L. S. Jordan, & D. A. Robin (Eds.), *Developmental apraxia of speech: Theory and clinical practice* (pp. 1–12). Austin, TX: Pro-Ed.

Hall, P. K. (2007b). Language disorders: Frequently co-occurring characteristics of children exhibiting DAS. In P. K. Hall, L. S. Jordan, & D. A. Robin (Eds.), *Developmental apraxia of speech: Theory and clinical practice* (pp. 87–108). Austin, TX: Pro-Ed.

Hall, P. K. (2007c). Speech characteristics of developmental apraxia of speech. In P. K. Hall, L. S. Jordan, & D. A. Robin (Eds.), *Developmental apraxia of speech: Theory and clinical practice* (pp. 13–66). Austin, TX: Pro-Ed.

Hanson, M. L. (1988). Orofacial myofunctional therapy: Historical and philosophical considerations. *International Journal of Orofacial Myology, 14,* 3–10.

Hanson, M. L., & Mason R. M. (2003). *Orofacial myology: International perspectives.* Springfield, IL: Charles C Thomas.

Haynes, W. O., & Pindzola, R. H. (2012). *Diagnosis and evaluation in speech pathology.* Boston, MA: Pearson.

Hegde, M. N. (2009). *Hegde's pocket guide to assessment in speech-language pathology.* San Diego, CA: Thompson.

Hegde, M. N. (2010). *A coursebook on scientific and professional writing for speech-language pathology.* Clifton Park, NY: Delmar Cengage Learning.

Hegde, M. N., & Freed, D. (2013). *Assessment of communication disorders in adults*. San Diego, CA: Plural.

Hegde, M. N., & Pomaville, F. (2013). *Assessment of communication disorders in children*. San Diego, CA: Plural.

Henry, C. E. (1990). The development of oral diadochokinesia and non-linguistic rhythmic skills in normal and speech-disordered young children. *Clinical Linguistics and Phonetics, 4*, 121–137.

Hobart, C., Frankel, J., & Wlaker, M. (2009). *A practical guide to child observation and assessment* (4th ed.). Cheltenham, UK: Stanley Thomas.

Howlin, P., & Cross, P. (1994). The variability of language test scores in 3 and 4 year old children of normal non-verbal intelligence: A brief research report. *European Journal of Disorders of Communication, 29*, 279–288.

Itoh, M., Horii, Y., Daniloff, R. G., & Binnie, C. A. (1982). Selected aerodynamic characteristics of deaf individuals during various speech and non-speech tasks. *Folia Phoniatrica et Logopaedica, 34*, 191–209.

Iwarsson, J. (2001). Effect of inhalatory abdominal wall movement on vertical laryngeal position during phonation. *Journal of Voice, 15*, 384–394.

Johnson, B. A. (1996). *Language disorders in children: An introductory clinical perspective*. Albany, NY: Delmar.

Jones, M. W., Morgan, E., Shelton, J. E., & Thorogood, C. (2007). Cerebral palsy: Introduction and diagnosis, part one. *Journal of Pediatric Health Care, 21*, 146–152.

Kamhi, A. G. (2006). Treatment decisions for children with speech-sound disorders. *Language, Speech, and Hearing Services in Schools, 37*, 271–279.

Karacay, S., Akin, E., Ortakoglu, K., & Bengi, A. O. (2006). Dynamic MRI evaluation of tongue posture and deglutitive movements in surgically corrected open bite. *Angle Orthodontist, 76*, 1057–1065.

Kent, R. D. (1994). *Reference manual for communicative sciences and disorders: Speech and language*. Austin, TX: Pro-Ed.

Knight, R. D. (2013). *Physics for scientists and engineers: A strategic approach*. Boston, MA: Pearson.

Knösel, W., Klein, S., Bleckmann, A., & Engelke, W. (2012). Coordination of tongue activity during swallowing in mouth-breathing children. *Dysphagia, 27*, 401–407.

Kummer, A. W. (2008). *Cleft palate and craniofacial anomalies: The effects on speech and resonance*. Clifton Park, NY: Delmar Cengage Learning.

Kummer, A. W., & Lee, L. (1996). Evaluation and treatment of resonance disorders. *Language, Speech, and Hearing Services in Schools, 27*, 271–281.

Lalla, F., Dingle, P., & Cheong, C. (2005). The antibacterial action of cloths and sanitizers and the use of environmental alternatives. *Journal of Environmental Health, 68*, 31–35.

Lane, H., & Perkell, J. S. (2005). Control of voice-onset time in the absence of hearing: A review. *Journal of Speech, Language, and Hearing Research, 48*, 1334–1343.

Lass, N. J. (2013). *Review of speech and hearing sciences*. St. Louis, MO: Elsevier.

Lebrun, Y. (1985). Tongue thrust, tongue tip position at rest, and stigmatism: A review. *Journal of Communication Disorders, 18*, 305–312.

Leder, S. B., Suiter, D. M., Murray, J., & Rademaker, A. W. (2013). Can an oral mechanism examination contribute to the assessment of odds of aspiration? *Dysphagia, 28*, 370–374.

Lewin, J. S., Hutcheson, K. A., Barringer, D. A., May, A. H., Roberts, D. B., Holsinger, C., & Diaz, E. M. (2008). Functional analysis of swallowing outcomes after supracricoid partial laryngectomy. *Head and Neck, 30*, 559–566.

Lippke, B. A., Dickey, S. E., Selmar, J. W., & Soder, A. L. (1997). *Photo Articulation Test* (3rd ed.). Austin, TX: Pro-Ed.

Lof, G., & Camarata, S. (2013, November). *Evidence-based practice: Science or pseudoscience*. Paper presented at the annual convention of the American Speech-Language Hearing Association, Chicago, IL.

Lowit, A., & Kent, R. D. (2011). *Assessment of motor speech disorders*. San Diego, CA: Plural.

Lundervold, A. J., Bergmann, N., & Wooton, C. (2005). Visual neglect in the first few weeks after stroke in the right hemisphere. *Scandinavian Journal of Psychology, 46*, 297–303.

Maclean, J., Cotton, S., & Perry, A. (2009). Postlaryngectomy: It's hard to swallow. *Dysphagia, 24*, 172–179.

Mann, G. (2002). *MASA: The Mann Assessment of Swallowing Ability*. Clifton Park, NY: Singular.

Marasa, F. K. (2007a). An explanation of the effect that two different swallowing patterns have on cranial articular motion: Part 1 of 3. *Journal of the American Academy of Gnathologic Orthopedics, 24*, 12–15.

Marasa, F. K. (2007b). An explanation of the effect that two different swallowing patterns have on cranial articular motion: Part 2 of 3. *Journal of the American Academy of Gnathologic Orthopedics, 24*, 8–12.

Marasa, F. K. (2008). An explanation of the effect that two different swallowing patterns have on cranial articular motion: Part 3 of 3. *Journal of the American Academy of Gnathologic Orthopedics, 25*, 10–12.

Martino, R., Silver, F., Teasell, R., Bayley, M., Nicholson, G., Streiner, D. L., & Diament, N. E. (2009). The Toronto Bedside Swallow Screening Test (TOR-BSST): Development and validation of a dysphagia screening tool for patients with stroke. *Stroke, 40*, 555–561.

Mason, R. (1988). Orthodontic perspectives on orofacial myofunctional therapy. *International Journal of Orofacial Myology, 14*, 49–55.

Mason, R., & Wickwire, N. (1978). Examining for orofacial variations. *Communiqué, 8*, 2–26.

McCullough, G. H., Rosenbek, J. C., Wertz, R. T., McCoy, S., Mann, G., & McCullough, K. (2005). Utility of swallowing evaluation measures for detecting aspiration post-stroke. *Journal of Speech and Hearing Research, 48*, 1280–1293.

Merrill, G. F. (2008). *Our marvelous bodies: An introduction to the physiology of human health.* New Brunswick, NJ: Rutgers University Press.

Miller, A. J. (2002). Oral and pharyngeal reflexes in the mammalian nervous system: Their diverse range in complexity and the pivotal role of the tongue. *International and American Associations of Dental Research, 13*, 409–425.

Mosheim, J. (2005). Infection control: Protocols protect the clinician and patient. *Advance for Speech-Language Pathologists and Audiologists, 15*, 7–9.

Nicolosi, L, Harryman, E., & Kresheck, J. (2004). *Terminology of communication disorders: Speech-language-hearing.* Philadelphia, PA: Lippincott Williams & Wilkins.

Oller, D. K. (1980). The emergence of the sounds of speech in infancy. In G. H. Yeni-Komshian, J. Kavanagh, & C. A. Ferguson (Eds.), *Child phonology: Vol. I. Production* (pp. 93–112). New York, NY: Academic Press.

Oller, D. K. (2000). *The emergence of speech capacity.* Mahwah, NJ: Lawrence Erlbaum.

Oller, D. K., Buder, E. H., Ramsdell, H. L., Warlaumont, A. S., Chorna, L., & Bakeman, R. (2013). Functional flexibility of infant vocalization and the emergence of language. *Proceedings of the National Academy of Science of the United States of America, 110*, 6318–6323.

Oller, D. K., Warlaumont, A. S., Ramsdell, H., Iyer, S., Franklin, B., Lee, C., . . . Patten, E. (2013, November). *Infant vocal development: The search for early identification of disorders.* Paper presented at the annual convention of the American Speech-Language-Hearing Association, Chicago, IL.

Overby, M., & Caspari, S. (2013, November). *Phonological development in children with CAS.* Paper presented

at the annual convention of the American Speech-Language-Hearing Association, Chicago, IL.

Ozanne, A. E. (1992). Normative data for sequenced oral movements and movements in context for children aged three to five years. *Australian Journal of Human Communication Disorders, 20*, 47–63.

Pannbacker, M., Middleton, G., Vekovius, G. T., & Sanders, K. L. (2001). *Report writing for speech-language pathologists and audiologists.* Austin, TX: Pro-Ed.

Parker, B. (2009). *Good vibrations: The physics of music.* Baltimore, MD: Johns Hopkins University Press.

Paskay, L. C. (2012). Orofacial myofunctional disorders: Assessment, prevention and treatment. *Journal of the American Orthodontic Society, 12*, 34–40.

Patel, R., Connaghan, K., Franco, D., Edsall, E., Forgit, D., Olsen, L., . . . Russell, S. (2013). "The Caterpillar": A novel reading passage for assessment of motor-speech disorders. *American Journal of Speech-Language Pathology, 22*, 1–9.

Pawar, P. V., Sayed, S. I., Kazi, R., & Jagade, M. V. (2008). Current status and future perspectives in prosthetic voice rehabilitation following laryngectomy. *Journal of Cancer Research Therapy, 14*, 186–191.

Peña-Brooks, A., & Hegde, M. N. (2007). *Assessment and treatment of articulation and phonological disorders in children.* Austin, TX: Pro-Ed.

Peng, C. L., Jost-Brinkmann, P. G., Yoshida, N., Chou, H.-H., & Lin, C.-T. (2004). Comparison of tongue functions between mature and tongue-thrust swallowing: An ultrasound investigation. *American Journal of Orthodontics and Dentofacial Orthopedics, 125*, 562–570.

Perri, M. A., & Halford, E. (2004). Pain and faulty breathing: A pilot study. *Journal of Bodywork and Movement Therapies, 8*, 297–306.

Poole, C., Miller, S. A., & Church, E. B. (2000). Ages and stages: Learning to follow directions. *Scholastic Early Childhood Today, 14*, 32–35.

Prater, R. J., & Swift, R. W. (1984). *Manual of voice therapy.* Boston, MA: Little, Brown.

Prendergast, P. M. (2012). Facial proportions. In A. Erian & M. A. Shiffman (Eds.), *Advanced surgical facial rejuvenation* (pp. 15–22). Berlin, Germany: Springer-Verlag.

Purves, D., Augustine, G. J., Fitzpatrick, D., Hall, W. C., LaMantia, A., McNamara, J. O., & Williams, S. M. (2004). *Neuroscience.* Sunderland, MA: Sinauer Associates.

Ramsay, D., Smithard, D., Donaldson, N., & Kalra, L. (2005). Is the gag reflex useful in the management of swallowing problems in acute stroke? *Dysphagia, 20*, 105–107.

Reiter, R., Brosch, S., Wefel, H., Schlömer, G., & Haase, S. (2011). The submucous cleft palate: Diagnosis and therapy. *International Journal of Pediatric Otorhinolaryngology, 75*, 85–88.

Riski, J. E. (n.d.). *Clinical skills for assessing velopharyngeal function* [PDF document]. Retrieved from http://www.choa.org/OurServices/craniofacial/programs/speech/speechpathology4.asp

Robin, N. H. (2008). *Medical genetics: Its application to speech, hearing, and craniofacial disorders.* San Diego, CA: Plural.

Ruda, J., Krakovitz, P., & Rose, A. S. (2012). A review of the evaluation and management of velopharyngeal insufficiency in children. *Otolaryngologic Clinics of North America, 45*, 653–669.

Rudebusch, J., & Weichmann, J. (2011, August 30). How to fit response to intervention into a heavy workload. *The ASHA Leader*, 10–12.

Schlenker, W. L., Jennings, B. D., Jeiroudi, M. T., & Caruso, J. M. (2000). The effects of chronic absence of active nasal respiration on the growth of the skull: A pilot study. *American Journal of Orthodontics and Dentofacial Orthopedics, 117*, 706–713.

Schmitter, M., Kress, B., Leckel, M., Henschel, V., Ohlmann, B., & Rammelsberg, P. (2008). Validity of temporalmandibular disorder examination procedures for assessment of temporalmandibular joint status. *American Journal of Orthodontics and Dentofacial Orthopedics, 133*, 796–803.

Schneider, S. L., & Sataloff, R. T. (2007). Voice therapy for the professional voice. *Otolaryngologic Clinics of North America, 40*, 1133–1149.

Secord, W. A., & Donohue, J. S. (2002). *Clinical assessment of articulation and phonology.* Greenville, SC: Super Duper Publications.

Seikel, J. A., King, D. W., & Drumright, D. G. (2010). *Anatomy and physiology for speech, language, and hearing.* Clifton Park, NY: Delmar.

Shipley, K. G., & McAfee, J. G. (2008). *Assessment in speech-language pathology: A resource manual* (4th ed.). Clifton Park, NY: Delmar Cengage Learning.

Shprintzen, R. J. (1997). *Genetics, syndromes, and communication disorders.* San Diego, CA: Singular.

Shprintzen, R. J., Schwartz, R. H., Daniller, A., & Hoch, L. (1985). Morphologic significance of bifid uvula. *Pediatrics, 753*, 553–561.

Singh, S., Prerna, B.. Dua, P., & Jain, S. (2011). Habit breaking appliance for tongue thrusting: A modification. *Indian Journal of Dental Sciences, 3*, 10–12.

Sivasankar, M., & Fisher, K. V. (2003). Oral breathing challenges in participants with vocal attrition.

Journal of Speech, Language, and Hearing Research, 46, 1416–1427.

Smithpeter, J., & Covell, D. (2010). Relapse of anterior open bites treated with orthodontic appliances with and without myofunctional therapy. *American Journal of Orthodontics and Dentofacial Orthopedics, 137*, 605–614.

Solomon, N. P., Clark, H. M., Makashay, M. J., & Newman, L. A. (2008). Assessment of orofacial strength in patients with dysarthria. *Journal of Medical Speech-Language Pathology, 16*, 251–158.

Stedman's medical dictionary for the health professions and nursing: Illustrated. (2005). Philadelphia, PA: Lippincott Williams & Wilkins.

Stein-Rubin, C., & Fabus, R. (2012). *Clinical assessment and professional report writing in speech-language pathology.* Clifton Park, NY: Cengage Learning.

Stern, I., & Greenberg, M. S. (2013). Clinical assessments of patients with orofacial pain and temporalmandibular disorders. *Dental Clinics of North America, 57*, 393–402.

St. Louis, K., & Ruscello, D. (2000). *The oral speech mechanism screening examination* (OSMSE). Baltimore, MD: University Park Press.

Strand, E. A. (2011, April). *Treatment of childhood apraxia of speech.* Paper presented at the North Carolina Speech-Hearing and Language Association, Raleigh, NC.

Strand, E. A., McCauley, R. J., Weigand, S. D., Stoeckel, R. E., & Baas, B. S. (2012). A motor speech assessment for children with severe speech disorders: Reliability and validity evidence. *Journal of Speech, Language, and Hearing Research, 56*, 505–520.

Strunk, W., Jr., & White, E. B. (1999). *Elements of style* (4th ed.). New York, NY: Macmillan.

Takeda, A., Baffi, J. Z., Kleinman, M. E., Cho, W. G., Nozaki, M., . . . Ambati, J. (2009). CCR3 is a target for age-related macular degeneration diagnosis and treatment. *Nature, 460*, 225–230.

Terré, R., & Mearin, F. (2006). Oropharyngeal dysphagia after the acute phase of stroke: Predictors of aspiration. *Neurogastroenterology and Motility, 18*, 200–205.

Thom, S. A., Holt, J. D., Hixon, T. J., & Smith, A. E. (2006). Velopharyngeal function during vocalization in infants. *The Cleft Palate–Craniofacial Journal, 43*, 539–546.

Tomblin, J. B., Morris, H. L., & Spriestersbach, D. C. (2002). *Diagnosis in speech-language pathology.* San Diego, CA: Singular.

Trapl, M., Enderle, P., Nowotny, M., Teuschl, Y., Matz, K., Dachenhausen, A., & Brainin, M. (2007). Dysphagia bedside screening for acute-stroke patients: The gugging swallowing screen. *Stroke, 38,* 2948–2952.

Trawick-Smith, J. W. (2013). *Early childhood development: A multicultural perspective* (6th ed.). Bloomington, MN: Pearson.

van der Meer, G., Ferreira, Y., & Loock, J. W. (2010). The s/z ratio: A simple and reliable clinical method of evaluating laryngeal function in patients after intubation. *Journal of Critical Care, 25,* 489–492.

Van Riper, C. (1963). *Speech correction: Principles and methods.* Englewood Cliffs, NJ: Prentice Hall.

Wadsworth, S. D., Maul, C. A., & Stevens, E. J. (1998). The prevalence of orofacial myofunctional disorders among children identified with speech and language disorders in grades kindergarten through six. *International Journal of Orofacial Myology, 24,* 1–19.

Waumbaugh, J. L. (2006). Treatment guidelines for apraxia of speech: Lessons for future research. *Journal of Medical Speech-Language Pathology, 14,* 317–322.

Waumbaugh, J. L., Duffy, J. R., McNeil, M. R., Robin, D. A., & Rogers, M. A. (2006). Treatment guidelines for acquired apraxia of speech: A synthesis and evaluation of the evidence. *Journal of Medical Speech-Language Pathology, 14,* 15–33.

Waumbaugh, J. L., Nessler, C., Cameron, R., & Mauszycki, S. C. (2013). Treatment for acquired apraxia of speech: Examination of treatment intensity and practice schedule. *American Journal of Speech-Language Pathology, 22,* 84–102.

Williams, P., & Stackhouse, J. (2000). Rate, accuracy and consistency: Diadochokinetic performance of young, normally developing children. *Clinical Linguistics and Phonetics, 14,* 267–293.

Wolfe, J., Garnier, M., & Smith, J. (2009). Vocal tract resonance in speech, singing, and playing musical instruments. *Human Frontier Science Program Journal, 3,* 6–23.

Wright, E. F., & North, S. L. (2009). Management and treatment of temporomandibular disorders: A clinical perspective. *Journal of Manual and Manipulative Therapy, 17,* 247–254.

Ylvisaker, M. (2004, May). *Evidence-based practice and rational clinical decision making.* Paper presented at the Evidence-Based Practice in Child Language Disorders Working Group, Austin, TX.

Ylvisaker, M., Coelho, C., Kennedy, M., Sohlberg, M. M., Turkstra, L., Avery, J., & Yorkston, K. (2002). Reflections on evidence-based practice and rationale for clinical decision making. *Journal of Medical Speech-Language Pathology, 10,* 25–33.

Yorkston, K. M., Beukelman, D. R., Strand, E. A., & Hakel, M. (2010). *Management of motor-speech disorders in children and adults.* Austin, TX: Pro-Ed.

Zafeiriou, D. I. (2004). Primitive reflexes and postural reactions in the neurodevelopmental examination. *Pediatric Neurology, 31,* 1–8.

Zemlin, W. R. (1998). *Speech and hearing science: Anatomy and physiology.* Englewood Cliffs, NJ: Prentice Hall.

Ziegler, W., Aichert, I., & Staiger, A. (2012). Apraxia of speech: Concepts and controversies. *Journal of Speech, Language, and Hearing Research, 55,* 1485–1501.

Zimmerman, I. L., Steiner, V. G., & Pond, R. E. (2011). *Preschool language scales* (5th ed.). Bloomington, MN: Pearson.

Zinsser, W. (2006). *On writing well: An informal guide to writing nonfiction.* New York, NY: Harper & Row.

Index